atlas of

pediatric
dermatology

atlas of

pediatric
dermatology

Bernard A. Cohen, MD

Director, Division of Pediatric Dermatology
The Johns Hopkins Medical Institutions
Baltimore, Maryland

Forewords by

Frank A. Oski, MD
Chairman and Given Professor of Pediatrics
The Johns Hopkins Medical Institutions

and

Thomas T. Provost, MD
Chairman and Professor of Dermatology
Noxell Professor of Dermatology
The Johns Hopkins Medical Institutions
Baltimore, Maryland

Ͷ WOLFE

London St. Louis Baltimore Boston Chicago Philadelphia Sydney Toronto

Published in 1993 by
Wolfe Publishing, an imprint of Mosby Europe Limited.

For full details of all Mosby Europe Limited titles
please write to Mosby Europe Limited, Brook House,
2-16 Torrington Place, London WC1E 7LT, England

Library of Congress Cataloging-in-Publication Data
Cohen, Bernard, 1951–
Atlas of pediatric dermatology / Bernard A. Cohen.
p.   cm.
Includes bibliographical references and index.
ISBN 1-56375-019-8
1. Pediatric dermatology.   I. Title.
[DNLM: 1. Skin Diseases—in infancy & childhood. 2. Skin
Manifestations—in infancy & childhood. WS   269   C678p]
RJ511.C63   1993
618.92'5—dc20
92–49298

British Library Cataloguing-in-Publication Data
A catalogue record for this book is available from the British Library.

Figure Credits
The following figures have been reprinted from Zitelli BJ, Davis HW, eds.,
Atlas of Pediatric Physical Diagnosis, 1st ed. (New York: Gower Medical Publishing, 1987):
1.6, 2.9, 2.13, 2.15, 2.17, 2.37, 2.58, 2.74, 3.14, 3.18, 3.28, 3.52, 4.2B, 4.8C, 5.22,
5.25, 6.13, 6.14, 7.9, 7.10, 7.11, 8.10, 8.14, 8.30, 8.38, 9.4, 9.6B, 9.9, 9.10, 9.11

Project Manager/Editor: Leah Kennedy
Editorial Assistant: David Yoon
Illustration Director: Laura Pardi Duprey
Illustrator: Patricia Gast
Art Director: Kathryn Armstrong
Designer: Anne Kenney
Junior Designer: Jennifer Bergamini

Printed in Singapore by Imago Productions Pte., Ltd.

10 9 8 7 6 5 4 3 2 1

To Sherry for her patience, love, and understanding during the preparation of this book.

To Michael, Jared, and Jennie for keeping me young.

ACKNOWLEDGMENTS

This book would not have been possible without the help of the children and parents who allowed me to photograph their skin rashes, and the practitioners who referred them to me. I am particularly indebted to the faculty at the Children's Hospital of Pittsburgh and the Johns Hopkins Children's Center for their inspiration and support.

I am grateful for the gentle but persistent prodding and sensitive guidance of editorial director Leah Kennedy who is responsible for the completion of this book in a timely fashion. I would also like to thank Tracy Shuford for keeping the communication lines open between the publisher and my office.

Special thanks go to Judy Liggett, the pediatric dermatology and cutaneous laser nurse who has assumed the gargantuan task of identifying and organizing the clinical slides. She continues to keep the kids smiling for pictures.

Finally, I would like to thank the residents in dermatology and pediatrics who by their questions and consultations have helped me to prioritize topics for inclusion in this book.

PREFACE

Since I began taking clinical photographs during my residency training 15 years ago, I have been impressed by the virtually unlimited variation in the expression of skin disease in children. However, with careful observation, clinical patterns that permit the development of a reasonable differential diagnosis begin to emerge. In this book I have been able to use over 500 illustrations to demonstrate both the diverse variations and common patterns that are fundamental to an understanding of rashes in children.

Atlas of Pediatric Dermatology is designed for the pediatrician with an interest in dermatology and for the dermatologist who cares for children. The text is organized around practical clinical problems, and most chapters end with an algorithm for developing a differential diagnosis. This book should not be considered an encyclopedic test of pediatric dermatology; it should be used in conjunction with the references suggested at the end of Chapter 1 and the more recent literature included in the chapters' Bibliographies.

During the last 20 years neonatology has grown into a respected pediatric discipline. This is reflected in Chapter 2, the longest chapter in the book, which is devoted to the dermatologic disorders of newborns and infants. A number of the chapters are organized by morphologic findings: Chapter 3, Papulosquamous Eruptions; Chapter 4, Vesiculopustular Eruptions; and Chapter 5, Lumps and Bumps. Disorders of pigmentation are summarized in Chapter 6, and disorders of the hair and nails in Chapter 8. Reactive Erythemas, Chapter 7, includes a series of descriptive diagnoses that are often confusing because of overlapping clinical features. Chapter 9, Factitial Dermatoses, concludes with several disorders that are triggered, exacerbated, or caused primarily by external factors.

Finally, the format of the text should be user friendly. I only hope that students of pediatric dermatology will enjoy reading the atlas as much as I enjoyed writing and illustrating it.

Bernard A. Cohen, MD

FOREWORDS

It is estimated that approximately 20 percent of all patients coming to visit a pediatrician, be they sick or well, have a dermatologic problem. The next best thing to having a dermatologist with you when you encounter these patients is to have your own working knowledge of pediatric dermatology. The more you see, the more you know, and just seeing the pictures in Bernard Cohen's *Atlas of Pediatric Dermatology* is one pleasant way to acquire a useful, working knowledge of this field.

Take this book, or at least a mental image of Cohen's clear and colorful pictures, with you every time you see a patient. It can make you a better pediatrician.

Frank A. Oski, MD
Chairman and Given Professor of Pediatrics
The Johns Hopkins Medical Institutions
Baltimore, Maryland

During the last 15 to 20 years, various subspecialties have developed in the field of dermatology. One of these successful areas is pediatric dermatology. Rapid progress has been achieved in this field by the dedicated, hard work of an academic cadre of men and women with specialized expertise in both pediatrics and dermatology. One of these leaders, Dr. Bernard Cohen, has compiled a well-written, concise atlas that pediatricians, dermatologists, medical students, and residents will find to be an immense help in the care of pediatric dermatology patients. The book is a labor of love by this highly dedicated and competent physician who has been a most effective advocate for this speciality.

Thomas T. Provost, MD
Chairman and Professor of Dermatology
Noxell Professor of Dermatology
The Johns Hopkins Medical Institutions
Baltimore, Maryland

CONTENTS

chapter one

INTRODUCTION

ANATOMY OF THE SKIN

Most of us think of our skin as a simple, durable covering for our skeleton and internal organs. However, the skin is actually a very complex and dynamic organ consisting of many parts and appendages (Fig 1.1). The outermost stratum corneum is an effective barrier against the penetration of irritants, toxins, and organisms; it is also a membrane that holds in body fluids. The remainder of the epidermis manufactures this protective layer. Melanocytes within the epidermis are important in protecting us from the harmful effects of ultraviolet light, and the Langerhans' cells are one of the body's first lines of immunologic defense.

The dermis, consisting largely of fibroblasts and collagen, is a tough, leathery, mechanical barrier against cuts, bites, and bruises. Its collagenous matrix also provides structural support for a number of cutaneous appendages. Hair, which grows from follicles deep within the dermis, is important for cosmetic reasons as well as for protection against sunlight and particulate matter. Sebaceous glands arise as an outgrowth of the hair follicles. Oil produced by these glands helps to lubricate the skin and contributes to the protective epidermal barrier. The nails are specialized organs of manipulation that also protect sensitive digits. Thermoregulation of the skin is accomplished by eccrine sweat glands as well as changes in the cutaneous blood flow regulated by glomus cells. The skin also holds specialized receptors for heat, pain, touch, and pressure. Sensory input from these structures helps to protect the skin surface against environmental trauma. Beneath the dermis, in the subcutaneous tissue, fat acts as stored energy and as a soft protective cushion.

EXAMINATION AND ASSESSMENT OF THE SKIN

The skin is the largest, most accessible, and most easily examined organ of the body, and the one of most frequent concern to the patient. Therefore, all physicians should be able to recognize basic skin diseases and dermatologic clues to systemic disease.

Optimal examination of the skin must be performed in a well-lit room. The physician should inspect the entire skin surface, including hair, nails, scalp, and mucous membranes. This may present particular problems in infants and teenagers, since examination of the skin in small segments may be necessary to prevent cooling or embarrassment. Although no special equipment is required, a hand lens and side lighting will aid in the assessment of skin texture and small discrete lesions.

Despite the myriad conditions affecting the skin, a systematic approach to the evaluation of a rash facilitates and simplifies the process of developing a manageable differential diagnosis. After assessing the general

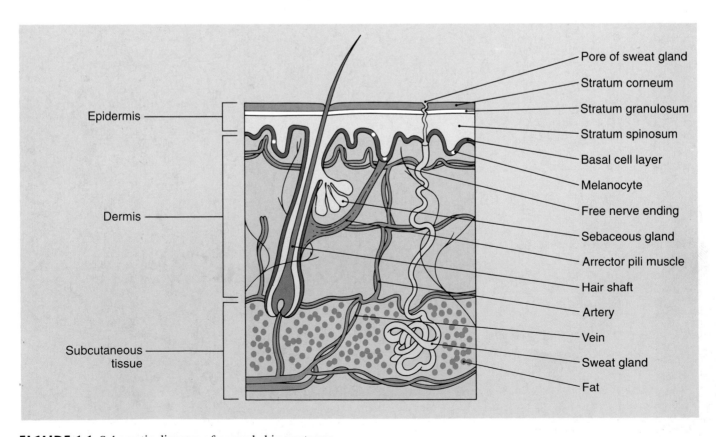

FIGURE 1.1 Schematic diagram of normal skin anatomy.

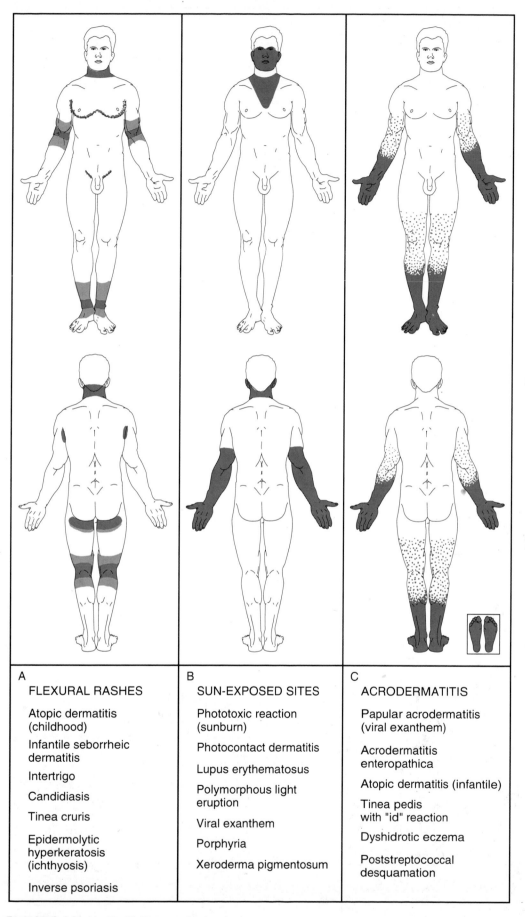

A FLEXURAL RASHES	B SUN-EXPOSED SITES	C ACRODERMATITIS
Atopic dermatitis (childhood)	Phototoxic reaction (sunburn)	Papular acrodermatitis (viral exanthem)
Infantile seborrheic dermatitis	Photocontact dermatitis	Acrodermatitis enteropathica
Intertrigo	Lupus erythematosus	Atopic dermatitis (infantile)
Candidiasis	Polymorphous light eruption	Tinea pedis with "id" reaction
Tinea cruris	Viral exanthem	Dyshidrotic eczema
Epidermolytic hyperkeratosis (ichthyosis)	Porphyria	Poststreptococcal desquamation
Inverse psoriasis	Xeroderma pigmentosum	

FIGURE 1.2 (**A, B, C**) Pattern diagnosis.

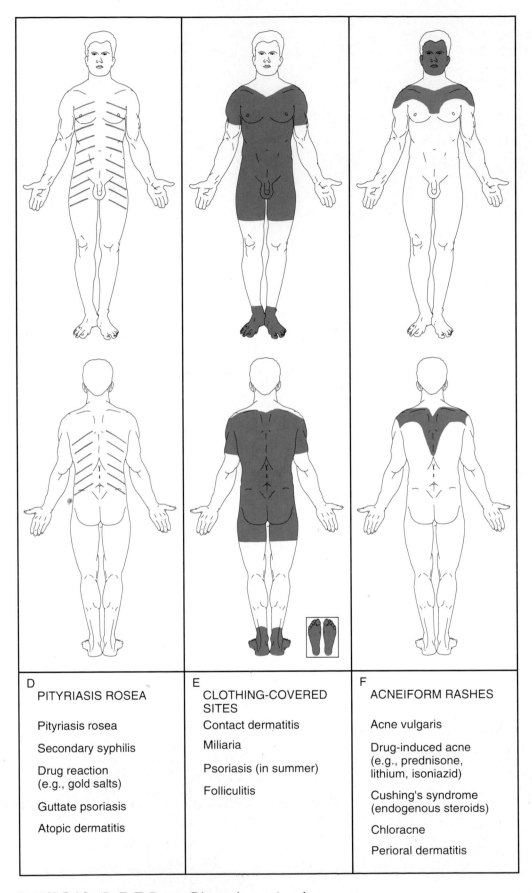

D PITYRIASIS ROSEA	E CLOTHING-COVERED SITES	F ACNEIFORM RASHES
Pityriasis rosea	Contact dermatitis	Acne vulgaris
Secondary syphilis	Miliaria	Drug-induced acne (e.g., prednisone, lithium, isoniazid)
Drug reaction (e.g., gold salts)	Psoriasis (in summer)	Cushing's syndrome (endogenous steroids)
Guttate psoriasis	Folliculitis	Chloracne
Atopic dermatitis		Perioral dermatitis

FIGURE 1.2 (D, E, F) Pattern Diagnosis, *continued.*

health of the child, the practitioner should obtain a detailed history of the cutaneous symptoms including date of onset, inciting factors, evolution of lesions, and the presence or absence of pruritus. Recent immunizations, infections, drugs, and allergies may be directly related to new rashes. The family history may suggest a hereditary or contagious process, and the clinician may need to examine other members of the family. Review of nursery records and photographs will help to document the presence of congenital lesions.

Attention should then turn to the distribution and pattern of the rash. The distribution refers to the location of the skin findings, while the pattern defines a specific anatomic or physiologic arrangement. For example, the distribution of a rash may include the extremities, face, or trunk, while the pattern could be flexural or intertriginous areas (Fig. 1.2A). Other common patterns include sun-exposed sites, acrodermatitis, pityriasis rosea, clothing-protected sites, and acneiform rashes (Fig 1.2B–F).

Next, the clinician should consider the local organization of the lesions, defining the relationship of primary and secondary lesions to one another in a given location (Fig 1.3). Are the lesions diffusely scattered or clustered (herpetiform)? Are they linear, serpiginous, annular, or dermatomal?

Depth of skin lesions, as noted by both observation and palpation, may also give further clues. Disruption

Figure 1.3 Organization of Lesions

Linear	Dermatomal	Serpiginous	Annular
Epidermal nevi	Herpes zoster	Psoriasis	Ringworm
Lichen striatus	Vitiligo	Erythema marginatum	Granuloma annulare
Contact dermatitis	Nevus depigmentosus	Cutaneous larvae migrans	Lupus
Warts	Becker's nevus	Elastosis perforans serpiginosa	Atopic dermatitis
Ichthyosis	Cafe-au-lait spot		Erythema annulare centrificum
Psoriasis	Port wine stain		
Porokeratosis			
Incontinentia pigmenti			

of the normal skin markings by scale, papules, vesicles, or pustules suggests the involvement of the epidermis. Changes in skin color with intact epidermal markings appear in dermal processes. Nodules and tumors deep in the dermis or subcutaneous tissue may also distort the surface markings.

Finally, the practitioner may develop a differential diagnosis using the morphology of the cutaneous lesions. Primary lesions (macule, papule, plaque, vesicle, bulla, pustule, wheal, nodule, and tumor) arise de novo in the skin (Fig. 1.4). Secondary lesions (scale, crust, ulcer, scar, excoriation, fissure) evolve from pri-

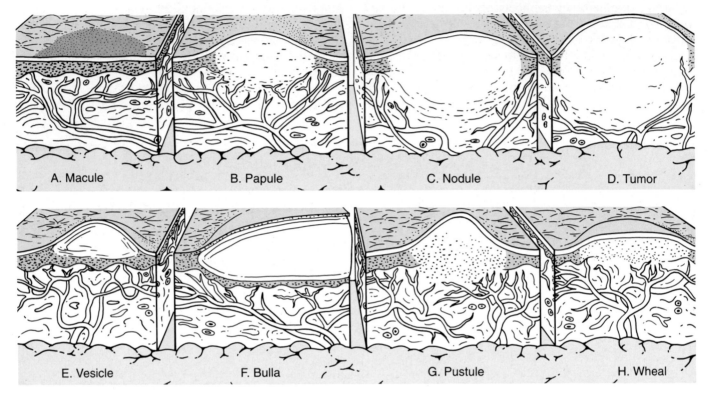

FIGURE 1.4 Primary skin lesions. **(A)** Macule: a small, flat lesion showing an alteration in color or tone. **(B)** Papule: a sharply circumscribed, somewhat elevated lesion. **(C)** Nodule: a soft or solid mass on or below the skin's surface. **(D)** Tumor; a localized and palpable mass of varied size and consistency. **(E)** Vesicle: a blister containing transparent free fluid. **(F)** Bulla: a large blister. **(G)** Pustule: a sharply circumscribed lesion containing free pus. **(H)** Wheal: an evanescent, edematous, circumscribed elevated lesion that appears and disappears rather quickly. (Adapted from CIBA.)

mary lesions or result from the patient's manipulation of primary lesions (Fig. 1.5).

The practitioner who becomes comfortable with dermatology will integrate all of these approaches into the evaluation of a child with a skin problem. This integrated approach will be reflected in the clinically focused format of this text. Each chapter will conclude with an algorithm summarizing the material in a differential diagnostic flow pattern. The limited bibliography includes insightful, historically significant, and/or well-organized reviews of the subject. General texts are listed at the end of this chapter.

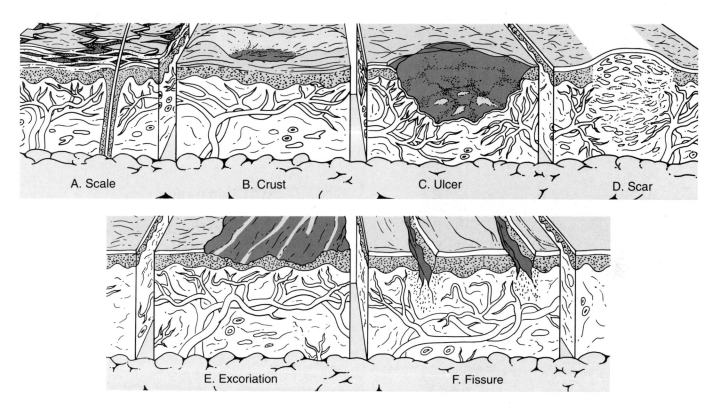

FIGURE 1.5 Secondary skin lesions. (**A**) Scale: a dry and greasy fragment of dead skin. (**B**) Crust: a dry mass of exudate from corrosive lesions consisting of serum, dried blood, scales, and dried pus. (**C**) Ulcer: a clearly defined, deep erosion of the epidermis and cutis. (**D**) Scar: a permanent skin change resulting in a new formation of connective tissue after destruction of the epidermis and cutis. (**E**) Excoriation: any scratch mark on the surface of the skin. (**F**) Fissure: any linear crack in the skin, usually accompanied by inflammation and pain. (Adapted from CIBA.)

DIAGNOSTIC TECHNIQUES

Potassium Hydroxide Preparation

There are a number of simple, rapid diagnostic techniques in dermatology. One of the most useful is to obtain a wet mount of skin scrapings for microscopic examination (Fig. 1.6A–C). Twenty percent potassium hydroxide (KOH) is used to change the optical properties of the material and make the scales more transparent. The technique requires practice and patience.

The first step is to obtain material by scraping loose scales at the margin of a lesion, nail parings, subungual debris, or the small pearly globules from a molluscum body. Short residual hair stubs (black dots in tinea capitis) may also be shaved off the scalp painlessly with a #15 blade. Scale is placed on the slide and moved to the center with a cover slip. One or two drops of KOH are applied and gently warmed with a match or the microscope light. Boiling the specimen will introduce artifact and should be avoided. Excess KOH can be removed with a paper towel applied to the edge of the cover slip. Thick specimens may be more easily viewed after gentle but firm pressure is applied to the cover slip with a pencil eraser. Thick scale will also dissolve after being set aside for 15 to 20 minutes.

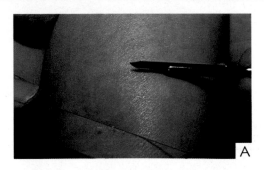
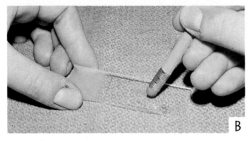
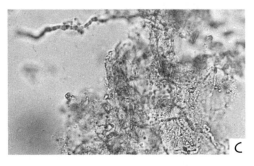

KOH Preparation

1. Obtain scales, hair, or nail fragments with a curved blade and place on a glass slide.

2. Place one or two drops of 10 percent to 20 percent potassium hydroxide on the specimen. Heat slide gently or set on the microscope stage with the light turned on. (Do not allow the KOH to boil.)

3. Absorb excess KOH with a paper towel, and apply pressure with a pencil eraser to flatten thick specimens.

4. Let slide sit 10 to 15 minutes to allow epithelial cells to dissolve, particularly if the specimen is thick.

5. Scan slide under low power for hyphae or yeast.

6. Examine suspicious areas under high power.

FIGURE 1.6 Potassium hydroxide (KOH) preparation. **(A)** Small scales are scraped from the edge of the lesion onto a microscopic slide. **(B)** The scales are crushed to make a thin layer of cells in order to visualize the fungus easily. **(C)** In this positive KOH prep of skin scrapings, fungal hyphae are seen as long, septate, branching rods at the margins and center of the scales.

View the preparation under a microscope, with the condenser and light at low levels to maximize contrast and with the objective at 10x. Focus up and down as the entire slide is rapidly scanned. True hyphae are long, branching, green hyaline rods of unifom width that cross the borders of epidermal cells. They often contain septa. False positives may be vegetative fibers, cell borders, or other artifacts. Yeast infections show budding yeast and pseudohyphae. Molluscum bodies are oval discs that have homogeneous cytoplasm and are slightly larger than keratinocytes. In hair fragments the fungi appear as small round spores packed within or surrounding the hair shaft. Hyphae are only rarely seen on the hair.

Scabies Preparation

A skin scraping showing a mite, egg, or feces is necessary to diagnose infestation with *Acarus scabei*, because many other skin rashes resemble scabies clinically (Fig. 1.7). The most important factor for obtaining a successful scraping is choice of site. Burrows and papules, which are most likely to harbor the mite, are commonly located on the wrists, fingers, and elbows. In infants primary lesions may also be found on the palms and soles.

A fresh burrow can be identified as a 5-mm to 10-mm elongated papule with a vesicle or pustule at one end. A small dark spot resembling a fleck of pepper may be seen in the vesicle. This spot is the mite, and it can be lifted out of the burrow with a needle or the point of a scalpel. Usually it is best to scrape the burrow vigorously while the skin is held taut between the thumb and index finger. Although this may induce a small amount of bleeding, if performed with multiple, short, rapid strokes, it is usually painless. A drop of mineral oil should be applied to the skin before scraping to ensure adherence of the scrapings to the blade. The scrapings are placed on the slide; another drop of mineral oil is added, and a cover slip applied. Gentle pressure with a pencil eraser may be used to flatten thick specimens. Mites are eight-legged arachnids easily identified with the scanning power of the microscope. Care must be taken to focus through thick areas of skin scrapings so as not to miss camouflaged mites. The presence of eggs (smooth ovals, approximately one-half the size of an adult mite) or feces (red-brown pellets, often seen in clusters) is also diagnostic. If eggs or feces are found first, perusal of the entire slide usually reveals the adult mite.

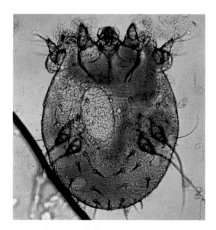

Scabies Preparation

1. Using a cotton-tip applicator, apply a drop of mineral oil on a suspicious lesion that has not been scraped.

2. Vigorously scrape the lesion with a curved blade while the skin is held taut between the opposite index finger and thumb.

3. Examine the slide under low power for the mite, eggs, and feces.

FIGURE 1.7 Microscopic appearance of the adult scabies mite. Note the small oval egg within the body.

Lice Preparation

Lice are six-legged insects visible to the unaided eye (Fig. 1.8). They are commonly found on the scalp, eyelashes, and pubic areas. Pubic lice are short and broad, with claws spaced far apart to grasp the sparse hairs on the trunk, pubic area, and eyelashes. Scalp lice are long and thin, with claws closer together to grasp the denser hairs found on the head. The lice are best identified close to the skin where eggs are more numerous and more obvious. Diagnosis can be made by identifying the louse, or by plucking hairs and confirming the presence of nits (eggs) by microscopic examination.

Tzanck Smear

The Tzanck smear is an important diagnostic tool in the evaluation of blistering diseases (Fig. 1.9). It is most commonly used to distinguish viral diseases, such as herpes simplex, varicella, and herpes zoster, from non-viral disorders. The smear is obtained by removing the roof of the blister with a curved scalpel blade or scissors, and scraping the base of the blister to obtain the moist, cloudy debris. The material is spread on a glass slide, air dried, and stained with Giemsa or Wright stain. The diagnostic finding of viral blisters is the multinucleated giant cell. The giant cell is a syncytium of epidermal cells, with multiple overlapping nuclei; it is much larger than other inflammatory cells. A giant cell may be mistaken for multiple epidermal cells piled on one another.

Wood's Light

Wood's light is an ultraviolet source that emits at a wavelength of 365 nanometers (nm). Formerly, its most common use was in screening patients for fungal alopecia, because the most common causative organism, *Microsporum audouinii*, was easily identified by its blue-green fluorescence under Wood's light. Today *Trichophyton tonsurans* is the most common fungus associated with tinea capitis, but it does not fluoresce. The only important fungus causing alopecia that fluoresces is *M. canis*.

Wood's light is still of value in diagnosing a number of other diseases. Erythrasma is a superficial bacterial infection of moist skin in the groin, axilla, and toe webs. It appears as a brown or red flat plaque, and is caused by a *Corynebacterium* that excretes a pigment containing a porphyrin. This pigment fluoresces coral, red, or pink under Wood's light. Tinea versicolor, a superficial fungal infection with hypopigmented macules and plaques on the trunk, also fluoresces under Wood's light with a green-yellow color. *Pseudomonas* infection of the toe web space and colonization of the skin in burn patients will fluoresce yellow-green. Patients with porphyria cutanea tarda excrete uroporphyrins in their urine, and examination of a urine specimen will show an orange-yellow fluorescence. Adequate blood levels of tetracycline produce yellow fluorescence in the opening of hair follicles, while lack of fluorescence indicates poor intestinal absorption or poor patient compliance.

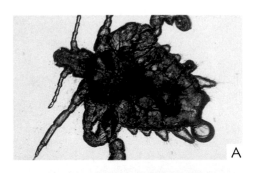
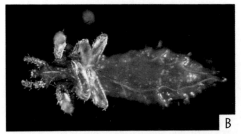

Lice Preparation

1. Search the involved area with the unaided eye or a hand lens.

2. Grasp any moving objects with a forceps, or snip hairs with nits and place on a glass slide under a piece of clear tape.

3. Examine under low power for viable organisms or unhatched nits.

FIGURE 1.8 Microscopic appearance of lice. **(A)** The crab louse has a short, broad body, with claws spaced far apart. **(B)** The head louse has a long, thin body, with claws closer together.

The Wood's light also emits purple light in the visible spectrum. This wavelength can be used to accentuate subtle changes in pigmentation. The purple light is absorbed by melanin in the skin, and variably reflected by patches of hypopigmentation and depigmentation. This may be particularly useful in evaluating light-pigmented individuals with vitiligo or ash leaf macules.

DERMATOLOGIC THERAPEUTICS

Topical Vehicles

Two variables are particularly important in the selection of effective topical therapy: the active medication and the vehicle. In general, ointments are occlusive and allow for high transcutaneous penetration of the active drug. Ointments are stable for long periods of time and require few preservatives and bacteriostatic additives. As a consequence, they are least likely to cause contact allergy or irritation. Creams are water washable and will take up water. They may be drying and occasionally sensitizing.

Open wet dressings (tap water, normal saline) provide symptomatic relief by cooling and drying acute inflammatory lesions. They cleanse the skin by loosening exudates and crusts that can be painlessly removed before the dressing dries. A Variety of astringents and antiseptics, such as vinegar or 5 percent aluminum acetate solution (e.g., Burrow's solution), may be added to com-

pression solutions, in a 1:20 to 1:40 dilution (see Scheman, 1990).

Powders promote drying and are especially useful in the intertriginous areas. Lotions are powders suspended in water (e.g., calamine lotion). When these preparations dry, they cool the skin and provide a uniform covering of the suspended agent.

Gels are aqueous preparations that liquefy on contact with the skin and leave a uniform film on drying. Gels are well tolerated in hair-bearing areas. Aerosols are also useful on the scalp. Traditional creams are suspensions of oil in water. As the proportion of oil increases, the preparation approaches the consistency of an ointment, which is the most lubricating vehicle. Pastes, which are mixtures of powder in ointment, are messy and may be difficult to remove from the skin. Used to protect areas prone to irritation, such as the diaper area, they can be removed with mineral oil.

Single-component generic preparations are often effective and inexpensive. Fixed multiple-component preparations are occasionally useful, but the practitioner must be aware of all the constituent agents and the increased risk of adverse drug reactions. Specially formulated medications are often prohibitively expensive and seldom indicated in general practice.

The practitioner must calculate the quantity of medication required so the patient can comply with the instructions. In a child, 15 g to 30 g of an ointment are

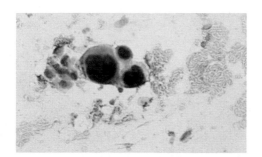

Tzanck Smear

1. Gently unroof blisters with a curved blade or scissors.

2. Blot fluid from vesicle.

3. Gently scrape base of blister or erosion with a curved blade.

4. Spread material thinly on glass slide.

5. Air dry and if possible fix for two minutes in 95 percent alcohol.

6. Cover slide with Wright's stain or Giemsa stain.

7. Scan slide under low power to find an area with epithelial cells, then examine under high power.

FIGURE 1.9 Tzanck preparation. Note the multinucleated giant cells characteristic of viral infection with herpes simplex and varicella/zoster.

Figure 1.10 Topical Steroids

Group	Generic name	Trade name	
1	Betamethasone dipropionate, augmented 0.05% Clobetasol propionate 0.05% Diflorasone diacetate 0.05%	Diprolene 0.05% Diprolene AF 0.05% Temovate 0.05% Psorcon 0.05%	High potency
2	Amcinonide Betamethasone dipropionate Diflorasone diacetate Halcinonide Fluocinonide Fluocinonide Diflorasone diacetate Desoximetasone	Cyclocort ointment 0.1% Diprosone ointment 0.05% Florone ointment 0.05% Halog cream 0.1% Lidex cream 0.05% Lidex ointment 0.05% Maxiflor ointment 0.05% Topicort cream 0.25%	
3	Betamethasone dipropionate Betamethasone benzoate Betamethasone valerate	Diprosone cream 0.05% Benisone gel 0.025% Valisone ointment 0.1%	
4	Triamcinolone acetonide Flurandrenolide Triamcinolone acetonide Fluocinolone acetonide	Aristocort ointment 0.1% Cordran ointment 0.05% Kenalog ointment 0.1% Synalar cream 0.025%	
5	Triamcinolone acetonide Flurandrenolide Fluocinolone acetonide Triamcinolone acetonide Fluocinolone acetonide Betamethasone valerate Hydrocortisone valerate	Aristocort cream 0.1% Cordran SP cream 0.05% Fluonid cream 0.01% Kenalog cream 0.1% Synalar cream 0.01% Valisone cream 0.1% Westcort cream 0.2%	
6	Hydrocortisone 1%, urea 10% Flumethasone pivalate Desonide	Alphaderm cream 1% Locorten cream 0.03% Tridesilon cream 0.05%	
7	Hydrocortisone 1% Hydrocortisone 1% Dexamethasone Methylprednisolone acetate Prednisolone	Hytone cream 1% Hytone ointment 1% Hexadrol cream 0.04% Medrol ointment 0.25% Meti-Derm cream 0.5%	
8	Hydrocortisone 0.5%	Cortaid cream	Low potency

needed to cover the entire skin surface once. This quantity will vary with the vehicle used and the experience of the individual applying the preparation.

Topical Corticosteroids

Topical steroids are available in every type of vehicle (see Scheman, 1990). A good rule is to become familiar with one or two products in each potency range (Fig. 1.10). A check of local pharmacies can determine the availability and cost of medications.

Most childhood skin eruptions requiring topical steroids can be readily managed with twice-daily applications of low- or medium-potency preparations. Only low-potency medications should be used on the face and intertriginous areas, because more potent preparations may produce atrophy, telangiectasias, and hypopigmentation. Regardless of the potency of their medication, patients should be followed carefully for steroid-induced changes, even though they are produced only rarely by therapy restricted to two to four weeks. Patients receiving chronic therapy should take frequent "time-outs" from their topical steroids (e.g., one week per month) and should taper them when possible. Tapering may be achieved by decreasing the frequency of application as well as by mixing the active preparation with a bland emollient such as petrolatum.

Steroids may mask infections and suppress local and systemic immune responses. Consequently, they are contraindicated in most patients with viral, fungal, bacterial, or mycobacterial infection.

Emollients (Moisturizers)

Any preparation that reduces friction and leaves a smooth, occlusive film that prevents drying is classified as a lubricant (see Scheman, 1990) (Fig. 1.11). In patients with chronic dermatitis, ointments (or water in oil-based products) provide the best lubrication, especially during the dry winter months. Less oily preparations (oil in water creams) are often preferred by patients during the spring and summer. Cultural preferences should also be taken into account when selecting a lubricant. Preparations containing topical sensitizers such as fragrance, neomycin, and benzocaine should be avoided, particularly by patients with inflamed skin.

A number of other topical and oral agents are used in the treatment of skin disorders. They will be discussed in detail in later chapters. The most commonly recommended agents are listed in Scheman (1990).

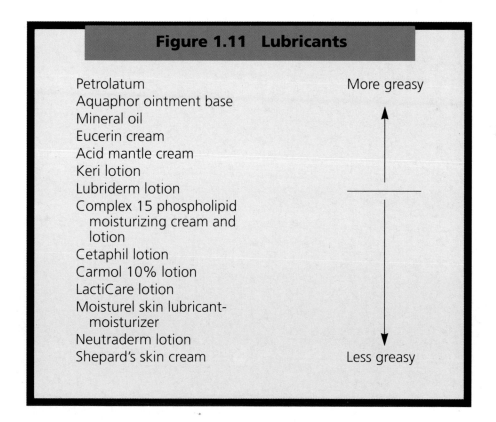

Figure 1.11 Lubricants

Petrolatum — More greasy
Aquaphor ointment base
Mineral oil
Eucerin cream
Acid mantle cream
Keri lotion
Lubriderm lotion
Complex 15 phospholipid moisturizing cream and lotion
Cetaphil lotion
Carmol 10% lotion
LactiCare lotion
Moisturel skin lubricant-moisturizer
Neutraderm lotion
Shepard's skin cream — Less greasy

BIBLIOGRAPHY

CIBA Information Services. *The basic skin lesions.* Summit, NJ: CIBA Pharmaceutical Company, n.d.

Fitzpatrick TB, Eisen AZ, Wolff K, Freedberg IM, Austen KF. *Dermatology in general medicine,* 3rd ed. New York: McGraw-Hill, 1987.

Hurwitz S. *Clinical pediatric dermatology.* Philadelphia: W.B. Saunders, 1981.

Lever WF, Schaumburg-Lever G. *Histopathology of the skin,* 7th ed. Philadelphia: J.B. Lippincott, 1990.

Meneghini CL, Bonifazi E. *An atlas of pediatric dermatology.* Chicago: Year Book Medical Publishers, 1986.

Ruiz-Maldonado R, Parish LC, Beare JM. *Textbook of pediatric dermatology.* Philadelphia: Grune and Stratton, 1989.

Schachner LA, Hansen RC. *Pediatric dermatology.* New York: Churchill Livingstone, 1988.

Scheman AJ. *Pocket guide to medications used in dermatology,* 2nd ed. Baltimore: Williams & Wilkins, 1990.

Verbov J, Morley N. *Color atlas of pediatric dermatology.* London: J.B. Lippincott, 1983.

Weinberg S, Leider M, Shapiro L. *Color atlas of pediatric dermatology.* London: McGraw-Hill, 1975.

Weston WL. *Practical pediatric dermatology.* Boston: Little, Brown, 1985.

chapter two

NEONATAL DERMATOLOGY

The skin of the newborn differs from adult skin in several ways (Fig. 2.1). It is less hairy, has less sweat and sebaceous gland secretion, is thinner, and has fewer intercellular attachments and fewer melanosomes.

CUTANEOUS PROBLEMS IN PRETERM NEONATES

In the preterm neonate, these skin differences are magnified. As a consequence, newborns are less well equipped to handle thermal stress and sunlight. They have increased transepidermal water loss and penetration of toxic substances and medications, and are more likely to develop blisters or erosions in response to heat, chemical irritants, mechanical trauma, and inflammatory skin conditions.

Barrier Properties and Use of Topical Agents

The barrier properties of the skin reside primarily in the stratum corneum, the compact layer of flattened keratinocytes that covers the surface. Although keratinization begins at 24 weeks, it is not complete until close to term. Transepidermal water loss and drug absorption through the epidermis at term is similar to those processes in older children and adults. Skin-barrier properties in babies of 36 weeks gestation approximate the same properties of term infants several days after birth. The development of these properties may be delayed by 14 to 21 days in children of less than 32 to 34 weeks gestational age. Barrier maturation may be further delayed when epidermal injury, inflammation, or hyperemia is present. Sepsis, ischemia, and acidosis in the severely ill newborn may also compromise barrier function. Moreover, even in healthy term infants, the surface-to-volume ratio, which is increased compared to older children and adults, may result in relatively high transcutaneous penetration of topical agents.

Percutaneous absorption of toxic substances in newborns, particularly preterm infants and term infants with disruption of barrier function, has been well documented.

Figure 2.1 Structural and Functional Differences of Adult, Term, and Preterm Infant Skin

	Adult	Term
Epidermal thickness	50 μm	50 μm
Cell attachments (desmosome, hemidesmosomes)	Normal	Normal
Dermis	Normal	↓Collagen and elastic fibers
Melanosomes	Normal	Fewer
Eccrine glands	Normal	Delayed activity for 1–7 days ↓Neurologic control for 2–3 yrs
Sebaceous glands	Normal	Normal
Hair	Normal	↓Terminal hair

Aniline dyes used to mark diapers, for instance, have caused methemoglobinemia and death. Topical steroids may produce adrenal suppression and systemic effects. Vacuolar encephalopathy has been demonstrated in infants bathed with hexachlorophene, particularly premature infants who have had repeated exposure.

Pentachlorphenol poisoning occurred in 20 infants who were accidentally exposed to this chemical in nursery linens. Topical application of povidone iodine to the perineum before delivery and the umbilical cord after delivery has resulted in elevated plasma iodine levels and thyroid dysfunction in the neonate. Other substances, including isopropyl alcohol, ethyl and methyl alcohol, and chlorhexidine, are readily absorbed and may produce toxic reactions.

In general, topical agents should only be used in newborns and infants if systemic administration of the agent is not associated with toxicity. Antiseptic agents should be used with great caution on limited areas of the skin, particularly in premature infants under 30 weeks gestation during the first several weeks of life. Injury to the skin induced by tape, monitors, adhesives, and cleansing agents should be kept to a minimum since they tend to compromise barrier function. When lubrication is necessary, small amounts of petrolatum or other fragrance-free bland emollients are adequate.

At birth the skin is covered with a greasy white material with a pH of 6.7 to 7.4. Although the function of this material, the vernix caseosa, is unknown, it may have lubricating and antibacterial properties. Beneath the vernix the skin has a pH of 5.5 to 6.0. Overwashing, particularly with harsh soaps, may result in irritation, alkaline pH, and a decrease in normal barrier function of the stratum corneum. Thus, bathing should be done gently several times a week with tap water, and mild soaps should be used only on areas where cutaneous bacteria are most numerous, such as the umbilicus, diaper area, neck, and axillae. In ill newborns bathing should be limited to saline compresses on irritated, macerated skin, common in intertriginous areas.

Figure 2.1 *continued*	
Preterm (30 wks)	**Significance**
27.4 μm	Permeability to topical agents ↑Transepidermal water loss
Fewer	↑Tendency to blister
↓↓Collagen and elastic fibers	↓Elasticity ↑Blistering
1/3 term infant	↑Photosensitivity
Total anhidrosis	↓Response to thermal stress
Normal	Barrier properties? Lubricant? Antibacterial?
Persistent lanugo	Helpful in assessing gestational age

Thermoregulation

Cold stress is the major risk to naked preterm infants nursed in a dry isolette. Decreased epidermal and dermal thickness results in increased heat loss from radiation and conduction. Minimal subcutaneous fat and an immature nervous system also decrease the premature's ability to respond to cooling. Heat loss may be minimized by increasing ambient humidity and temperature and covering the child with a plastic bubble. Maintenance of normal body temperature should develop with advancing postnatal age and a weight level that approaches 2000 g.

In growing preemies and full-term infants, hyperthermia may be a problem in warm climates, particularly when additional thermal stresses such as insulated clothing and phototherapy are present. Although sweat glands are anatomically complete at 28 weeks gestation, they may not be fully functional until several weeks after delivery, even in the full-term neonate. At birth, sweating has been demonstrated in response to thermal stress in term babies; however, it may not be detectable in infants of less than 35 weeks gestation for several weeks. Consequently, sweating may not be an effective mechanism for thermoregulation in term or premature infants for at least several weeks, and thermal stress should be minimized.

Pigmentation and Photoprotection

Although melanocytes are actively synthesizing and transferring pigment to epidermal keratinocytes by 20 to 24 weeks of intrauterine life, the skin surface tends to be less pigmented during the first few postnatal months than later. As a consequence, infants have less natural protection from sunlight and are more likely to develop sunburn.

Several investigators have expressed concern about using sunscreens in children under six months of age. However, these infants are not ambulatory, and sun avoidance and protective clothing are effective barriers to excessive sun exposure for them.

Certain children are particularly sensitive to sun-light, and prolonged sun avoidance beyond infancy as well as aggressive use of sunscreens may be mandatory (see Chapter 7). Hereditary porphyrias, xeroderma pigmentosum, Bloom's syndrome, Cockayne's syndrome, and a number of other photosensitivity disorders may present with exaggerated sunburn reactions in infancy. In some infants, tingling and burning of the skin may occur after sun exposure, without obvious physical findings. In neonatal lupus erythematosus the skin rash is often triggered by sun exposure. Although some of these children will benefit from broad-spectrum sunscreens (e.g., Photoplex) or sunscreens with sun protective factors above 15, photoreactions may be caused by wavelengths of light that are not absorbed by currently available sunscreens. In some patients, oral beta-carotene may provide additional protection.

CUTANEOUS COMPLICATIONS OF THE INTENSIVE CARE NURSERY

Scars and burns are inevitable complications of nursery care and monitoring. Careful management of the skin in the nursery and after discharge will minimize the risk of serious functional impairment and cosmetic disfigurement.

Surgical Scars

Wounds from subclavian and jugular venous lines generally heal with barely noticeable scars. Occasionally, scars will be more obvious, but they will usually fade over the first two years of life, particularly if the wounds conform to the normal skin lines. However, dimpling may result from sutures used to keep the lines in place (Fig. 2.2). Scarring and dimpling may also be minimized by gentle massage of the area.

Frequently, chest tubes are placed in such an emergent setting that little time is taken to consider optimal site selection. Lateral placement beyond the breast tis-

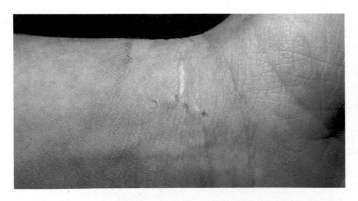

FIGURE 2.2 Scar from an arterial cut. Recurrent drainage ended after a small fistulous tract in the scar was excised from the wrist of this two-year-old girl.

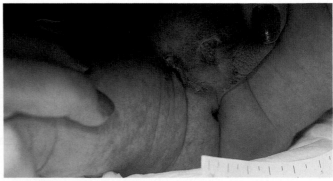

FIGURE 2.3 Several hours after an umbilical artery catheter was removed from this infant, a purple area developed unilaterally on the scrotum, perineum, and perirectal skin. One day later the area became ulcerated. Note the formation of granulation tissue and early scarring one week later.

sue may eliminate the need for later surgical repair. Gentle massage after removal may prevent the formation of adhesions and dimpling. As with other surgical scars, these lesions will tend to improve spontaneously over the first several years of life.

Arterial Catheters

In addition to local scarring, arterial catheters may be associated with serious systemic and cutaneous complications in the areas distal to their placement. Extensive ischemia and necrosis of the genital and buttock skin are unusual complications of umbilical artery spasm and thromboembolism. Ensuing ulcerations may take months to heal and may require surgical repair (Fig. 2.3). Radial artery catheters have rarely been associated with the necrosis of digits. However, more subtle findings, such as discrepancies in hand size, may not be evident for a year.

Chemical and Thermal Burns

Infiltration of the soft tissues by intravenous fluids often produces cutaneous inflammation and necrosis. Hypertonic fluids such as glucose and calcium may result in full-thickness sloughing of the skin and contractures (Fig. 2.4). These lesions usually heal over weeks to months, and may require splinting, physical therapy, and surgical repair, particularly if they are located over joints.

Removal of monitor leads, endotracheal and nasotracheal tubes, and adhesives with dressings results in extensive trauma to the skin. Although full-thickness sloughs rarely develop, postinflammatory hyperpigmentation and hypopigmentation are common. Pigmentary changes may persist for years, particularly in dark-pigmented individuals, but usually fade markedly within the first year of life. Other topical agents, such as iodophors, soaps, detergents, and solvents, may produce severe irritant reactions, particularly in premature infants or children with antecedent cutaneous injuries (Fig. 2.5).

Accidental thermal burns have been reported after exposure to heated water beds, radiant warmers, transcutaneous oxygen monitors, and heated humidified air. Although cold stress must be minimized in the small premature infant, extensive burns with cutaneous and airway involvement may be prevented by close monitoring of these devices.

Heel Stick Nodules

Repeated blood sampling from the heel leads to the formation of 3-mm to 5-mm deep-seated papules and nodules in many graduates of the neonatal intensive care unit (Fig. 2.6). Although the most prominent lesions are noted in children who have had frequent heel sticks, these scars are also detected in infants who have had only a few. Lesions may be palpable at the time of discharge from the nursery. Over a period of several months they generally become more superficial and resemble milia. Papules typically calcify over the ensuing months and resolve spontaneously in 18 to 30 months. During this time the infants are asymptomatic, and walking is not delayed.

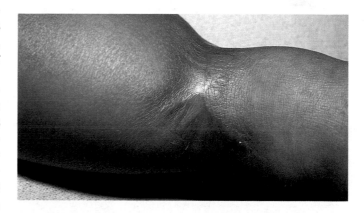

FIGURE 2.4 Infiltration of the antecubital skin with 20 percent glucose resulted in an ulcer that healed with severe scarring. The scar was surgically revised at four years of age.

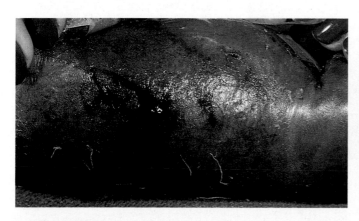

FIGURE 2.5 Application of a topical iodophor-containing solution produced an erosive irritant dermatitis on the flank of a premature infant in the intensive care nursery. Fortunately, this area healed with only minimal scarring.

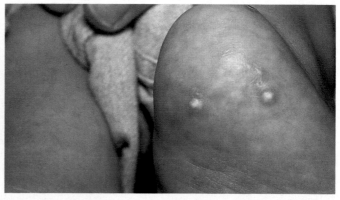

FIGURE 2.6 Heel-stick papules on the feet of this graduate of the intensive care nursery resolved without treatment.

TRANSIENT ERUPTIONS OF THE NEWBORN

A number of innocent rashes occur in infants. Although they are usually transient, they may be dramatic and cause parental anxiety. Early recognition is important to distinguish these lesions from more serious disorders and to provide appropriate counseling to parents.

Transient Vascular Phenomena

During the first two to four weeks of life, cold stress may be associated with *acrocyanosis* and *cutis marmorata* (Fig. 2.7). In acrocyanosis the hands and feet become variably and symmetrically blue in color, without edema or other cutaneous changes. Cutis marmorata is identified by the characteristic reticulated cyanosis or marbling of the skin, which symmetrically involves the trunk and extremities. Both patterns usually resolve with warming of the skin, and recurrence is unusual after one month of age. Acrocyanosis is readily differentiated from persistent central cyanosis (cyanosis of the lips, face, and/or trunk), that occurs in association with pulmonary or cardiac disease. Cutis marmorata that persists beyond the neonatal period may be a marker for trisomy 18, Down's syndrome, Cornelia de Lange syndrome, or hypothyroidism. Cutis marmorata telangiectatica congenita (CMTC or congenital phlebectasia) (Fig. 2.8) may mimic cutis marmorata. However, the lesions are persistent in a localized patch on the trunk or extremities. The eruption may extend in a dermatomal pattern, and occasionally widespread lesions and reticulated cutaneous atrophy are present. Although congenital phlebectasia may be an isolated cutaneous finding, it may also occur in association with other mesodermal and neuroectodermal anomalies.

The *harlequin color change* is noted when the infant is lying horizontally, and the dependent half of the body turns bright red in contrast to the pale upper half (Fig. 2.9). The color shifts when the infant is rolled from side to side. This phenomenon lasts from seconds to 20 minutes, and recurrences are common until three to four weeks of life. The cause is unknown, and it is not associated with serious underlying disease.

Benign Pustular Dermatoses

Several innocent pustular eruptions must be differentiated from potentially serious infectious dermatoses. *Erythema toxicum neonatorum* (ETN) is the most common pustular rash, occurring in up to 70 percent of full-term infants (Fig. 2.10). Although lesions usually appear on the second or third day of life, onset has been reported up to two to three weeks of age. ETN typically begins with 2-mm to 3-mm erythematous blotchy macules and papules, which may evolve over several hours to pustules on a broad erythematous base, giving affected infants a "flea-bitten" appearance. Lesions may be isolated or clustered on the face, trunk, and proximal extremities, and usually fade over five to seven days. Recurrences, however, may be noted for several weeks. A Wright's stain of the pustule contents reveals sheets of eosinophils and occasional neutrophils, and 15 percent to 20 percent of patients will have a circulating eosinophilia.

Transient neonatal pustular melanosis (TNPM) occurs in 4 percent of newborns, particularly black male infants (Fig. 2.11). Unlike ETN, lesions are usually present at birth, and probably evolve in many children prenatally. TNPM characteristically appears as 2-mm to 5-mm pustules on a nonerythematous base on the chin,

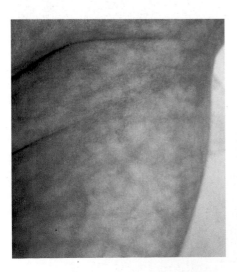

FIGURE 2.7 Cutis marmorata. Note the reticulated bluish-purple mottling of this infant's thigh.

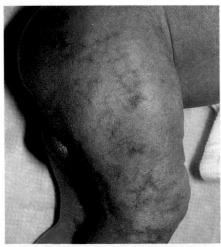

FIGURE 2.8 Cutis marmorata telangiectatica congenita was associated with some cutaneous atrophy on the left leg of a newborn. A careful medical evaluation failed to reveal any associated anomalies.

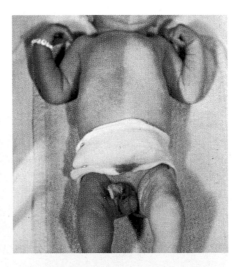

FIGURE 2.9 The dependent side is bright red in this infant with the harlequin color change.

neck, upper chest, sacrum, abdomen, and thighs. Over several days, lesions develop a central crust, which then desquamates, leaving a hyperpigmented macule with a collarette of fine scale. Lesions in different stages of development may be present simultaneously. Often the only manifestation of the eruption is the presence of brown macules with a rim of scale at birth. A Wright's stain of the pustular smear shows numerous neutrophils and rare eosinophils.

Acropustulosis of infancy is a chronic recurrent pustular eruption that appears on the palms and soles but may also involve the scalp, trunk, buttocks, and extremities (Fig. 2.12). Onset may occur during the newborn period or early infancy, and episodes typically last from one to three weeks with intervening remissions for one to three weeks. Disease-free periods tend to lengthen until the rash resolves by two to three years of age. During flares infants are usually fussy, and pruritus is severe. Histopathology of the lesions reveals sterile intraepider-

mal pustules. A Wright's stain shows numerous neutrophils and occasional eosinophils. Although oral Dapsone (1–3 mg/kg/d) will suppress lesions and symptoms in 24 to 48 hours, brief courses of moderate or high-potency topical steroids to the palms and soles may provide safe temporary relief.

Benign pustular dermatoses may be differentiated from herpes simplex infection by the absence of multinucleated giant cells on Wright's stained smears of pustular contents. Negative Gram-stain and potassium hydroxide preparations will exclude bacterial and candidal infection. In seriously ill infants, however, viral and bacterial cultures may be required to confirm the clinical impression. Serologic studies for syphilis and scrapings for ectoparasites will exclude syphilis and scabies in children with acropustulosis.

The benign pustular dermatoses may also be confused with several other innocent papulopustular rashes, including sebaceous gland hyperplasia, miliaria, milia, and acne.

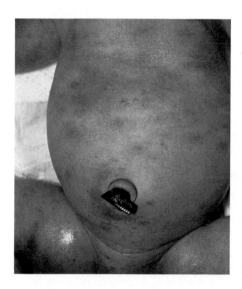

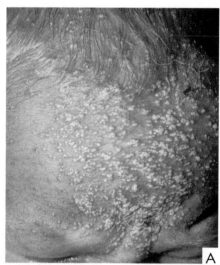

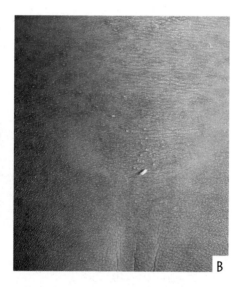

FIGURE 2.10 Erythema toxicum neonatorum. Numerous yellow papules and pustules are surrounded by large, intensely erythematous rings on the trunk of this infant.

FIGURE 2.11 Transient neonatal pustular melanosis. (**A**) Numerous tiny pustules dot the forehead and scalp of this neonate. (**B**) Healing pustules and

brown macules dot the lower back and sacrum of a two-day-old boy. Note the Mongolian spot on his gluteal cleft.

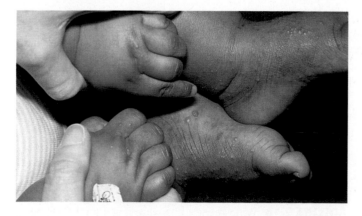

FIGURE 2.12 Acropustulosis of infancy. Multiple 2-mm to 3-mm pustules covered the hands and feet of this otherwise healthy infant. Lesions recurred episodically until this child was three years old.

Sebaceous gland hyperplasia is a common finding over the nose and cheeks of term infants (Fig. 2.13). Lesions consist of multiple 1-mm to 2-mm yellow papules that result from maternal or endogenous androgenic stimulation of sebaceous gland growth. Parents should be counseled that the eruption resolves within four to six months.

Miliaria results from obstruction to the flow of sweat and rupture of the eccrine sweat duct. In miliaria crystallina, superficial 1-mm to 2-mm vesicles appear on noninflamed skin when the duct is blocked by keratinous debris just beneath the stratum corneum (Fig. 2.14). Small papules and pustules are typical of milliaria rubra (prickly heat), in which the obstruction occurs in the mid-epidermis (Fig. 2.15). Deep-seated papulopustular lesions of miliaria profunda occur only rarely in infancy, when the duct ruptures at the dermal-epidermal junction.

Miliaria occurs frequently in term and preterm infants after the first week of life, in response to thermal stress. Lesions erupt in crops in the intertriginous areas, scalp, face, and trunk. In older infants, lesions appear most commonly in areas of skin occluded by tight-fitting clothing. Cooling the skin and loosening clothing result in prompt resolution of the rash.

Milia appear as pearly yellow 1-mm to 3-mm papules on the face, chin, and forehead of 50 percent of newborns (Fig. 2.16). Occasionally they erupt on the trunk and extremities. Although milia usually resolve without treatment during the first month of life, they may persist for several months. Histology demonstrates miniature epidermal inclusion cysts, which arise from the pilosebaceous apparatus of vellus hairs. Large numbers of lesions distributed over a wide area or persistence beyond several months of age suggest the possibility of oral-facial-digital syndrome or trichodysplasia. Increasing numbers of lesions, particularly in areas of normal trauma, such as the hands, knees, and feet, may occcur in patients with mild variants of scarring epidermolysis bullosa, where blistering is subtle.

Mild *acne* develops in up to 20 percent of newborns. Lesions may be present at birth or appear in early infancy (Fig. 2.17). Although closed comedones (whiteheads) predominate, open comedones (blackheads), red papules, pustules, and rarely cysts may also occur. As in sebaceous hyperplasia, maternal and endogenous androgens probably play a role in the pathogenesis of neonatal acne. Treatment is usually unnecessary since lesions involute spontaneously within one to three months. Risk of acne in adolescence does not seem to be increased.

Occasionally, the onset of acne is delayed until three to six months of age. Lesions tend to be more pleiomor-

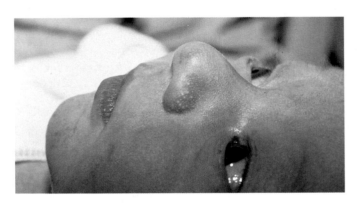

FIGURE 2.13 Sebaceous gland hyperplasia. Note the yellow papules on the nose of this newborn.

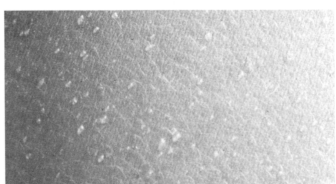

FIGURE 2.14 Miliaria crystallina. Tiny thin-walled vesicles quickly desquamated when this child was placed in a cooler environment.

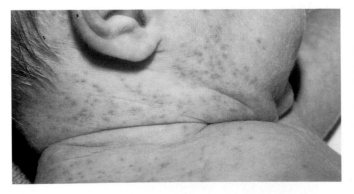

FIGURE 2.15 Miliaria rubra. The red papules of prickly heat are readily visible on this infant.

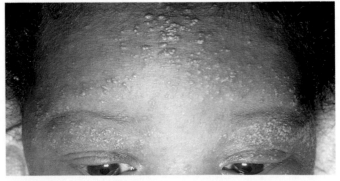

FIGURE 2.16 Widespread milia were noted on the forehead and eyelids of this vigorous newborn. The white papules resolved spontaneously before the two-month pediatric check-up.

phic, and inflammatory papules and pustules are common. Although infantile acne usually resolves by three years of age, lesions may persist up to 11 years. As with neonatal acne, infantile acne is probably triggered by endogenous androgens. Children with early onset, persistent disease, and a positive family history of severe acne tend to have a more severe course, with resurgence at puberty. Severe infantile acne should prompt a search for other signs of hyperandrogenism and an abnormal endogenous or exogenous source of androgens.

Subcutaneous Fat Necrosis of the Newborn

Fat necrosis is a benign, self-limited process that usually occurs in otherwise healthy infants (Fig. 2.18). Discrete red or hemorrhagic nodules and plaques up to 3 cm in diameter appear most commonly over areas exposed to trauma, such as the cheeks, back, buttocks, arms, and thighs, during the first few weeks of life. Lesions are usually painless, but marked tenderness may be present. Although the cause is unknown, difficult deliveries, hypothermia, perinatal asphyxia, and maternal diabetes predispose the newborn to the development of fat necrosis.

Nodules usually resolve without scarring in one to two months. However, lesions occasionally become fluctuant, drain, and heal with atrophy. When calcification

occurs, infants should be evaluated for primary hyperparathyroidism, and calcium levels must be monitored.

Histopathology demonstrates necrosis of fat with a foreign-body giant-cell reaction. Remaining fat cells contain needle-shaped clefts, and calcium deposits are scattered throughout the subcutis.

Occasionally, early lesions of scleredema neonatorum are confused with subcutaneous fat necrosis. However, scleredema is usually differentiated from fat necrosis by the presence of diffuse waxlike hardening of the skin in a severely ill newborn. Unlike subcutaneous fat necrosis, skin results shows only minimal inflammation in the fat. Thickening of the skin results from increased size of fat cells and interlacing bundles of collagen in the dermis and subcutis.

MINOR ANOMALIES

Minor anomalies occur in up to half of all newborns and are of no physiologic consequence. Their presence, particularly in association with other minor anomalies, should prompt an evaluation for more serious multisystem disease.

Dimpling is a common finding over bony prominences, particularly the sacral area (Fig. 2.19). Although

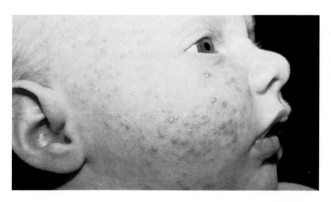

FIGURE 2.17 Neonatal acne. Red papules and pustules are present over the nose and cheeks of this infant. This eruption cleared without treatment by three months of age.

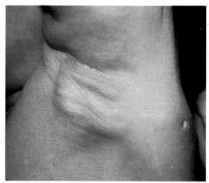

FIGURE 2.18 Subcutaneous fat necrosis. Red nodules are evident on the arm of this neonate. Lesions resolved without atrophy by two months of age.

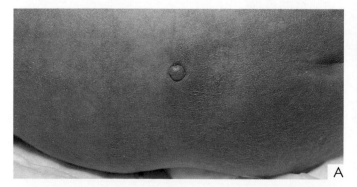

FIGURE 2.19 (A) A sacral dimple was noted in this healthy infant. CT scan of the lumbosacral spine was normal. (B) At birth a spongy mass was palpable in the sacral area of this

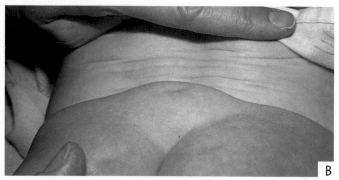

baby. A magnetic resonance image of this tumor revealed a lipoma and a normal spine.

skin dimples may be the first sign of several dysmorphic syndromes, these lesions are usually of only cosmetic consequence. Spinal anomalies should be excluded when deep dimples, sinus tracts, or other cutaneous lesions such as lipomas, hemangiomas, nevi, tufts of hair, or sinus tracts involve the lumbosacral spine.

Periauricular sinuses, pits, tags, and cysts occur when brachial arches or clefts fail to fuse or close normally (Fig. 2.20). Defects may be unilateral or bilateral and are occasionally associated with other facial anomalies. Although occult lesions may be discovered when they present with secondary infection, many of these anomalies are noted at birth and are readily excised during childhood.

Supernumerary digits appear most commonly as rudimentary structures at the base of the ulnar side of the fifth finger (Fig. 2.21). They are usually familial and asymptomatic. Histology demonstrates bundles of peripheral nerves extending in various directions, sharply demarcated from dermal connective tissue. A good cosmetic result is best achieved by local surgical excision.

Supernumerary nipples may appear unilaterally or bilaterally anywhere along a line from the mid axilla to the inguinal area (Fig. 2.22). Accessory nipples may develop without areolae, resulting in their misdiagnosis as congenital nevi. Malignant degeneration rarely occurs. Most accessory nipples are excised for cosmetic purposes.

Umbilical granulomas occur commonly during the first few weeks of life. Normally the cord dries and separates in seven days. The open surface epithelializes and scars down in an additional one to two weeks. Excessive moisture and low-grade infection may result in the growth of exuberant granulation tissue, forming an umbilical granuloma (Fig. 2.23). Cauterization with silver nitrate or dessication with repeated applications of isopropyl alcohol will usually produce rapid healing of the granuloma.

Umbilical granulomas must be differentiated from umbilical polyps which result from persistence of the omphalomesenteric duct or urachus. There may be a mucoid discharge at the tip of the firm red polyp which, upon histologic examination, demonstrates gastrointestinal or urinary tract mucosa. Surgical excision is necessary.

THE SCALY NEWBORN

At delivery the skin is smooth, moist, and velvety. Desquamation begins at 24 to 36 hours of age and may not be complete for three weeks (Fig. 2.24). As peeling progresses, the underlying skin appears normal; cracking and fissuring are absent. Desquamation at birth or in the first day of life is abnormal and suggests postmaturity, intrauterine stress, or congenital icthyosis.

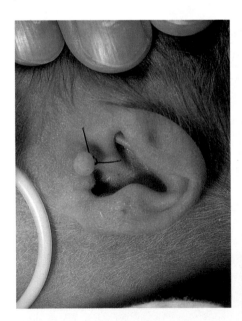

FIGURE 2.20 This preauricular skin tag was tied off in the nursery.

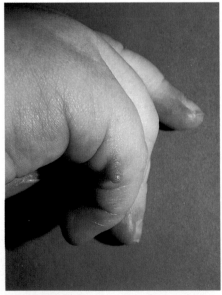

FIGURE 2.21 This rudimentary supernumerary digit was present at birth. It was surgically excised at six months of age.

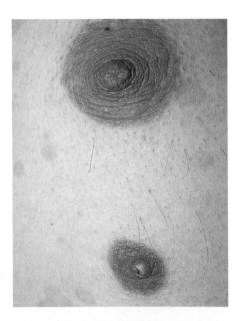

FIGURE 2.22 This accessory nipple was an incidental finding on a healthy teenager.

Collodion Baby

These infants are born encased in a thick cellophane-like membrane (Fig. 2.25). Although the collodian membrane may desquamate, leaving normal skin, 60 percent to 70 percent of these infants go on to develop congenital ichthyosiform erythroderma. Less commonly, this membrane is a prelude to lamellar ichthyosis, Netherton's syndrome, or Conradi's syndrome. The association with other variants of ichthyosis is less clear.

Although the horny layer is markedly thickened in collodian babies, barrier function is compromised by cracking and fissuring. Increased insensible water loss, heat loss, and risk of cutaneous infection and sepsis are minimized by placing affected newborns in a high-humidity, neutral-thermal environment. Debridement of the membrane is contraindicated, and topical applications should be restricted to bland emollients such as petrolatum. Desquamation is usually complete by two to three weeks of life.

A severe variant of ichthyosis, the *harlequin baby*, occurs rarely (Fig. 2.26). Although these infants appear normal at birth, within minutes they develop a thick generalized membrane, deep cracks and fissures, and marked ectropian and eclabian. Most infants succumb to respiratory distress or infection, but children who survive the neonatal period may develop scales reminiscent of lamellar ichthyosis.

Ichthyosis

The icthyoses are a heterogenous group of scaling disorders, which may be differentiated by mode of inheritance, clinical features, histology, and biochemical markers (Fig. 2.27). Rarely, icthyosis is a marker of multisystem disease in the newborn (Fig. 2.28).

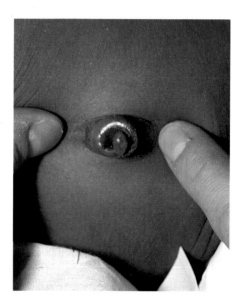

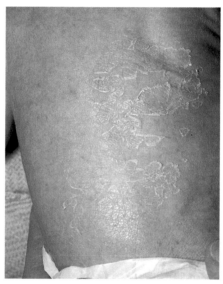

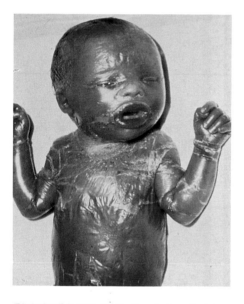

FIGURE 2.23 An umbilical granuloma responded to cautery with silver nitrate. Note the bright-red, friable nodule at the umbilical stump.

FIGURE 2.24 Scaling was marked at one week of age in this healthy infant. A week later the scaling had resolved completely.

FIGURE 2.25 Collodian baby. A shiny transparent membrane covered this baby at birth. She later developed lamellar ichthyosis. Note the ectropian and eclabian.

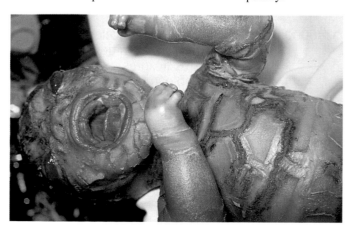

FIGURE 2.26 Harlequin baby. This baby developed thick plate-like scales immediately after drying in the delivery room. Respiratory failure resulted in death during the first week.

suprapubic area, and thighs. Secondary candidiasis or impetigo may mask the underlying process.

The cause of seborrheic dermatitis is unknown. However, the yeast *Pityrosporum* has been implicated in adult seborrhea, and has been identified in the scalp of infants with cradle cap. This organism tends to proliferate in areas where sebaceous glands are most numerous and active, which probably explains the timing and distribution of the eruption. Seborrheic dermatitis may clear without treatment by two to three months of age but often persists until eight to 12 months. Mild keratolytics found in antiseborrheic shampoos (zinc pyrithione, sulfur, and salicylic acid) are helpful in managing cradle cap. Emollients and low-potency topical steroids will hasten the resolution of cutaneous lesions. Topical antifungals have been approved for treating adult seborrheic dermatitis and may be useful in infants, particularly in patients with associated candidiasis.

Severe multisystem disease may begin with a pro-gressive diaper dermatitis. A seborrheic dermatitis-like eruption is characteristic of *histiocytosis X* (Fig. 2.39). However, the rash tends to become hemorrhagic and erosive, particularly in the diaper area. Scaly, crusted, purpuric plaques also develop on the scalp, trunk, and extremities. Diagnostic skin biopsies demonstrate infiltrates of atypical histiocytes containing Langerhans' cell granules. Similar infiltrates may involve the liver, lungs, kidneys, and nervous system, resulting in severe organ dysfunction and death.

Several benign variants of histiocytosis have been described in newborns and infants (Fig. 2.40). Reddish-yellow patches and papules erupt most commonly on the head and neck, but lesions may involve the trunk and extremities. There is no evidence of systemic disease. The histologic findings are indistinguishable from histiocytosis X, although Langerhans' cell markers have been absent in some patients. Cutaneous lesions generally involute without therapy within several years.

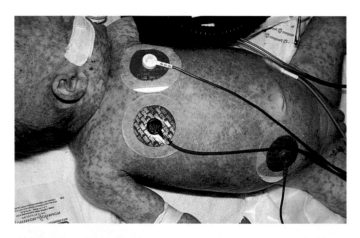

FIGURE 2.39 Histiocytosis X. A hemorrhagic diaper dermatitis rapidly generalized to the entire skin surface in this three week-old infant with diarrhea, poor weight gain, lymphadenopathy, and hepatosplenomegaly. This child died of disseminated histiocytosis at six weeks of age.

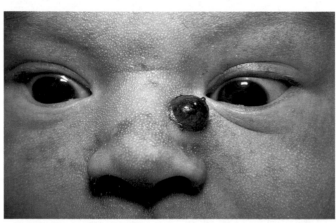

FIGURE 2.40 Benign cephalic histiocytosis. Although this nodule demonstrated typical microscopic changes of histiocytosis X, this infant developed no evidence of systemic disease, and several other skin nodules resolved without treatment.

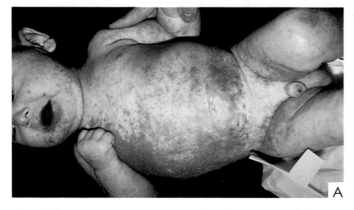

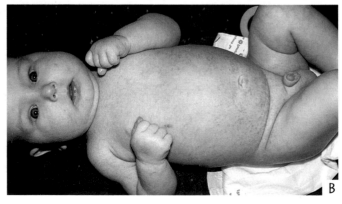

FIGURE 2.41 Acrodermatitis enteropathica. **(A)** A bright-red scaling dermatitis spread to the intertriginous areas, face, and extremities of this four-week-old infant. **(B)** After four

days of zinc supplementation, many lesions were healing with desquamation.

However, infants should receive long-term pediatric follow-up, because histiocytosis X occasionally presents with self-limited skin disease in infancy and systemic complications in later childhood or adolescence.

Acrodermatitis enteropathica (AEP) classically presents with an erosive diaper dermatitis, diarrhea, and hair loss during the first few months of life (Fig. 2.41A and B). Weeping, crusted, erythematous patches also appear in a periorificial, acral, and intertriginous distribution. Affected infants are irritable, grow poorly, and are prone to infection and septicemia.

AEP is an autosomal recessive disorder of zinc metabolism. Affected infants have either a defect in or low levels of a zinc-binding protein in the gastrointestinal tract, with resultant zinc malabsorption. Breast milk contains a compensatory zinc-binding ligand that facilitates absorption. Consequently, breast-fed infants do not develop symptoms until nursing is discontinued. Zinc is stored in the fetal liver, particularly during the last month of gestation. As a result, affected premature infants who are not breast fed become zinc deficient quickly. Normal infants who require hyperalimentation, as well as those with zinc losses from other malabsorption states (e.g., cystic fibrosis, chronic infectious diarrhea, short bowel syndrome), will also develop an AEP-like rash if they do not receive zinc supplementation. Similar rashes have also been reported with biotin deficiency, essential fatty acid deficiency, and urea enzyme cycle defects which result in essential amino acid deficiency.

AEP responds within several days to high doses of oral or intravenous zinc. Although dietary zinc without supplementation may be adequate in older children with AEP, these patients require close monitoring of growth and development. Some patients will require lifelong zinc supplements.

Congenital Syphilis

Although the incidence of neonatal syphilis decreased in the 1970s and 1980s, there has been a recent resurgence, particularly in urban centers. Infants born to mothers who have syphilis late in their pregnancy are at high risk for contracting the disease.

Although clinical manifestations of syphilis may be delayed until several years of age, common findings in the newborn include mucocutaneous lesions, prematurity, poor growth, and hepatosplenomegaly. Occasionally, severe systemic disease presents with generalized lymphadenopathy, pneumonitis, nephritis, enteritis, pancreatitis, osteochondritis, hematologic abnormalities, and meningitis.

Mucocutaneous lesions usually appear between two and six weeks of age. The most common finding in the skin is a maculopapular eruption, beginning on the palms and soles and spreading over the extremities and trunk (Fig. 2.42A). These lesions are comparable to the secondary syphilitic eruption of adults, and may be associated with vesiculation, ulceration, and desquamation. Moist, warty excrescences may develop in the intertriginous and periorificial areas. Smooth, round, moist mucous patches are characteristic of early neonatal syphilis, and commonly involve the mouth and perianal area. These lesions are highly infectious and readily demonstrate treponemes on dark-field examination. "Snuffles," or rhinitis with profuse and occasionally bloody rhinorrhea, is invariably present in symptomatic babies (Fig. 2.42B).

Diagnosis may be confirmed by dark-field examination of mucocutaneous lesions and serologic studies of the serum and cerebrospinal fluid. Screening of babies at risk for syphilis should include both specific treponoma (FTA-Abs) and nontreponemal (RPR or Veneral

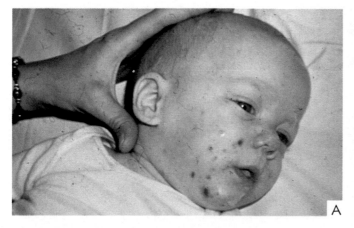
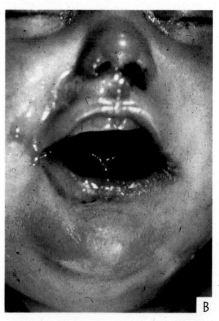

FIGURE 2.42 Neonatal syphilis. (**A**) A scaly eruption reminiscent of the lesions of secondary syphilis appeared on the face, trunk, and extremities of this infant. (**B**) "Snuffles," mucous patches, and condyloma lata were present in this infant.

Disease Reasearch Laboratories) studies. Early diagnosis and treatment with high-dose penicillin will prevent late complications of syphilis, including skeletal and dental anomalies, neurologic deterioration, eighth nerve deafness, and ophthalmologic disease.

VESICULOPUSTULAR DERMATOSES

Vesiculobullous and pustular eruptions may present a confusing clinical picture. Their diagnosis is critical, and early therapeutic intervention may be lifesaving.

Infections and Infestations

Viral infections, including *herpes simplex* and *varicella-zoster*, produce characteristic vesiculopustular eruptions. Herpes simplex is a common cause of self-limited oral and cutaneous lesions in toddlers and older children. However, in neonates there is a high risk of dissemination. Varicella is less common, but if lesions appear during the first week of life, the risk of mortality approaches 30 percent.

Herpes simplex infection occurs in one out of 3500 deliveries. Innoculation occurs from lesions on the cervix or vaginal area in most cases. However, the disease may be acquired postnatally from nursery personnel or family members. The incubation period varies from two to 21 days and peaks at six days. Consequently, infants may appear normal in the nursery but develop lesions after discharge. Manifestations vary from subclinical disease to widely disseminated infection and death. Skin rash develops in 70 percent of infected babies, and 90 percent of these children go on to develop systemic disease with involvement of the lungs, liver, gastrointestinal tract, and brain.

Cutaneous lesions typically begin as 1-mm to 2-mm clustered red papules and vesicles, which may become pustular, denuded, and hemorrhagic over the following two to three days (Fig. 2.43A). The first lesions commonly develop on the scalp after head deliveries, and on the feet or buttocks after breech presentation.

Suspicious blisters will reveal multinucleated giant cells when their contents are prepared on a glass slide with Giemsa or Wright's stain (Fig. 2.43B). Viral cultures from blister fluid or denuded areas of skin often demonstrate cytopathic effect within 24 to 36 hours. Early intervention with parenteral vidarabine and acyclovir may decrease the risk of disseminated disease, as well as morbidity and mortality when dissemination has already occurred. Skin lesions should be gently cleansed and excess blister fluid absorbed with a gauze pad to reduce cutaneous spread. Skin lesions may recur for up

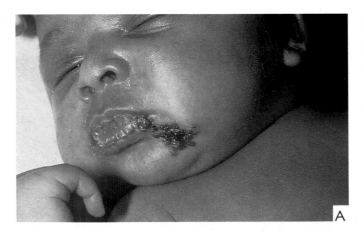
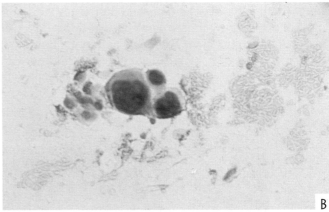

FIGURE 2.43 Herpes simplex. (**A**) The eroded vesicles at the corner of the mouth were the first sign of herpes infection in this neonate. (**B**) Tzanck preparation. Note the multinucleated giant cells characteristic of viral infection.

to five years, prompting a trial of oral acyclovir, particularly when recurrences are frequent.

When a mother has varicella within three weeks of delivery, her baby has a 25 percent risk of acquiring the disease during the neonatal period. Early exposure during the first trimester occasionally leads to the development of the neonatal varicella syndrome with linear scars, limb anomalies, ocular defects, and central nervous system involvement (Fig. 2.44).

As in herpes simplex, infants are usually well at birth but develop vesicles at three to ten days of life. Dissemination may result in pneumonitis, encephalitis, and purpura fulminans, with widespread bleeding, hypotension, and death. Children with chicken pox before three days of life and after ten days often have mild disease because of the presence of protective transplacental antibody.

Varicella-zoster immune globulin and parenteral acyclovir may improve the outcome, and should be considered early in the course. As with herpes simplex, the Tzanck smear will show multinucleated giant cells. These two viral infections can be definitively differentiated only by culture of the blister contents.

Several common bacterial infections present with vesiculopustular eruptions in infancy. The rash tends to be localized in *impetigo* and generalized in *staphylococcal scalded skin syndrome (SSSS)* (see Chapter 4).

In *classic streptococcal impetigo*, honey-colored crusts are found overlying infected insect bites, abrasions, and other skin rashes such as diaper dermatitis. *Bullous impetigo*, however, is characterized by slowly enlarging blistering rings surrounding central umbilicated crusts. Lesions may appear anywhere on the skin surface. However, in young infants, areas prone to trauma, such as the diaper area, circumcision wound, and umbilical stump, are frequent sites of primary infection. Bullous lesions are caused by certain epidermal toxin-producing types of *Staphylococcus*. Although lesions may remain localized, they are highly infectious and may be inoculated to multiple sites on the patient as well as other family members. In newborns and young infants, dissemination of the toxin may result in widespread erythema and blistering typical of SSSS (Fig. 2.45). Gentle presure on the skin causes the upper epidermis to slide off, leaving a denuded base (Nikolsky sign).

In localized impetigo, bacteria are identified in Gram-stained material obtained directly from the rash. In SSSS, the practitioner may be unable to identify a primary cutaneous site of infection. In these children, noncutaneous sources, including lungs, bone, meninges, and ears, must be sought.

Small patches of impetigo respond well to topical antibiotic therapy (e.g., mupirocin, bacitracin, bacitracin-

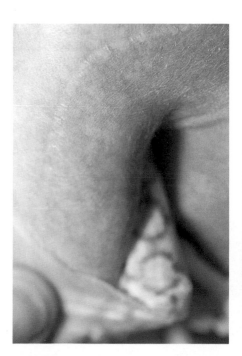

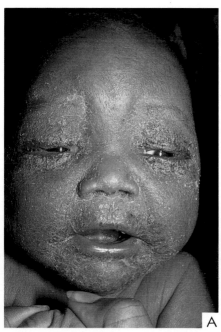

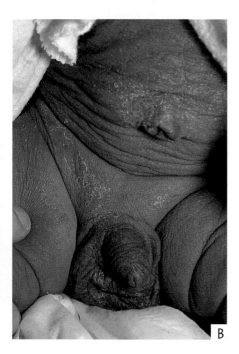

FIGURE 2.44 Varicella. A linear scar was evident on the arm of this newborn whose mother developed chicken pox during the first trimester.

FIGURE 2.45 Staphylococcal scalded skin syndrome developed in this neonate who was being treated for mastitis.

Erosive patches were most marked on the face (**A**) and diaper areas (**B**).

polymixin B) and normal saline compresses. Healthy infants with recalcitrant or widespread impetigo require oral antibiotics with broad-spectrum Gram-positive coverage (erythromycin, dicloxacillin, cephalexin, trimethoprin-sulfamethoxazole, amoxicillin/clavulanate potassium). Neonates and young infants may not localize infection to the epidermis and superficial dermis. Any signs of progressive cellulitis or visceral dissemination should prompt immediate hospitalization, treatment with parenteral antibiotics, and supportive care. When infants develop infection in the first two to three weeks of life, even after discharge from the hospital, a nursery source should be suspected. Breaches in nursery hygiene and skin colonization of nursery personnel should be investigated.

Disseminated candidiasis in the newborn may be confused with bacterial infection. In congenital candidiasis, which develops during the first day of life, generalized erythematous papules, vesicles, and pustules may slough, leaving large denuded areas reminiscent of

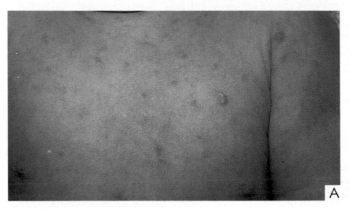

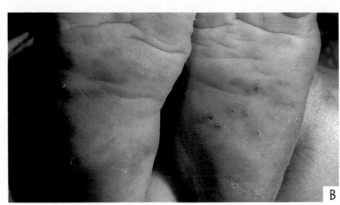

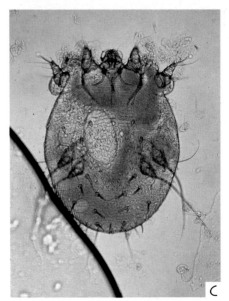

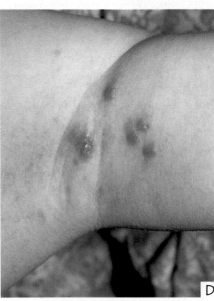

FIGURE 2.46 Burrows were present on the trunk (**A**), hands, and feet (**B**) of this infant with widespread scabies. (**C**) A gravid adult scabies mite was identified in a scraping of material from a burrow. (**D**) Scabies nodules in the axillae of this infant persisted for four months.

SSSS. The organism is acquired by ascending vaginal or cervical infection. Diagnostic features include the presence of oral thrush in some infants at birth and the identification of pseudohyphae and spores from pustules and scale. When infants acquire infection at delivery, the onset of lesions may be delayed by seven to ten days, and erosive patches with satellite pustules are usually limited to intertriginous areas. Full-term infants often go on to heal with desquamation without treatment, although topical antifungals may be helpful. Preterm infants are at high risk for dissemination, and early diagnosis and initiation of parenteral amphotericin may be lifesaving.

Scabies is a common, well-characterized, infectious dermatosis produced by the *Sarcoptes scabei* mite. The impregnated female burrows through the outer epidermis to deposit her eggs. The resulting diagnostic rash consists of pruritic linear burrows on the finger webs, wrists, elbows, belt line, areola, scrotum, and penis. In infants, burrows are widespread, with involvement of the trunk, scalp, and extremities, including the palms and soles (Fig 2.46A and B). Although infants may be otherwise healthy and well grown, chronic infestation may result in poor feeding, fussiness, and failure to thrive. Chronic and recurrent infection with pustules, crusting, and cellulitis are frequent complications.

This diagnosis should be considered in any infant with a widespread dermatosis that involves the palms and soles, particularly if other family members are involved. The presence of burrows is pathognomonic, and an ectoparasite preparation will be confirmatory. After a drop of mineral oil is applied to a burrow, the skin surface should be stretched between the examiner's thumb and index finger. Vigorous scraping with a #15 blade should be performed until the burrow is no longer palpable. This may leave a small bleeding point at the center of the burrow. The material is subsequently spread with the blade on a glass slide and pressed under a cover slip. The female mite, eggs, and fecal material are readily visualized under a scanning 10x lens (Fig 2.46C).

Until recently, topical 1 percent lindane (gamma benzene hexachloride) has been the mainstay of treatment. Although the risk of toxicity with lindane is low when it is used appropriately in the medical setting, severe central nervous system reactions have been reported in young infants, particularly wasted, chronically ill children. Alternative agents are either ineffective (crotamiton, benzyl benzoate), potentially toxic (sulfur ointment, benzyl benzoate), or cosmetically unacceptable (sulfur ointment). In 1989, Herbert Laboratories introduced permethrin 5 percent cream. Studies have shown that permethrin has a higher cure rate than lindane and that it may be used safely in children as young as two months.

At the start of therapy parents should be carefully instructed and given limited quantities of the scabicide. The entire family and any others who have contact with the infant, such as babysitters, should be treated simultaneously. Topical lubricants will be necessary for several weeks after treatment to counteract drying and irritation produced by the scabicides and to resolve cutaneous lesions. Persistent pruritic nodules may arise from some burrows, particularly in intertriginous areas (Fig. 2.46D). Nodular scabies requires only symptomatic treatment, unless new inflammatory lesions appear. Secondary infection responds to tap water compresses and antibiotics as indicated.

Mechanobullous diseases (epidermolysis bullosa) are a heterogenous group of blistering dermatoses characterized by the development of lesions after trauma to the skin. Epidermolysis bullosa (EB) variants are differentiated on the basis of their inheritance pattern, clinical presentation, histopathology, and biochemical markers (Fig. 2.47). Although blisters may appear at birth or in the neonatal period, in mild localized forms, onset of lesions is often delayed until later childhood or adult life.

EB may be classified into three major types based upon the cleavage plane of the blister (see Fig. 2.47). In EB simplex, blisters are intraepidermal, and the clinical

Figure 2.47 Mechanobullous Disorders

I	Variant	Site of Blister	Inheritance
	Epidermolysis bullosa simplex EBS generalized (Koebner)	Intraepidermal (basal cell cytolysis)	Autosomal dominant
	EBS localized (Weber–Cockayne)	Intraepidermal (suprabasal)	Autosomal dominant
	EB Ogna	Intraepidermal	Autosomal dominant
II	Junctional EB atrophicans generalized gravis (letalis, Herlitz)	Lamina lucida (reduced number, abnormal hemidesmosomes)	Autosomal recessive
	EB atrophicans generalized mitis	Lamina lucida	Autosomal recessive
	EB atrophicans localized	Lamina lucida	
	EB atrophicans inversa	Lamina lucida	Autosomal recessive
III	Dystrophic Epidermolysis Bullosa EBD Cockayne–Touraine	Dermis (↓anchoring fibrils)	Autosomal dominant
	EBD albulopapuloid (Pasini)	Dermis (rudimentary anchoring fibrils)	Autosomal dominant
	EBD recessive (Hallopeau–Siemens)	Dermis (↓or absence of anchoring fibrils)	Autosomal recessive

Figure 2.47 *continued*

Onset	Clinical Features
Birth to early infancy	Nonscarring generalized blisters worse on hands and feet
Infancy to adulthood	Nonscarring blisters on hands and feet; hyperhidrosis
Infancy	Linkage to erythrocyte GPT locus
Birth	Often lethal by 2 years; nonscarring widespread blisters. Dysplastic nails, teeth; severe oral lesions
Birth	Blisters heal with atrophy; dysplastic nails; enamel dysplasia
Nail changes—birth Skin changes—school age	Localized blistering of hands, feet; nails dystrophic; enamel dysplasia
Infancy, early childhood	Milia, scar formation; dystrophy or loss of nails
Birth	Healing with scars, milia; nail dystrophy; albulopapuloid lesions on trunk
Birth	Generalized blisters healing with scars, milia, dystrophic nails, digital fusion, severe oral lesions; dysplastic teeth; esophageal strictures, conjunctival and corneal erosion; ↑collagenase in blisters

course is usually mild (Fig. 2.48). In junctional EB, blisters form at the dermal–epidermal junction, usually through the lamina lucida in the basement membrane zone. Although patients may have mild disease comparable to EB simplex, in some children progressive blistering with involvement of the mucous membranes and gastrointestinal tract can lead to inanition, sepsis, and death in the first two years of life (Fig. 2.49). Dystrophic EB is characterized by scarring blisters that form in the dermis beneath the basement membrane zone. Blisters may be localized to the hands and feet or be widespread with involvement of the dentition, nails, airway, and esophagus (Fig. 2.50).

EB should be considered in infants with recurrent blistering when infection has been excluded. Family history and examination of other family members will aid in clinical diagnosis. A skin biopsy with electron microscopy will provide precise identification of the cleavage plane in the skin. Genetic counseling and prenatal diagnosis should be discussed with the family, particularly in severe variants.

In children without a family history of EB, it may be difficult to determine a prognosis in the newborn period. Infants with dystrophic EB may do very well, while children with junctional disease may develop a downhill course after a period of stabilization. In this setting the practitioner should be reassuring and postpone discussion of prognosis until after a period of observation.

Treatment is dependent on the severity of EB. In mild variants, patients will learn to avoid traumas that trigger bullae formation. Pain and progression of large blisters may be controlled by gently unroofing lesions, or cutting a square skin window and covering with a topical antibiotic ointment and sterile gauze. Adhesives should be applied from dressing to dressing, and kept out of direct contact with the skin.

For severely affected children, the practitioner must orchestrate a multidisciplinary approach to management. The dermatologist, ophthalmologist, gastroenterologist, otolaryngologist, plastic surgeon, thoracic surgeon, dentist, and physical therapist may be involved in care. Preventive care includes avoidance of trauma to

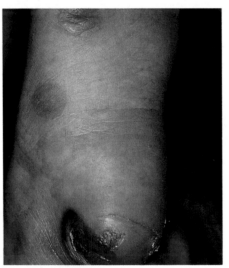

FIGURE 2.48 Epidermolysis bullosa simplex. Numerous blisters form easily in pressure areas.

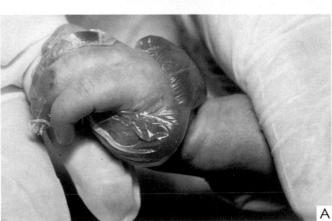

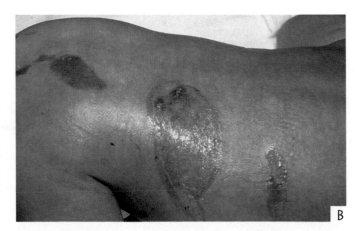

FIGURE 2.49 Junctional epidermolysis bullosa. Widespread involvement was seen in this infant at birth. **(A)** Note the erosions and the large, intact blister over the thumb and dorsum of the hand. **(B)** Large, denuded areas are noted over the back and buttocks.

the skin and mucous membranes, and early treatment of infection with topical and oral antibiotics. Iron may be required to replace chronic blood losses through the skin. Adaptic, Vaseline gauze, and Telfa dressings help to retain moisture, reduce pain, and facilitate healing of erosions and ulcers. Topical dressings should be gently held in place by clean wraps such as gauze or Kling, and soaked off without tearing at fresh granulation tissue. New semipermeable dressings (N-ter-face, Ensure, Vigilon) and occlusive dressings (Duoderm, Comfeel) may be useful in the treatment of recalcitrant wounds. Good nutrition is mandatory for cutaneous healing and general growth and development.

Aplasia cutis congenita is a heterogenous group of disorders whose common feature is congenital absence of the skin. Although the cause is unknown, this entity has been recognized for over 150 years. In the classic form, one or several erosions or ulcerations covered with a crust or thin membrane involve the vertex of the scalp (Fig. 2.51). Healing with atrophic hairless scars

may take two to six months, depending on the size and depth of the ulceration, which may extend through the soft tissue into bone. This benign variant is usually inherited as an autosomal dominant trait. Less commonly, the trunk and extremities are involved, and lesions may be associated with limb defects, epidermolysis bullosa, and chromosomal aberrations.

In uncomplicated aplasia cutis congenita, the defect is amenable to simple excision during later childhood or adult life. Large lesions may require staged excision and the use of tissue expanders (Fig. 2.52). In the newborn, care must be taken to evaluate the depth of the defect, prevent further tissue damage and infection, and search for associated anomalies. Gentle normal saline compresses, topical antibiotics, and sterile dressings are adequate for most patients. Large defects may respond to occlusive dressings (Duoderm, Comfeel). Occasionally, early surgical intervention is necessary.

Perinatal trauma to the scalp may result in similar defects noted at birth or within the first month of life.

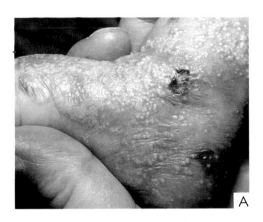
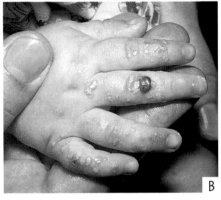
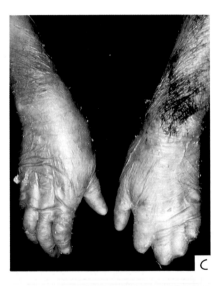

FIGURE 2.50 Dystrophic epidermolysis bullosa. **(A)** Blisters, erosions, and hundreds of milia are seen on the foot and ankle and **(B)** hand of this newborn. **(C)** In this child, severe scarring encased the fingers, resulting in syndactyly.

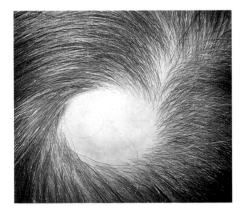
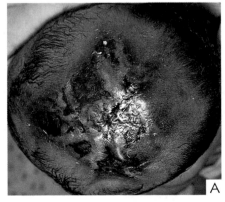
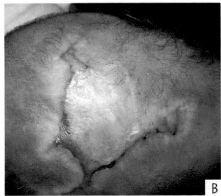

FIGURE 2.51 Aplasia cutis congenita. This child, his mother, and his grandfather had similar hairless, atrophic plaques on the occiput. A thin hemorrhagic membrane was noted at birth.

FIGURE 2.52 (A) An extensive area of aplasia cutis was noted on the scalp of this newborn. **(B)** Five months later the scalp was almost completely healed.

When the child was five years old, the residual scar was repaired following tissue expansion.

common sites of involvement, but dermoids occasionally present on the mid chest, sacrum, perineum, and scrotum (Fig. 2.71).

Dermoid cysts are lined by an epidermis that contains mature adnexal structures, including sebaceous glands, eccrine glands, and apocrine glands. Although there is no risk of malignancy, lesions on the head may extend to periosteum and cause erosion of the underlying bone. Cysts may be surgically excised during infancy or childhood.

Lesions on the head must be differentiated from hematomas, encephaloceles, and malignant tumors. A CT scan and magnetic resonance imaging of the head will demonstrate the cystic nature of the dermoid and exclude the possibility of communication with the central nervous system or infiltrative tumor.

Dermoids overlying the sacrum may be associated with occult defects of the vertebral column and spinal cord. Magnetic resonance imaging will visualize the tumor and associated anomalies.

In *recurrent infantile digital fibroma*, single or multiple fibrous nodules appear on the fingers and toes (Fig. 2.72). Although these tumors may occur in older children, 85 percent are diagnosed before one year of age, and many are noted at birth or in the first month of life. Lesions rarely exceed 2.0 cm in diameter. Skin biopsy demonstrates numerous fibroblasts and interlacing collagen bundles. The presence of perinuclear intracytoplasmic inclusion bodies was thought to suggest a viral etiology. However, this has been refuted by studies using electron microscopy. Although excision is followed by recurrence in 75 percent of cases, most digital fibromas involute spontaneously within several years.

Infantile myofibromatosis, also referred to as congenital fibromatosis, usually presents as a solitary, firm, red or blue, mobile subcutaneous tumor (Fig. 2.73). However, multiple tumors may involve muscle and bone, and visceral lesions may produce organ dysfunction, especially in the lungs. On histologic examination these well-circumscribed tumors contain fibroblasts and smooth muscle cells without cytologic atypia. Solitary lesions are usually excised without recurrence, but new tumors may erupt for the first several months of life. In the

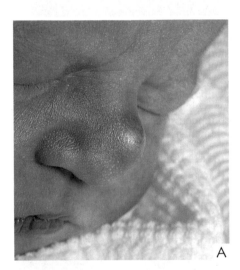 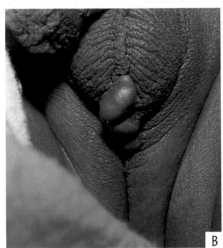

FIGURE 2.71 Dermoid cyst. (A) This partially compressible mass was present on the nose at birth. A CT scan of the head to exclude a communication with the underlying central nervous system was normal. (B) This cyst on the median raphe of the scrotum of a four-month-old had not changed since birth.

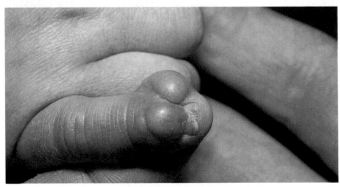 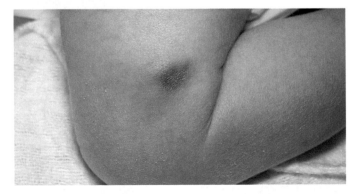

FIGURE 2.72 Recurrent infantile digital fibroma. This tumor on the finger of a seven-month-old boy recurred after local excision. However after an initial growth phase, it began to involute without further therapy.

FIGURE 2.73 Myofibromatosis. An infiltrating subcutaneous tumor on the thigh of a one-month-old demonstrated histologic features of myofibromatosis. Other benign and malignant tumors, including neuroblastoma, leukemia, and lymphoma, should be included in the differential diagnosis.

majority of infants without severe visceral disease, spontaneous involution occurs in the first year of life.

Malignant tumors rarely present at birth or in the newborn period.

Fifty percent of patients with neuroblastoma are diagnosed in the first two years of life, and many develop clinical disease before six months. Although cutaneous metastases are seen in only about 3 percent of all patients with neuroblastoma, nearly a third of affected newborns present with skin lesions as their initial manifestation. Metastases usually appear as 0.5-cm to 2.0-cm, firm, bluish-red papules and nodules on the trunk and extrem-ities. Stroking results in blanching and a red halo, probably from the release of catecholamines from tumor cells. These "blueberry muffin" lesions must be distinguished from areas of extramedullary hematopoiesis seen in infants with congenital infections such as rubella, cytomegalovirus, and toxoplasmosis (Fig. 2.74).

Cutaneous plaques and tumors may also be the earliest finding in newborns with leukemia (Fig. 2.75), rhabdomyosarcoma (Fig. 2.76), lymphoma, and a number of other carcinomas and sarcomas. Skin biopsy of rapidly growing or infiltrative lesions may lead to early diagnosis and therapy.

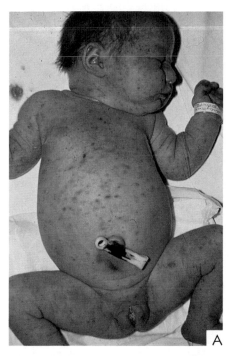 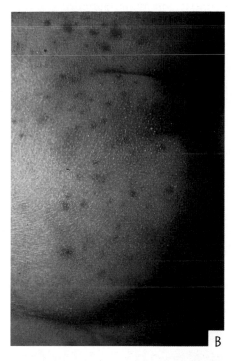

FIGURE 2.74 (A, B) Blueberry muffin rash. This infant with congenital rubella demonstrated the typical cutaneous lesions of extramedullary hematopoiesis.

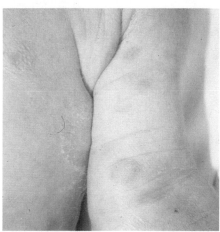

FIGURE 2.75 Congenital leukemia cutis. This newborn presented with a hemoglobin of 5.0 g percent and infiltrative, pale-pink, annular plaques on the extremities.

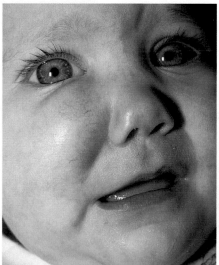

FIGURE 2.76 Rhabdomyosarcoma. This rapidly growing congenital mass was part of an infiltrating rhabdomyosarcoma involving the cheek, orbit, nose, and sinuses of this infant. This child was treated with surgical debulking of the mass and chemotherapy.

REACTIVE ERYTHEMAS

Reactive erythema refers to a group of disorders characterized by erythematous macules, plaques, and nodules that vary in size, shape, and distribution. Unlike specific dermatoses, they represent reaction patterns in the skin triggered by a number of different endogenous and environmental factors. In infants, erythema multiforme, erythema nodosum, urticaria, and vasculitis occur after exposure to various infections and drugs. Just as in older children and adults, management of affected infants involves identification and elimination of the offending agent and supportive care. Several reactive erythemas, however, are peculiar to infancy.

Neonatal lupus erythematosus is the most common cause of congenital heart block. Although cutaneous lesions may not appear until several months of age, they are frequently present at birth. Affected infants demonstrate annular erythematous plaques with a central scale, telangiectasias, atrophy, and pigmentary changes (Fig. 2.77). Lesions typically range from 0.5 cm to 3.0 cm in diameter, and may spread from the scalp and face to the neck, upper trunk, and upper extremities. Although the development of the cutaneous rash does not require sunlight, it may be triggered or exacerbated by exposure to the sun.

The cause of neonatal lupus is unknown. However, the presence of transplacentally acquired ssA(Ro) and ssB(La) antibodies is thought to play a primary role in the pathogenesis of the disorder. In adults, ssA and ssB antibodies are associated with Sjögren's syndrome and a photosensitive variant of systemic lupus known as subacute cutaneous lupus erythematosus.

In addition to conduction defects and structural cardiac anomalies, affected infants may develop hepatosplenomegaly, anemia, leukopenia, thrombocytopenia, and lymphadenopathy. With the exception of cardiac involvement, neonatal lupus usually resolves spontaneously in six to twelve months as transplacentally derived antibody wanes. The use of low- and medium-potency topical steroids on intensely inflammatory cutaneous lesions for several weeks may reduce the risk of scarring. Subtle atrophy and pigmentary changes may persist indefinitely. Rarely, infants will require systemic corticosteroids and supportive care. Parents should be instructed to protect children with sunscreens and avoid direct exposure to the sun for at least four to six months. Mothers without clinical signs of lupus also require careful follow-up because they are at increased risk of developing overt disease.

Annular erythema of infancy is an innocent gyrate erythema which presents during the first six months of life with red papules and plaques that enlarge in a centrifugal pattern (Fig. 2.78). Lesions may develop a dusky center and exceed 10 cm in diameter over one to three weeks. Plaques periodically fade, only to recur for months to years. Although this reaction may be triggered by infections, drugs, and malignancy, evaluation for an underlying disease is usually unrevealing. Fortunately, infants generally continue to thrive, and lesions eventually resolve without treatment.

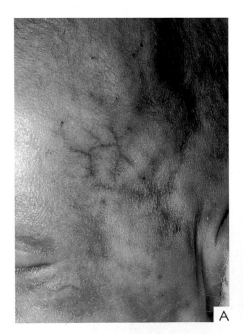
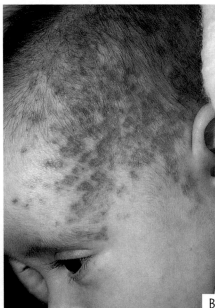
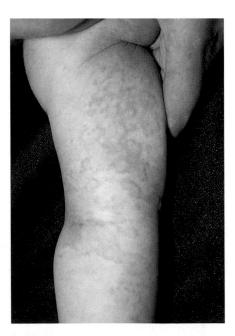

FIGURE 2.77 Neonatal lupus erythematosus. (**A**) This newborn presented with extensive cutaneous atrophy facial telangiectasias, hepatosplenomegaly, and thrombocytopenia. (**B**) At one month of age this infant developed an extensive eruption of annular red plaques with central atrophy. Lesions first appeared on the scalp and face, and subsequently spread to the neck and trunk.

FIGURE 2.78 Annular erythema of fancy. This eruption persisted for months on the trunk and extremities of an otherwise healthy infant.

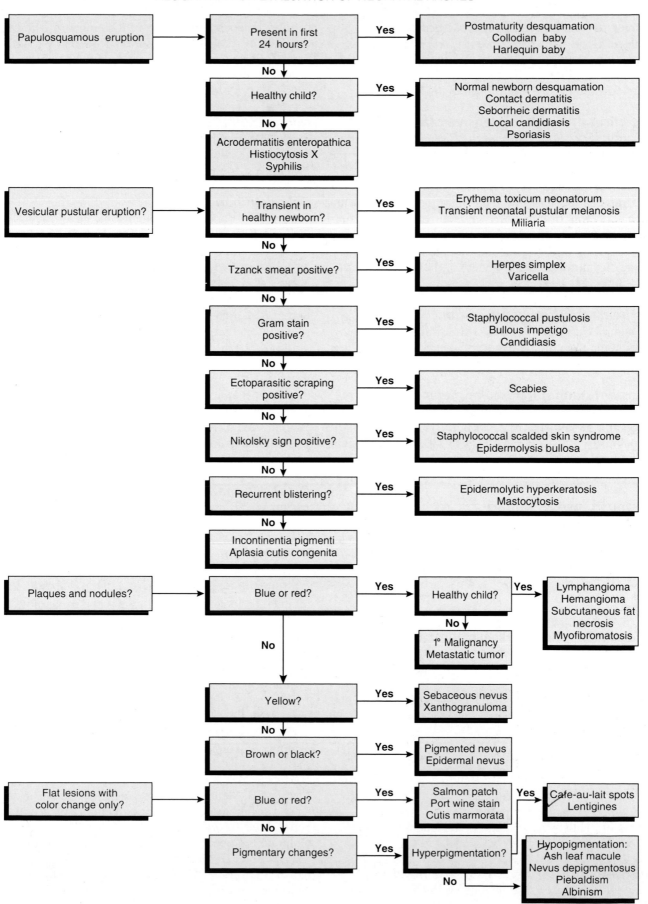

BIBLIOGRAPHY

Barrier properties and topical agents
Maibach HI, Boisits EK. *Neonatal skin structure and function.* New York: Marcel Dekker, 1982.
Nachman RL, Esterly NB. Increased skin permeability in preterm infants. *J Pediatr* 79:628–632, 1971.

Complications of the intensive care nursery
Ballard RA. *Pediatric care of the ICN graduate.* Philadelphia: Saunders, 1988.

Cutis marmorata
Fitzsimmons JS, Starks M. Cutis marmorata telangiectatica congenita or congenital generalized phlebectasia. *Arch Dis Child* 45:724–726, 1970.
Powell ST, Su WPD. Cutis marmorata telangiectatica: report of nine cases and review of the literature. *Cutis* 34:305–312, 1984.

Erythema toxicum neonatorum
Freeman RG, Spiller R, Knox JM. Histopathology of erythema toxicum neonatorum. *Arch Dermatol* 82:586,1960.

Transient neonatal pustular melanosis
Barr RJ, Globerman LM, Werber FA. Transient neonatal pustular melanosis. *Int J Dermatol* 18:636–638, 1979.
Ramamurthy RS, Reveri M, Esterly MB, et al. Transient neonatal pustular melanosis. *J Pediatr* 88:831–835, 1976.

Acropustulosis of infancy
Jarratt M, Ramsdell W. Infantile acropustulosis. *Arch Dermatol* 115:834–836, 1979.
Kahn G, Rywlin AM. Acropustulosis of infancy. *Arch Dermatol* 115:831–834, 1979.

Miliaria
Holzle E, Kligman AM. The pathogenesis of miliaria rubra: role of the resident microflora. *Br J Dermatol* 99:117–137,1978.

Milia
Epstein W, Kligman AM. The pathogenesis of milia and benign tumors of the skin. *J Invest Dermatol* 26:1–11, 1956.

Newborn acne
Forest MG, Cathaird AM, Bertrand JA. Evidence of testicular activity in early infancy. *J Clin Endocrinol Metab* 37:148, 1973.
Ginkis FL, Hall WK, Tolman MM. Acne neonatorum. *Arch Dermatol* 66:717–721, 1952.

Subcutaneous fat necrosis of the newborn
Norwood-Galloway A, Lebwohl M, Phelps RG, et al. Subcutaneous fat necrosis of the newborn with hypercalcemia. *J Am Acad Dermatol* 16:435–439, 1987.
Tsuji T. Subcutaneous fat necrosis of the newborn. Light and electron microscopic studies. *Br J Dermatol* 95:407–416, 1976.

Minor anomalies
Steele MW, Golden WL. Syndromes of congenital anomalies. In: Kelley VC, ed. *Practice of Pediatrics.* Philadelphia: Lippincott, 1984.

Collodion baby
Baden HP, Kubilus J, Rosenbaum K, Fletcher A. Keratinization in the harlequin fetus. *Arch Dermatol* 118:14–18, 1982.
deDobbeleer G, Heenen M, Song M, Achten G. Collodion baby skin. Ultrastructural and autoradiographic study. *J Cutan Pathol* 9:196–202, 1982.
Lareque M, Gharbi R, Daniel J, et al. Le bebe collodion evolution a propos de 29 cas. *Ann Dermatol Venereol* 103:31, 1976.

Ichthyosis
Rand RE, Baden HP. The icthyoses—a review. *J Am Acad Dermatol* 8: 285–305,1983.
Williams ML. The ichthyoses—pathogenesis and prenatal diagnosis: a review of recent advances. *Pediatr Dermatol* 1:1–24, 1983.

Diaper dermatitis
Jordan WE, Blaney TL. Factors influencing diaper dermatitis. In: Maibach HI, Boisits EK, eds. *Neonatal Skin Structure and Function.* New York: Marcel Dekker, 1982:217.
Neville EA, Finn OA. Psoriasiform napkin dermatitis—a follow-up study. *Br J Dermatol* 92:279–285, 1975.
Stein H. Incidence of diaper rash when using cloth and disposable diapers. *J Pediatr* 101:721–723, 1982.

Seborrheic dermatitis
Skinner RB Jr, Noah PW, Taylor RM, et al. Double blind treatment of seborrheic dermatitis with 2% ketoconazole cream. *J Am Acad Dermatol* 12:852–856, 1985.
Yates VM, Kerr EI, Mackie RM. Early diagnosis of infantile seborrheic dermatitis and atopic dermatitis—clinical features. *Br J Dermatol* 108:633–645, 1983.

Histiocytosis X
Esterly NB, Maurer HS, Gonzales-Crussi F. Histiocytosis X: a seven year experience at a children's hospital. *J Am Acad Dermatol* 13:481–496, 1985.
Gianotte F, Caputo R. Histiocytic syndromes: a review. *J Am Acad Dermatol* 13:383–404, 1985.
Roper SS, Spraker MK. Cutaneous histiocytosis syndromes. *Pediatr Dermatol* 3:19–30, 1985.

Acrodermatitis enteropathica

Campo AG Jr, McDonald CJ. Treatment of acrodermatitis enteropatica with zinc sulfate. *Arch Dermatol* 112: 687–689, 1976.

Danbolt N, Closs K. Akrodermatitis enteropathica. *Acta Derm Venereol* (Stockholm) 23:127–169, 1942.

Gonzalez JR, Botet MV, Sanchez JL. The histopathology of acrodermatitis enteropathica. *Am J Dermatopathol* 4:303–311, 1982.

Congenital syphilis

Dorfman DH, Glaser JH. Congenital syphilis presenting in infants after the newborn period. *N Engl J Med* 323: 1299–1301, 1990.

Mascola L, Pelosi R, Blount JH, et al. Congenital syphilis revisited. *Am J Dis Child* 139:575, 1985.

McIntosh, K. Editorial: congenital syphilis—breaking through the safety net. *N Engl J Med* 323:1339–1340, 1990.

Rathbun KC. Congenital syphilis. *Sex Transm Dis* 10:93, 1983.

Herpes simplex

Jenista JA. Perinatal herpesvirus infections. *Semin Perinatol* 7:9, 1983.

Whitley R, Arvin A, Prober C, et al. A controlled trial comparing vidarabine with acyclovir in neonatal herpes simplex infection. *N Engl J Med* 324:444–449, 1991.

Whitley R, Arvin A, Prober C, et al. Predictors of morbidity and mortality in neonates with herpes simplex virus infections. *N Engl J Med* 324:450–454, 1991.

Varicella

Glickman FS, Albanese P, Kuhnlein E. Congenital varicella. *Cutis* 28:578, 1981.

Herrmann KL. Congenital and perinatal varicella. *Clin Obstet Gynecol* 25:605, 1982.

La Foret E, Lynch CL. Multiple congenital defects following maternal varicella. *N Engl J Med* 236:534–537, 1947.

Staphylococcal scalded skin syndrome

Elias PM, Fritsch P, Epstein EH Jr. Staphylococcal scalded skin syndrome (review). *Arch Dermatol* 113: 207–219, 1977.

Ginsburg CM. Staphylococcal toxin syndromes. *Pediatr Infect Dis J* 2(Suppl):23, 1983.

Lyell A. Toxic epidermal necrolysis (the scalded skin syndrome): a reappraisal. *Br J Dermatol* 100:69–86, 1979.

Candidiasis

Chapel TA, Gagliardi C, Nichols W. Congenital cutaneous candidiasis. *J Am Acad Dermatol* 6:926–928, 1982.

Johnson DE, Thompson TR, Ferrieri P. Congenital candidiasis. *Am J Dis Child* 135:273–275, 1981.

Scabies

Estes SA. The diagnosis and management of scabies. Piscataway, NJ: Reed & Carnrick, 1988.

Taplin D, Meinking TL, Chen JA, Sanchez R. Comparison of crotamiton 10% cream (Eurax) and permethrin 5% cream (Elimite) for the treatment of scabies in children. *Pediatr Dermatol* 7:67–73, 1990.

Epidermolysis bullosa

Fine JD. Editorial: changing clinical and laboratory concepts in inherited epidermolysis bullosa. *Arch Dermatol* 124:523–526, 1988.

Hintner H, Stingl G, Schuler G, et al. Immunofluorescence mapping of antigen determinants within the dermal-epidermal junction in mechanobulous diseases. *J Invest Dermatol* 76: 113–118, 1981.

Pessar A, Verdicchio JF, Caldwell D. Epidermolysis bullosa. The pediatric dermatologic management and therapeutic update. *Adv Dermatol* 3:99, 1988.

Thiers BH. Journal club—the mechanobullous diseases, hereditary epidermolysis bullosa and epidermolysis bullosa acquisita. *J Am Acad Dermatol* 5:745–748, 1981.

Aplasia cutis congenita

Frieden IJ. Aplasia cutis congenita: a clinical review and proposal for classification. *J Am Acad Dermatol* 14: 646–660, 1986.

Levin DL, Nolan KS, Esterly NB. Congenital absence of the skin. *J Am Acad Dermatol* 2:203, 1980.

Mastocytosis

Caplan RM. The natural course of urticaria pigmentosa. *Arch Dermatol* 87:146–157, 1983.

Guzzo C, Lavker R, Roberts LJ, Fox K, Schechter N, Lazarus G. Urticaria pigmentosa: systemic evaluation and successful treatment with topical steroids. *Arch Dermatol* 127:191–196, 1991.

Simon RA. Treatment of mastocytosis. *N Engl J Med* 302:231–232, 1980.

Smith ML, Orton PW, Chu HM, Weston W. Photochemotherapy of dominant, diffuse, cutaneous mastocytosis. *Pediatr Dermatol* 7:251–255, 1990.

Soter NA, Austen KF, Wasserman SL. Oral sodium cromoglycate in the treatment of systemic mastocytosis. *N Engl J Med* 301:465–469, 1979.

Incontinentia pigmenti

Carney RG. Incontinentia pigmenti, a world statistical analysis. *Arch Dermatol* 112:535–542, 1976.

Cohen BA. Incontinentia pigmenti. *Neurol Clin N Am* 5:361, 1987.

Vascular nevi

Cohen BA. Hemangiomas in infancy and childhood. *Pediatr Ann* 16:17, 1987.

Cohen BA. Management of vascular lesions in adolescents. *Adolesc Med* 1:385, 1990.

Reyes BA, Geronemus. Treatment of port-wine stains during childhood with flashlamp-pumped pulsed dye laser. *J Am Acad Dermatol* 23:1142–1148, 1990.

Tan OT, Carney JM, Margolis R, et al. Histologic response of port wine stains treated by argon, carbon dioxide, and tuneable dye lasers. *Arch Dermatol* 122: 1016–1022, 1986.

Lymphangiomas

Hilliard RI, Mckendry JBJ, Phillips MJ. Experience and reason—briefly recorded: congenital abnormalities of the lymphatic system: a new clinical classification. *Pediatrics* 86:988, 1990.

Levine C. Primary disorders of the lymphatic vessels: a unified concept. *J Pediatr Surg* 24:233–240, 1989.

Epidermal nevus

Basler RSW, Jacobs SI, Taylor WB. Ichthyosis hystrix. *Arch Dermatol* 114:1059–1060, 1978.

Eichler C, Flowers FP, Ross J. Epidermal nevus syndrome: case report and review of clinical manifestations. *Pediatr Dermatol* 6:316–320, 1989.

Sebaceus nevus

Domingo J, Helwig EB. Malignant neoplasms associated with nevus sebaceus of Jadassohn. *J Am Acad Dermatol* 1:545, 1979.

Morioka S. The natural history of nevus sebaceus. *J Cutan Pathol* 12:200–213, 1985.

Smooth muscle nevus

Bronson DM, Fretzin DF, Farrell LN. Congenital pilar and smooth muscle nevus. *J Am Acad Dermatol* 8:111–114, 1983.

Connective tissue nevus

Schorr WF, Opitz JM, Reyes CN. The connective tissue nevus—osteopoikilosis syndrome. *Arch Dermatol* 106: 208–214, 1972.

Verbov J, Graham R. Buschke–Ollendorff syndrome—disseminated dermatofibrosis with osteopoikilosis. *Clin Exp Dermatol* 11:17–26, 1986.

Pigmented nevi

Everett MA. Histopathology of congenital pigmented nevi. *Am J Dermatopathol* 11:11–12, 1989.

Rhodes AR, Sober AJ, Day CL, et al. The malignant potential of small congenital nevocellular nevi. *J Am Acad Dermatol* 6:230–241, 1982.

Silvers DN, Helwig EB. Melanocytic nevi in neonates. *J Am Acad Dermatol* 4:166–179, 1981.

Juvenile xanthogranuloma

Cohen BA, Hood A. Xanthogranuloma: report on clinical and histologic findings in 64 patients. *Pediatr Dermatol* 6:262, 1989.

Dermoid cyst

Kennard CD, Rasmussen JE. Congenital midline nasal masses: diagnosis and management. *J Dermatol Surg Oncol* 16:1025–1036, 1990.

Recurrent infantile digital fibroma

Iwasaki H, Kiruchi M, Mori R, et al. Infantile digital fibromatosis. *Cancer* 46:2238–2247, 1980.

Infantile myofibromatosis

Spraker MK, Stack C, Esterly NB. Congenital generalized fibromatosis. *J Am Acad Dermatol* 10:365–371, 1984.

Venecie PV, Bigel P, Desgruelles C, et al. Infantile myofibromatosis. *Br J Dermatol* 117:255–259, 1987.

Malignant tumors

Abdesalam AR, Heyn R, Tefft M, Hays D, Newton WA Jr, Beltangady M. Infants younger than 1 year of age with rhabdomyosarcoma. *Cancer* 58:2606–2610, 1986.

Francis JS, Sybert VP, Benjamin DR. Congenital monocytic leukemia: report of a case with cutaneous involvement, and review of the literature. *Pediatr Dermatol* 6:306–311, 1989.

Schneider KM, Becker GM, Krasna IH. Neonatal neuroblastoma. *Pediatrics* 36:359, 1965.

Neonatal lupus erythematosus

Lee LA, Weston WL. New findings in neonatal lupus syndrome. *Am J Dis Child* 138:233–236, 1984.

Watson RM, Lane AT, Barnett NK, et al. Neonatal lupus erythematosus. A clinical, serological and immunogenetic study with review of the literature. *Medicine (Baltimore)* 63:362, 1984.

Annular erythema of infancy

Peterson AQ Jr, Jarratt M. Annular erythema of infancy. *Arch Dermatol* 117:145–148, 1981.

chapter three

PAPULOSQUAMOUS
ERUPTIONS

Papulosquamous eruptions comprise a group of disorders characterized by the presence of superficial papules and scale. These conditions account for a large number of patients in both pediatric dermatology and pediatric primary care practice. In disorders of keratinization (psoriasis, pityriasis rubra pilaris, keratosis follicularis, ichthyosis, hyperkeratosis of the palms and soles, and porokeratosis) cutaneous lesions develop as a result of genetically programmed increased production or retention of scale at the surface. In the inflammatory dermatoses (dermatitides, pityriasis rosea, pityriasis lichenoides, lichenoid dermatoses, and fungal infections), the clinical signs are caused by epidermal response to dermal inflammation.

DISORDERS OF KERATINIZATION

Psoriasis

Psoriasis is a common disorder characterized by red, well-demarcated plaques with a dry, thick, silvery scale (Fig. 3.1). The condition affects 1 percent to 3 percent of Americans, of whom almost 20 percent develop the rash before the age of 20.

Psoriasis is a multifactorial disorder with both hereditary and environmental components. In more than one third of patients, other family members are affected. A number of HLA types have been associated with psoriasis in different populations.

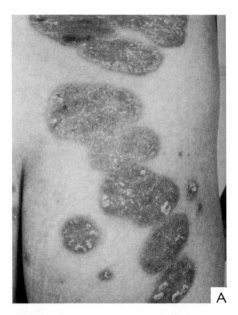

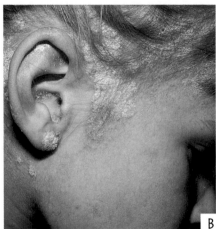

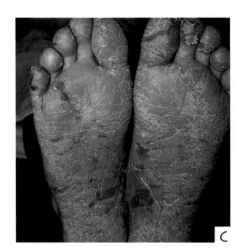

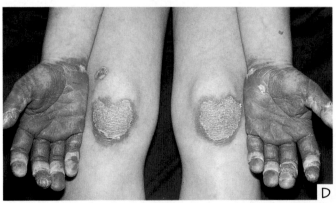

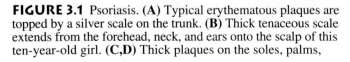

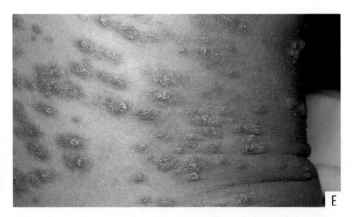

FIGURE 3.1 Psoriasis. **(A)** Typical erythematous plaques are topped by a silver scale on the trunk. **(B)** Thick tenaceous scale extends from the forehead, neck, and ears onto the scalp of this ten-year-old girl. **(C,D)** Thick plaques on the soles, palms, elbows, and knees of this eight-year-old boy caused severe pain when he attempted to walk or use his hands. **(E)** Widespread guttate lesions erupted on the trunk and extremities of this child one week after a streptococcal pharyngitis.

Cutaneous lesions tend to locate on the scalp, the sacrum, and the extensor surfaces of the extremities. About 50 percent of children present with large plaques over the knees and elbows. Thickening and fissuring of the skin of the palms and soles may also be present. In a third of children, many drop-like lesions (guttate psoriasis) are scattered over the body, including the face, trunk, and extremities. In infancy psoriasis may present as a persistent diaper dermatitis. In older children the eyelids, genitals, and periumbilical area are commonly involved (Fig. 3.2). Scalp disease may develop as an isolated finding but is often seen with other variants. Itchy red plaques with thick, tenacious scale are often evident at the frontal hairline and around the ears. Nail changes include onycholysis (separation of the nail plate from the nail bed producing "oil drop changes"), pitting, yellowing, increased friability, and subungual hyperkeratosis.

Eight percent of patients suffer from psoriatic arthritis, one of the seronegative spondyloarthropathies. In half of these individuals arthritis develops before the skin rash. Examination of the joints characteristically demonstrates heat, pain, and swelling of multiple joints of the hands and feet, particularly the distal interphalangeal joints. The arthritis tends to be progressive, with the eventual development of flexure deformities and contractures. In addition to the typical lesions of plaque psoriasis, patients often demonstrate severe psoriatic involvement of the hands, feet, and nails. The HLA B-27 antigen is usually positive.

Rarely, children develop erythrodermic psoriasis with acute widespread erythema and scaling or pustular psoriasis with generalized erythema and pustule formation (Fig. 3.3). These variants are associated with high fevers, chills, arthralgias, myalgias, and severe cutaneous tenderness. Fluid and electrolyte loss and leukocytosis may be marked. Secondary bacterial infection and sepsis can occur.

Although the factors initiating rapid turnover in epidermal cells that contribute to psoriatic plaques are unknown, a hereditary predisposition is suspected, and upper respiratory tract and streptococcal infections are known to precipitate outbreaks. Psoriatic lesions are often induced in areas of local injury such as scratches, surgical scars or sunburn, a response termed the Koebner phenomenon (Fig. 3.4). In areas of thick scale, tortuous capillary loops proliferate close to the surface. Gentle

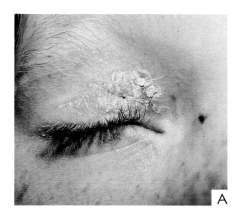 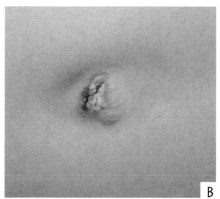 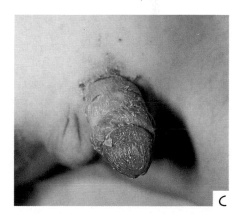

FIGURE 3.2 (A,B,C) These lesions were present on the penis, eyelids, and periumbilical area of this five-year-old for six months before the diagnosis of psoriasis was considered.

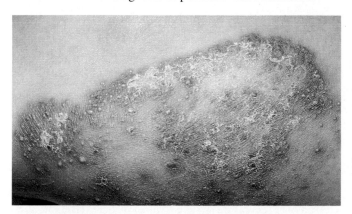

FIGURE 3.3 Generalized pustulation developed suddenly within psoriatic plaques on this eight-year-old. Skin lesions were associated with fever, chills, and arthralgias.

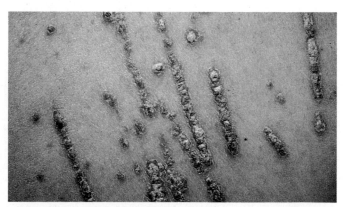

FIGURE 3.4 Koebner phenomenon in psoriasis. Pruritus was severe in this child who developed linear plaques in excoriations.

removal of the scale causes multiple small bleeding points, referred to as the Auspitz sign (Fig. 3.5).

The diagnosis is usually made by identifying the typical morphology and distribution of skin lesions. Confirmatory skin biopsy findings include regular thickening of the epidermal rete ridges, elongation and edema of the dermal papillae, thinning of the epidermis overlying tortuous dermal capillaries, absence of the granular layer, parakeratosis, spongiform pustules, and Munro microabscesses.

The course of psoriasis is chronic and unpredictable, marked by remissions and exacerbations. A number of different topical agents including lubricants, corticosteroids, tar, anthralen, and keratolytics are useful in managing cutaneous lesions. Chronic or recalcitrant disease and psoriatic arthritis may require ultraviolet light therapy [UVB (sunburn wavelengths) and/or PUVA (psoralen photosensitizer+UVA) or long-wavelength ultraviolet light]. Life-threatening erythrodermic and pustular psoriasis and psoriatic arthritis usually respond to oral retinoids and antimetabolites. However, the use of systemic agents requires close laboratory and clinical monitoring.

Pityriasis Rubra Pilaris

Pityriasis rubra pilaris (PRP) is an uncommon disorder of keratinization characterized by small follicular papules, widespread orange-red scaly plaques surrounded by islands of spared skin, and marked thickening of the skin on the palms and soles (Fig. 3.6). Onset most commonly occurs in prepubertal children and in adults after age 50, and has been associated with trauma and acute, self-limited illness. Most cases are sporadic and acquired, but a familial variant has been reported. Overall, 75 percent of cases resolve spontaneously within three to four years, but in familial disease persistence is the rule.

In childhood, the circumscribed variant, which accounts for a majority of the cases, begins with the development of coalescing hyperkeratotic papules on the elbows and knees and a palmoplantar keratoderma (Fig. 3.7). Superficial red, scaly plaques occasionally appear on the face and trunk. Less commonly, children develop a pattern that mimics the classic adult variety. The eruption begins with follicular, hyperkeratotic patches on the back, chest, and abdomen, which expand to involve interfollicular skin. Lesions on the scalp and other sebaceous areas develop simultaneously or soon thereafter, and may disseminate.

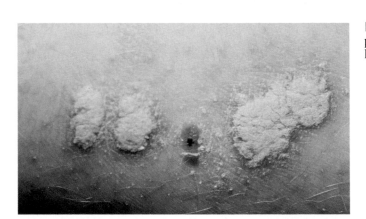

FIGURE 3.5 Auspitz sign. Removal of the thick scale from a psoriatic plaque produces small points of bleeding from underlying tortuous capillaries.

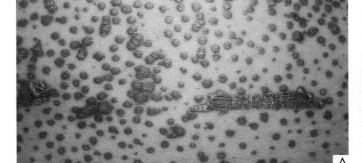

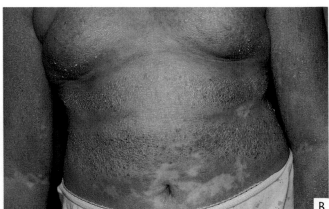

FIGURE 3.6 PRP. **(A)** Discrete hyperkeratotic follicular papules on the trunk and extremities of this ten-year-old girl progressed over several weeks to confluent plaques. **(B)** Note several discrete areas of sparing on the abdomen and arm flexures.

Even in widespread disease, islands of spared, normal-appearing skin are characteristic. Discrete hyperkeratotic papules may also remain over the knuckles, wrists, elbows, and knees. In erythrodermic PRP, facial edema and scale may lead to ectropian formation. Nail dystrophy with subungual hyperkeratoses may also be present.

The clinical presentation, particularly with keratoderma of the hands and feet and follicular papules, helps to distinguish PRP from psoriasis, seborrheic dermatitis, atopic dermatitis, and pitryiasis rosea. A skin biopsy demonstrating interfollicular orthohyperkeratosis and perifollicular parakeratosis is typical but not diagnostic.

Although PRP is usually self-limited in childhood, severe, disabling disease may require systemic therapy with retinoids or methotrexate.

Keratosis Follicularis (Darier's Disease)

This autosomal dominant disorder typically presents in children from eight to 15 years old and is characterized by hyperkeratotic follicular papules on the face, scalp, neck, and seborrheic areas of the trunk (Fig. 3.8). Although the onset is usually insidious, a rapidly progressive course may follow an inciting event such as intense exposure to the sun or a viral infection. Red, scaly papules

coalesce to form widespread thick, odoriferous, greasy plaques, particularly on the scalp, forehead, around the ears, shoulders, mid-chest, and mid-back. Flexures may also be involved with moist vegetating plaques.

Other characteristic lesions include flat-topped warty papules on the dorsum of the hands and tiny hyperkeratotic papules and pits on the palms and soles. Subtle pebbly papules on the oral mucosa may simulate leukoplakia. Nail dystrophy with thickening or thinning of the nail plate, fracture of the distal nail plate, longitudinal white and red streaks, and subungual hyperkeratosis may also be present.

Although the cause of Darier's disease is unknown, the identification of various T-cell abnormalities by several investigators suggests an immunologic basis. The tendency of affected individuals to develop disseminated herpes simplex (Kaposi's varicelliform eruption) and recurrent staphylococcal infections has been recognized for years.

The characteristic clinical picture should permit easy differentiation of Darier's disease from other papulosquamous disorders such as seborrheic dermatitis, PRP, and psoriasis. Classic histologic changes on skin biopsy, including dyskeratosis with the formation of corps ronds

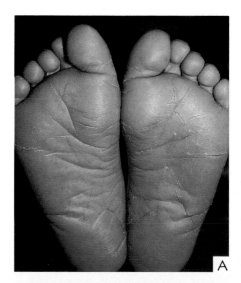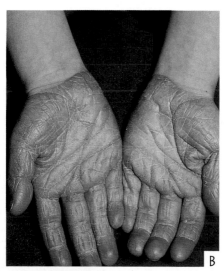

FIGURE 3.7 PRP. (**A,B**) This child developed a salmon-colored keratoderma of the palms and soles.

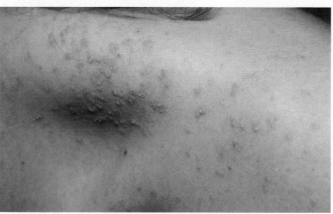

FIGURE 3.8 Keratosis follicularis. Hyperkeratotic follicular papules erupted progressively on the trunk and face of this nine-year-old girl. Some of the most prominent lesions are seen on her shoulder.

and corps grains, suprabasal acantholysis leading to the formation of suprabasal clefts, and the formation of villi by upward-proliferating dermal papillae, will confirm the diagnosis.

Although Darier's disease tends to persist throughout life, many patients experience episodic flares and remissions in disease activity. Topical vitamin A acid (retinoic acid) may be helpful in managing early lesions. However, its use is limited by a high risk of irritation. Recent experience with oral retinoids has been promising, but prolonged use may be associated with unacceptable complications including hyperostoses, epiphyseal plate changes, increased skin fragility, and teratogenicity. Aggressive protection from the sun and treatment of secondary bacterial and viral infections will also control exacerbations.

Figure 3.9   Variants of Palmoplantar Keratoderma (PPK)

Disorder	Genetics	Onset
Diffuse PPK		
Unna–Thost	AD (1/200–1/40,000)	Infancy
Keratoderma hereditaria mutilans (of Vohwinkel)	AD (Rare)	Infancy
Mal de Meleda	AR	Infancy
Howel–Evans syndrome	AD	Adolescence
Papillon–Lefèvre	AR	Birth–2 or 3 yrs
Focal PPK		
Punctate PPK	AD (2–5% of blacks)	Childhood
PPK Striata	AD	Adolescence
Tyrosinemia Type II (Richner–Hanhart Syndrome)	AR	Infancy through adulthood
Porokeratosis	AD (Rare)	Childhood through adulthood

AD = autosomal dominant; AR = autosomal recessive.

Ichthyoses

The ichthyoses are a heterogeneous group of scaling disorders characterized by retention hyperkeratosis (ichthyosis vulgaris, X-linked ichthyosis) or increased epidermal cell proliferation (lamellar ichthyosis, epidermolytic hyperkeratosis). These diseases can be distinguished on the basis of clinical findings, histopathology, and biochemical markers, as outlined in Chapter 2.

Hyperkeratosis of the Palms and Soles

This condition comprises a heterogeneous group of keratodermas characterized by focal or generalized thickening of the skin of the palms and/or soles, and occasionally by more widespread cutaneous lesions associated with systemic disease (Fig. 3.9). Unna–Thost dermatosis, the most common variant which is inherited in an autosomal dominant pattern, presents in the first year

Figure 3.9 *Continued*

Involvement	Hyperhidrosis	Associated Findings
Palms, soles	Severe	
Honeycombed keratoderma Star shaped plaques on hands, feet, elbows, knees.	+/-	Digital constriction band Deafness Alopecia

Palms, soles, elbows, knees,
  including dorsal surfaces
  (transgridiens)
	+/-	Flexion contractures
		Constriction bands
		Koilonychia

Soles, sometimes palms	+/-	Esophageal carcinoma Epidermal cysts Thin lateral eyebrows Follicular papules

Soles more severe than palms,
  intense erythema, wrists,
  ankles, elbows, knees,
  follicular hyperkeratoses
	+/-	Nail dystrophy
		Periodontitis
		Calcification of falx cerebri
		Mental retardation
		Arachnodactyly

Palms, soles		Variable
Palms, fingers		Variable
Fingertips, palms		Corneal ulcerations Mental retardation
Extremities, trunk		Squamous cell carcinoma

of life with diffuse hyperkeratosis restricted to the palmar and plantar surfaces (Fig. 3.10). Although lesions may be asymptomatic, hyperhidrosis may lead to maceration and the formation of painful fissuring, blisters, and bacterial superinfection. Unna–Thost must be distinguished from a number of unusual keratodermas associated with hyperkeratoses extending to the dorsal surfaces of the hands and feet, elbows, knees and other distant sites (Fig. 3.11).

Focal keratoderma with discrete papules and plaques on the palms and soles also appears as an isolated phenomenon or in association with widespread cutaneous findings and systemic disease. A mild autosomal dominant variant with pits and hyperkeratotic papules in the hand and foot creases occurs in 2 percent to 5 percent of blacks (Fig. 3.12). Occasionally this keratoderma is painful and requires surgical treatment.

Neurosensory deafness, carcinoma of the esophagus (Howel–Evans syndrome), and peripheral neuropathy (Charcot–Marie–Tooth disease) are rarely associated with palmoplantar keratoderma and can be excluded by auditory screening and a careful family history. Hyperkeratosis of the extremities presenting as part of a diffuse disorder of keratinization, such as psoriasis or PRP, can be distinguished by a thorough examination of the integument.

Porokeratosis

This is a disorder of keratinization characterized by annular, sharply demarcated plaques with raised hyperkeratotic borders (Fig. 3.13). The four known variants are distinguished on the basis of morphology and distribution of the lesions, time of onset, triggering factors, and mode of inheritance.

Porokeratosis of Mibelli This condition invariably develops in childhood as subtle brown scaly papules that slowly enlarge to form irregularly shaped plaques with hypopigmented atrophic centers and raised, grooved borders. Lesions are usually unilateral and vary in size from a few millimeters to several centimeters. One to three

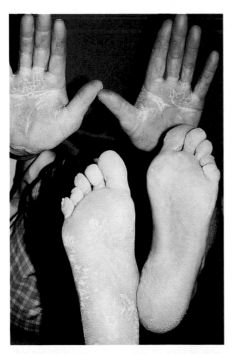

FIGURE 3.10 Progressive hyperkeratosis of the palms and soles began at five months of age in this ten-year-old whose father and sister had similar symptoms.

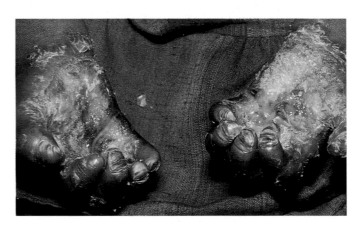

FIGURE 3.11 Olmsted syndrome. Severe scarring keratoderma of the palms and soles was associated with perioral and perigenital hyperkeratosis, hyperhidrosis, recurrent cutaneous infections, and poor growth in this five-year-old girl. Treatment with oral retinoids resulted in some decrease in the palmar and plantar lesions.

FIGURE 3.12 Focal keratoderma. Asymptomatic hyperkeratotic papules and pits on the hand creases of a black teenager.

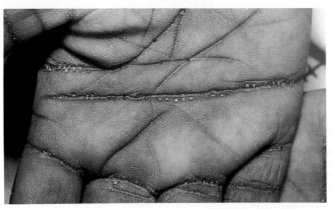

lesions are usually present. This rare autosomal dominant variant appears most commonly on the extremities, thighs, and perigenital skin, although any area, including mucous membranes, can be involved. Biopsies of the longitudinal furrow in the border demonstrate the diagnostic coronoid lamella, consisting of a parakeratotic column filling a deep epidermal invagination. Squamous cell carcinoma may arise within these slowly progressive lesions. Although excision or carbon dioxide laser surgery can be useful, recurrrences have been reported. Linear porokeratosis presents much like the Mibelli variant. However, plaques are linearly arranged on the distal extremities and trunk, where they demonstrate a zosteriform pattern. Onset is also in early childhood, but the mode of inheritance has not been established.

Disseminated Superficial Actinic Porokeratosis Disseminated superficial actinic porokeratosis (DSAP) is a common autosomal dominant variant with delayed expression, occurring primarily in lightly pigmented individuals of Celtic extraction. Many small, 2-mm to 4-mm hyperkeratotic papules appear symmetrically on sun-exposed surfaces of the extremities during the second and third decades. These brown, red, or skin-colored lesions may coalesce to form irregular circinate patterns. Progression of papules, which occurs particularly during the summer months, may be slowed by aggressive use of sun protection.

Punctate Porokeratosis This condition, affecting the palms and soles, has been described as a separate entity. However, it usually presents in association with the Mibelli or linear variant. Punctate porokeratosis may also occur as a widely disseminated form, reminiscent of DSAP but with involvement of both sun-exposed and sun-protected areas. It should be included in the differential diagnosis of punctate keratoderma.

Dermatitides

Many of these disorders demonstrate changes of both acute (erythema, edema, vesiculation, crusts) and chronic (scaling, lichenification, hypopigmentation, hyperpigmentation) inflammation. Microscopically, dermatitis is recognized by the presence of intercellular edema (spongiosis), variable epidermal thickening (acanthosis), and the presence of dermal inflammatory cells, usually lymphocytes. Various dermatitic disorders can be distinguished on the basis of their clinical features and specific histologic patterns.

A reasonable way to think of the dermatitides is as exogenous ("outside job") versus endogenous ("inside job") phenomena. Exogenous disorders include irritant and allergic contact dermatitis and photodermatitis. Endogenous dermatitides include atopic dermatitis, dyshidrotic eczema, nummular dermatitis, and seborrheic dermatitis. Juvenile palmar and plantar dermatosis and perioral dermatitis are triggered by a combination of inside and outside factors. Pityriasis rosea and parapsoriasis present with distinctive dermatitic patterns, but their causes are unclear.

Contact Dermatitis This term refers to a group of conditions in which an inflammatory reaction in the skin is triggered by direct contact with environmental agents. In the most common form, irritant contact dermatitis, changes in the skin are induced by caustic agents such as acids, alkalis, hydrocarbons, and other primary iritants. Anyone exposed to these agents in a high enough concentration for a long enough period of time will develop a reaction. The rash is usually acute (occurring within minutes) with itching or burning, well-demarcated erythema, edema, blister formation, and/or crust formation.

In contrast, allergic contact dermatitis is a T-cell-mediated immune reaction to an antigen that comes into

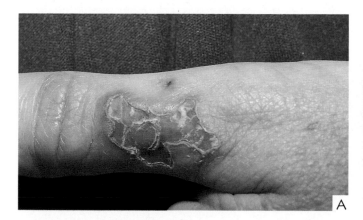

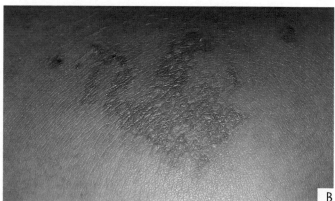

FIGURE 3.13 (A) Porokeratosis of Mibelli on the thumb and (B) upper thigh. Note the hyperkeratotic borders, which demonstrated a coronoid lamella on skin biopsy. Both lesions were slowly progressive.

contact with the skin. Although it frequently presents with dramatic onset of erythema, vesiculation, and pruritus, the rash may become chronic with scaling, lichenification, and pigmentary changes (Fig. 3.14). Sometimes the allergen is obvious, such as poison ivy or nickel-containing jewelry. Often, however, some detective work is required to identify the inciting agent. The initial reaction occurs after a seven- to 14-day period of sensitization in susceptible individuals. Once sensitization has occurred, re-exposure to the allergen will elicit a more rapid reaction, sometimes within hours. This is a classic example of a type IV delayed hypersensitivity response.

The most common allergic contact dermatitis in the United States is poison ivy or rhus dermatitis (Figs. 3.15 and 3.16). This typically appears as linear streaks of erythematous papules and vesicles. However, with heavy exposure or in especially sensitive individuals, the rash may appear in large patches. When lesions involve the skin of the face or genitals, impressive swelling can occur and may obscure the primary eruption. Direct contact with the sap of the plant (poison ivy, poison oak, or poison sumac), whether from leaves, stems, or roots, will produce the dermatitis. Indirect contact with clothing or pets that have brushed against the plant, with logs or railroad ties on which the vine has been growing, or with smoke from a fire in which the plant is being burned is another means of exposure. Areas of skin exposed to the highest concentration of rhus antigen will develop changes first. Other sites that have received lower doses will then react in succession, giving the illusion of spreading. However, once on the skin the allergen becomes fixed to epithelial cells within about 20 minutes and cannot spread further. Thorough washing within minutes of exposure can prevent or reduce the eruption. Other common contact allergens include nickel, rubber, glues and/or dyes in shoes, ethylenediamine in topical lubricants, neomycin in topical antibiotics, and topical anesthetics.

Some allergens known as photosensitizers require sunlight to become activated. Photocontact dermatitis caused by drugs (e.g., tetracyclines, sulfonylureas, and thiazides) characteristically erupts in a symmetric distribution on the face, the "V" of the neck, and the arms distal to the ends of the shirt sleeves. Topical photosensitizers (e.g., dyes, furocoumarins, halogenated salicylanilides, para-aminobenzoic acid) produce localized patches of dermatitis when applied to sun-exposed sites. These agents are found in cosmetics, sunscreens, dermatological products, germicidal soaps, and woodland and house plants (see Chapter 7).

Occasionally the local reaction in a contact dermatitis is so severe that the patient develops a widespread secondary eczematous dermatitis. When the dermatitis appears at sites that have not been in contact with the offending agent, the reaction is referred to as "autoeczematization" or an "id" reaction.

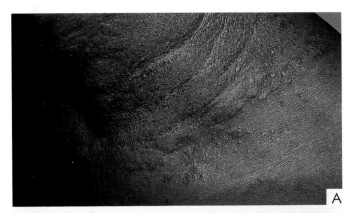

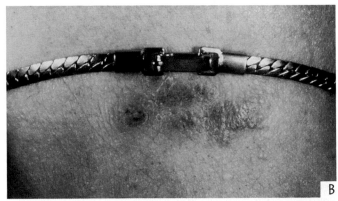

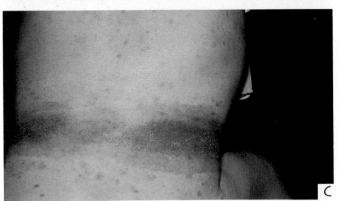

FIGURE 3.14 (**A**) Allergic contact dermatitis from application of Lanacaine demonstrates sharply demarcated, hyperpigmented, lichenified patches on the neck. (**B**) The location of the rash is helpful in determining the cause of a contact dermatitis, such as in this girl with a nickel allergy. (**C**) This child became sensitized to the elastic waistbands of his underwear.

Although localized patches of contact dermatitis are best treated topically, widespread reactions require, and respond within 48 hours, to a tapering two- to three-week course of systemic corticosteroids, beginning at 0.5 to 1.0 mg/kg/day. Patients may experience rebound of the rash when treated with a shorter course. Oral steroids may also be indicated in severe local reactions involving the eyelids, extensive parts of the face, the genitals, and/or the hands, where swelling and pruritus may become incapacitating.

Atopic Dermatitis Also known as eczema, this is a chronically recurrent, genetically influenced skin disorder of early infancy, childhood, and occasionally adult

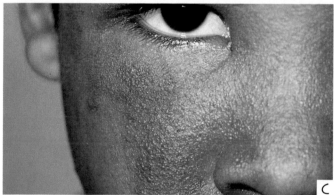

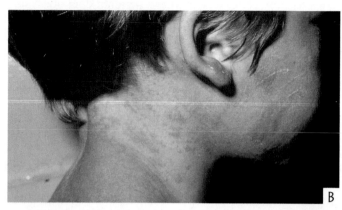

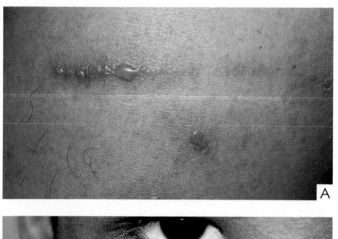

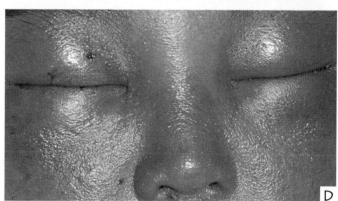

FIGURE 3.15 Poison ivy or rhus dermatitis. **(A)** Linear streaks of pruritic papules and vesicles are typical of contact dermatitis to a plant. **(B,C)** With heavier exposure, however, the eruption can develop into large patches. Note the tiny vesicles in the facial lesion in the child shown in C. **(D)** Reactions involving the face and genitals can provoke impressive swelling.

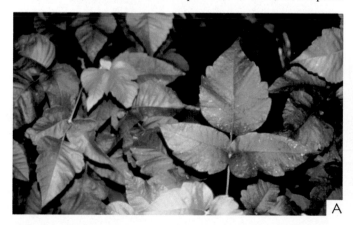

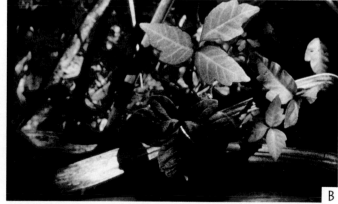

FIGURE 3.16 (A) Poison ivy. The plant has characteristic shiny leaves in groups of three. It may grow as a vine, low shrub, or bush. **(B)** Poison oak. This, too, has leaves in groups of three, although the edges tend to be more scalloped than those of poison ivy. (Part B courtesy of Dr. Mary Jelks.)

life. Although it was initially described in the 19th century, it was not until 1935 that Hill and Sultzberger first characterized the clinical entity. The term atopy, derived from a Greek word which means "not confined to a single place," was introduced in 1923 by Coca and Cooke to describe a cohort of patients with asthma and allergic rhinitis who demonstrated immediate wheal and flare reactions on skin testing with a variety of environmental allergens. The sera of these patients contained skin sensitizing antibodies that were subsequently characterized as IgE immunoglobulins. It was later recognized that these atopic individuals also frequently manifested the itchy, eczematous dermatitis that was labeled as atopic dermatitis.

Although data are not precise, recent surveys reveal that atopic dermatitis is rather common, with an incidence of 7 per 1000 individuals in the United States. The prevalence is highest among children, affecting 3 percent to 5 percent of all children between six months and ten years of age. Subtle findings may be present during the first few months of life, and almost 60 percent of patients can be expected to have an initial outbreak by their first birthday. Another third develop disease between one and five years. Onset of eczema in adolescence and adulthood is unusual and should alert the clinician to the possibility of other diagnoses.

In families with a history of allergic rhinitis or asthma, nearly one third of children can be expected to develop skin lesions of atopic dermatitis. Inversely, in patients with atopic dermatitis, one third can be expected to have a personal history of allergic rhinitis or asthma, with two thirds having a family history of these disorders. Half of those who manifest the dermatologic condition in infancy or childhood ultimately develop allergic respiratory symptoms. Atopic dermatitis does not appear to be linked to the histocompatability locus antigen, as has been described in allergic rhinitis. Rather, it seems to be inherited as an autosomal trait with multifactorial components.

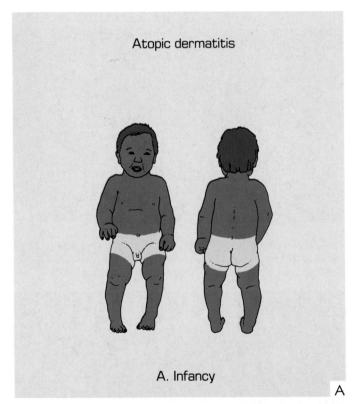

Atopic dermatitis

A. Infancy

A

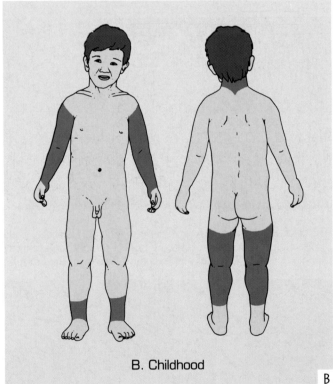

B. Childhood

B

FIGURE 3.17 Characteristic distribution of lesions of atopic dermatitis in infancy, childhood, and adulthood. (**A**) In infancy, widespread lesions may be generalized, sparing only the diaper area. The head and neck, as well as the flexural and extensor surfaces of the distal extremities, are often severely involved.

(**B**) In older childhood, lesions tend to involve the flexural surfaces of the upper and lower extremities, as well as the neck. With severe flares of disease activity, the rash may become more generalized.

The term *eczema*, which means "boil over," is used by many physicians when referring to atopic dermatitis. However, most dermatologists use the word eczematous as a morphologic term to describe the clinical findings in various sorts of acute (erythema, scaling, vesicles, and crusts) and chronic (scaling, lichenification, and pigmentary changes) dermatitis. Both acute and chronic dermati-

tis may be present in atopics at different sites at the same time and the same site at different times during the course of the disease.

The distribution and morphology of skin lesions in atopic dermatitis are diagnostic, and the clinical findings show a characteristic pattern of evolution (Fig. 3.17). The infantile phase begins between one and six

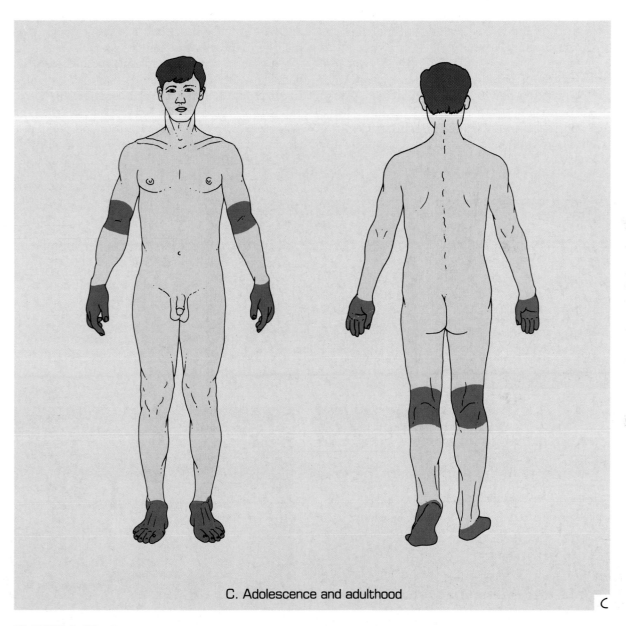

C. Adolescence and adulthood

FIGURE 3.17 (C) In adults, the lesions are usually restricted to the flexural creases. In some patients, however, involvement of the palms and soles may become particularly prominent.

months of age and lasts about two or three years (Fig. 3.18). Typically, the rash is composed of red, itchy papules and plaques, many of which ooze and crust. Lesions are symmetrically distributed over the cheeks, forehead, scalp, trunk, and the extensor surfaces of the extremities. The diaper area is usually spared.

The childhood phase of atopic dermatitis occurs between the age of four and ten years. Circumscribed erythematous, scaly, lichenified plaques are symmetrically distributed on the wrists, ankles, and flexural surfaces of the arms and legs (Fig. 3.19). These areas develop frequent secondary infection, probably because of the introduction of organisms by intense scratching. Although the eruption may become chronic and, rarely, generalized, remissions can occur at any time. Most children experience improvement during the warm, humid summer months and exacerbations during the fall and winter.

Seventy-five percent of children with atopic dermatitis improve by the age of ten to 14 years; the remaining individuals may go on to develop chronic adult disease. Major areas of involvement include the flexural creases of the arms, neck, and legs. Chronic dermatitis may be restricted to the hands or feet, but some patients develop recurrent, widespread lesions.

Nummular Eczematous Dermatitis Although this disorder was initially described as distinct from atopic dermatitis, clinicians frequently use this term to describe the discrete, coin-shaped red patches seen on many patients with atopic dermatitis. Lesions typically appear as tiny papules and vesicles which form confluent patches on the arms and legs (Fig. 3.20). Nummular lesions may be extremely pruritic, and they are difficult to treat, particularly during the winter months when the incidence seems to peak.

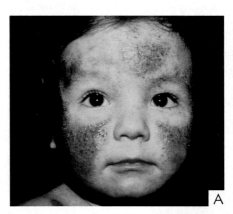
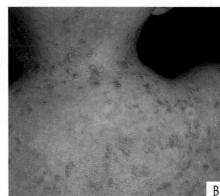

FIGURE 3.18 Infantile eczema. **(A)** This infant has an acute, weeping dermatitis on the cheeks and forehead. Involvement of **(B)** the trunk and **(C)** the extremities, with erythema, scaling, and crusting, are evident. **(D)** Usually, the diaper area is the only portion of the skin surface that is spared.

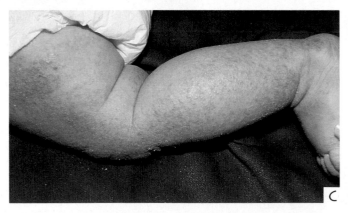
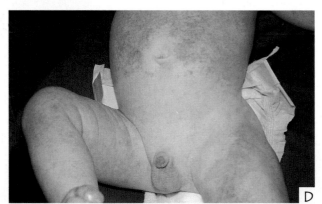

Prurigo Nodularis   Whereas chronic rubbing leads to lichenification and scratching to linear excoriations, picking and gouging at the itchy, irritated skin tends to produce markedly thickened papules known as prurigo nodules (Fig. 3.21). Although prurigo nodularis is not specific to atopic dermatitis, many patients with these nodules also have an atopic diathesis, manifesting allergic rhinitis, asthma, or food allergy. Frequently there are other stigmata of atopic dermatitis as well. Prurigo lesions tend to localize to the extremities, although widespread cutaneous involvement can be observed in some cases.

Follicular Eczema   Although a few atopics initially present with a predominance of follicular papules, virtually all patients develop these 2-mm to 4-mm follicular

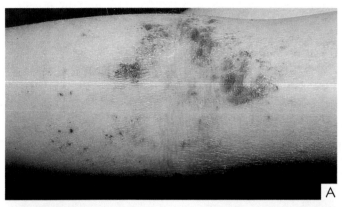

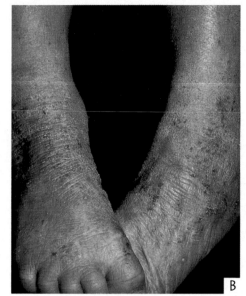

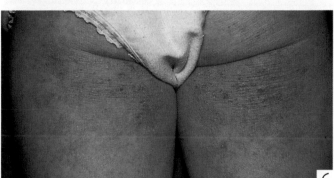

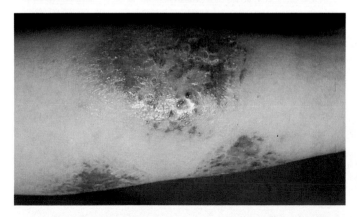

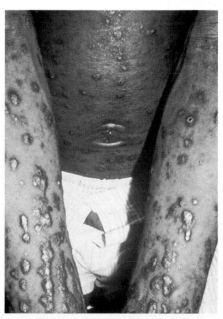

FIGURE 3.19 Atopic dermatitis of childhood, with lesions on (**A**) the arm, (**B**) the legs, and (**C**) the creases of the buttocks. In childhood, dermatitis involves the flexural surfaces of the upper and lower extremities. The neck, ankles, wrists, and posterior thighs may be severely affected.

FIGURE 3.20 Nummular eczema. Acute, vesicular, and crusted coin-shaped patches erupt on the extremities of individuals with this disease. The term *nummular eczema* is also used to describe chronic circular patches on the extremities and trunks of atopic patients.

FIGURE 3.21 Prurigo nodularis. Widespread, lichenified nodules involve the trunk and extremities of an adolescent with severe atopic dermatitis. Lesions may be particularly resistant to treatment.

lesions sometime during their clinical course (Fig. 3.22). Lesions are usually widespread on the trunk, but careful observation also reveals their presence on the extremities, particularly early in flares of disease activity. In children with chronic disease, discrete papules may be obscured by excoriations and lichenification, particularly in the flexural creases.

Ichthyosis Vulgaris Hyperlinearity of the palms and soles typical of ichthyosis vulgaris is a common finding in patients with atopic dermatitis. Retained polygonal scales are usually evident on the distal lower extremities, but they may also show a generalized distribution (Fig. 3.23). Xerosis associated with ichthyosis may contribute to the pruritus associated with atopic dermatitis.

Keratosis Pilaris Although keratosis pilaris (KP) is often an isolated finding, it is commonly associated with atopic dermatitis and/or ichthyosis vulgaris. KP results from localized perifollicular retention of scales. Clinically, this is characterized by horny follicular papules and erythema on the upper arms, medial thighs, and cheeks (Fig. 3.24).

Infraorbital Folds Often referred to as Dennie's lines or Morgan folds, extra infraorbital folds are suggestive of atopy (Fig. 3.25). In many patients, they represent current or past local inflammation produced by persistent scratching and rubbing of these tissues. Although not specific for atopic dermatitis, they may be a useful finding when they are associated with other diagnostic physical signs.

Pigmentary Changes Postinflammatory hypopigmentation and hyperpigmentation occur commonly in atopics, especially in the setting of chronic disease (Fig. 3.26). Although pigmentary changes may be quite prominent, this is not always the case; subtle and poorly demarcated areas of hypopigmentation in atopics are referred to as

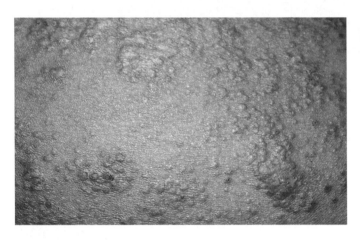

FIGURE 3.22 Follicular eczema. In certain cases, follicular papules may be the only manifestation of atopic dermatitis. These lesions occur in most atopics at some time during the course of their disease, as in this adolescent with follicular eczema on his back.

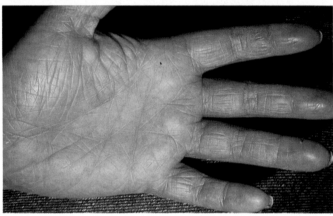

FIGURE 3.23 Ichthyosis vulgaris. Hyperlinearity of the palms and soles was marked in this woman with atopic dermatitis and ichthyosis vulgaris. She had two children with mild atopic dermatitis, showing similar manifestations on the palms and soles, and thick scaling on the anterior surfaces of their lower legs.

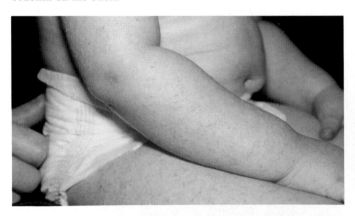

FIGURE 3.24 Keratosis pilaris. Fine follicular papules are symmetrically distributed over the extensor surfaces of the arms and legs of this toddler.

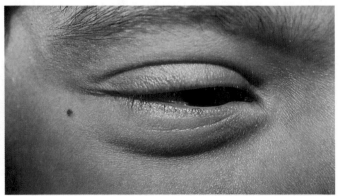

FIGURE 3.25 Edema of the infraorbital folds. Eyelid edema and lichenification due to chronic rubbing resulted in the development of an extraorbital fold. Although not specific to atopic dermatitis, this feature should suggest such a diagnosis when seen in association with other, more pathognomonic findings.

pityriasis alba (Fig. 3.27). Changes are most marked in darkly pigmented individuals or lighter-skinned patients after tanning. The extremities and face are the areas most commonly involved. Although some postinflammatory pigmentary changes persist indefinitely, fading of hyperpigmentation and repigmenting of lightened areas usually occur during prolonged remissions.

Hand (and Foot) Dermatitis Involvement of the hands and feet is common at all ages and may be the only manifestation of disease in adolescents and adults. The rash is commonly triggered by contact irritants. Clinical findings include dry, scaly patches on the palms and soles and frequent fissuring of the palms, soles, and digits. The term *dyshidrotic eczema* is reserved for patients with atopic dermatitis who develop intensely pruritic, deep-seated inflammatory vesicles of the sides of the palms, soles and/or digits (Fig. 3.28). This is actualy an inaccurate name, because histopathology of these lesions demonstrates spongiotic vesicles, typical of an acute dermatitis, and normal sweat glands. Involvement of the paronychial skin may lead to separation of the nail from the underlying nail bed (onycholysis), as well as yellowing and pitting of the nail plate (Fig. 3.29).

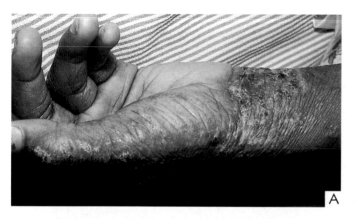
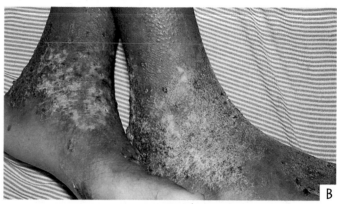

FIGURE 3.26 Postinflammatory pigmentary changes of atopic dermatitis. Changes in pigmentation are marked on (**A**) the hands and (**B**) the feet of this nine-year-old girl with severe, chronic atopic dermatitis. In this child, the pigmentary changes are associated with lichenification and crust formation.

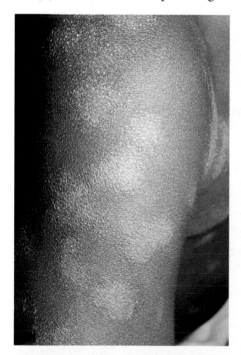
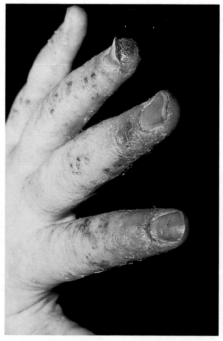
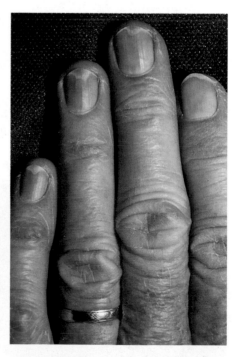

FIGURE 3.27 Pityriasis alba. In some atopics, subtle inflammation may result in poorly demarcated areas of hypopigmentation known as pityriasis alba. Lesions are most prominent in darkly pigmented individuals.

FIGURE 3.28 Dyshidrosis. Chronic cracking, oozing, and scaling develop after the tiny pruritic vesicles have been scratched.

FIGURE 3.29 Nail dystrophy. Nail changes including onycholysis and pitting may occur when chronic dermatitis affects the fingertips, as in this 45-year-old woman.

Secondary bacterial infection is the most frequent complication of atopic dermatitis. Since it may also trigger an acute exacerbation of clinical disease, early recognition and treatment are mandatory. Crusted exudative patches should suggest superinfection (Fig. 3.30). Although Group A β-hemolytic streptococci are frequently present in these infected areas, investigators have recently found a predominance of *Staphylococcus aureus*.

Eczema Herpeticum Primary herpes simplex may produce widespread cutaneous and, on rare occasions, disseminated visceral disease in patients with atopic dermatitis. The acute development of multiple, grouped 2-mm to 3-mm vesicles or crusts associated with high fever and worsening pruritus should suggest the diagnosis of eczema herpeticum (Fig. 3.31). Tzanck smears and viral cultures will confirm the diagnosis, and acyclovir should be started immediately.

A number of other organisms including human papillomaviruses (warts), the virus that causes molluscum contagiosum, and dermatophytes such as *Trichophyton rubrum* may produce chronic, recalcitrant infections in atopic patients.

The cause of atopic dermatitis remains elusive. An immunologic etiology is suggested by the chronic elevation of immunoglobulin E seen in most patients and by the association with rare immunodeficiency states. Some investigators have proposed a primary role for an aberrant response to histamine and other mediators of inflammation in the skin. A number of other immunologic parameters have been studied in patients with atopic dermatitis. However, laboratory findings vary from patient to patient and also in the same patient at different times in the course of disease.

Pathophysiologically, many external factors, including dry skin, soaps, wool fabrics, foods, infectious agents,

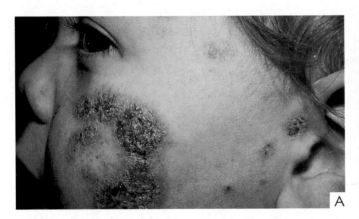
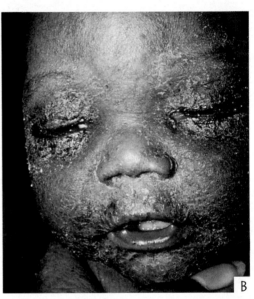

FIGURE 3.30 Secondary bacterial infection in atopic dermatitis. **(A)** Honey-colored crusts on an erythematous base are typical of impetigo in a child with eczema. Group A β-hemolytic streptococci were cultured from the facial crusts. **(B)** Staphylococcal scalded skin syndrome is evident in this infant with chronic infantile eczema. *Staphylococcus aureus* was cultured from the facial crusts.

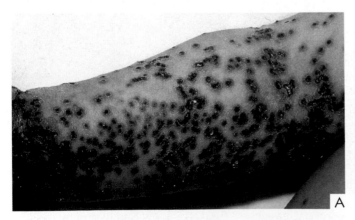
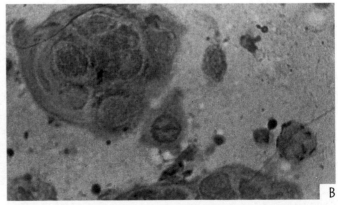

FIGURE 3.31 Herpes simplex. **(A)** Eczema herpeticum, the primary cutaneous manifestation of herpes simplex in an atopic, spread rapidly over the trunk and extremities of this ten-month-old girl. **(B)** A Tzanck smear from an intact vesicle demonstrated multinucleated giant cells typical of herpes simplex. The giant cell is surrounded by acantholytic epidermal cells. This finding is specific for blisters caused by herpes simplex and varicella zoster infections. However, these two blistering viral eruptions can only be differentiated from one another by viral culture.

and environmental antigens, can act in concert to produce pruritus in susceptible individuals. The resultant scratching leads to acute and chronic changes diagnostic of atopic dermatitis (Fig. 3.32).

Although the histopathology of affected skin is characteristic (scale, acanthosis, spongiosis, lymphocytic dermal inflammation), skin biopsies are not diagnostic. Atopic dermatitis is a clinical diagnosis. Characteristic cutaneous findings in a patient with a family history of atopy should suggest the disorder. To aid in diagnosis, several investigstors have proposed a number of primary and secondary criteria (Fig. 3.33).

A number of conditions may mimic the clinical findings of atopic dermatitis. It can be distinguished from infantile seborrheic dermatitis by the distribution of lesions, since atopic dermatitis spares moist intertriginous areas such as the axillae and perineum, where seborrhea is prominent. Exposure history and distribution help to differentiate contact dermatitis, as do the discreteness of lesions, pattern, and lack of symptoms in pityriasis rosea. Thick, silvery scale and the Koebner phenomenon help to distinguish psoriasis, and central clearing with an active scaly, vesiculopustular border helps to differentiate tinea corporis. The eruption in his-

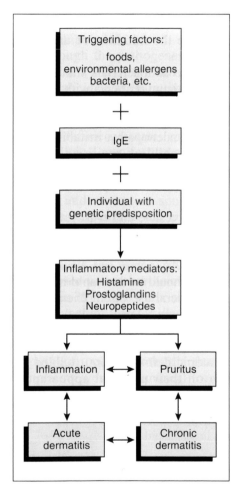

FIGURE 3.32 Schematic representation of the processes by which external factors including foods, bacteria, and environmental allergens trigger the release of cutaneous inflammatory factors, resulting in pruritus and inflammation of the skin of susceptible individuals. Secondary manipulation of the skin (i.e., rubbing and excoriation) produces many of the symptoms of acute and chronic dermatitis. Dermatitic changes in the skin result in further pruritus, thus potentiating an escalating cycle of increasing clinical findings, particularly during flare periods.

Figure 3.33 Diagnostic Criteria for Atopic Dermatitis*

Major Criteria (all required for diagnosis)	Common Findings (at least two)	Associated Findings (at least four)
Pruritus	Personal or family history of atopy	Ichthyosis, xerosis, hyperlinear palms
Typical morphology and distribution of rash	Immediate skin test reactivity	Pityriasis alba
		Keratosis pilaris
	White dermographism	Facial pallor, infraorbital darkening
	Anterior subcapsular cataracts	Dennie–Morgan folds
		Keratoconus
		Hand dermatitis
		Repeated cutaneous infections

*Adapted from Hanifin JM, Lobitz WC. New concepts of atopic dermatitis. *Arch Dermatol* 113:663, 1977.

Some children develop asymptomatic red papules, pustules, and nodules on either a normal-appearing or a red, scaly base on the chin and nasolabial folds (Fig. 3.37). Lesions may extend to the cheeks, eyelids, and forehead. Although initially reported in association with the use of fluorinated topical corticosteroids on the face, this type of perioral dermatitis occurs more frequently in children with no history of topical agents. Interestingly, histopathology demonstrates features of dermatitis, folliculitis, and occasionally granulomatous inflammation consistent with rosacea or sarcoidosis. However, affected children are otherwise healthy, and the rash responds

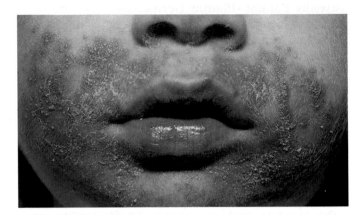

FIGURE 3.37 Perioral dermatitis with bright red papules, pustules, and scale erupted on the cheeks, chin, and upper lip of this four-year-old boy. Lesions subsequently appeared around the nose and eyes. The rash vanished after two weeks of treatment with oral erythromycin and noncomedogenic moisturizers.

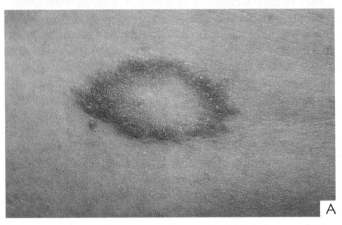

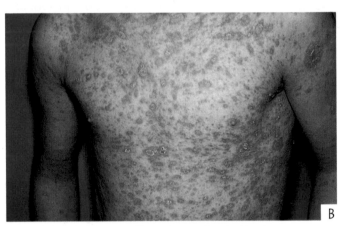

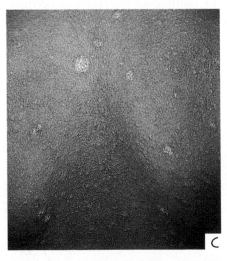

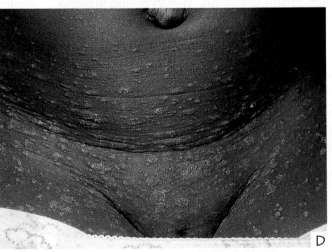

FIGURE 3.38 Pityriasis rosea. (A) The large herald patch on the chest of this ten-year-old girl shows central clearing, mimicking tinea corporis. (B) Many oval lesions are seen on the chest of a white teenager. (C) Note the Christmas tree pattern on the back of a black adolescent. (D) Small papular lesions as well as larger scaly patches were most prominent on the abdomen and thighs of this five-year-old girl.

well to oral antibiotics such as erythromycin and tetracycline (for children over 12 years of age). Topical antibiotics, benzoyl peroxide, vitamin A acid, and other keratolytics may also be useful. Topical steroids should be used with extreme caution because of the risk of precipitating a superimposed folliculitis, telangiectasias, and atrophy, particularly with long-term exposure.

Pityriasis Rosea Pityriasis rosea (PR) is an innocent, self-limited disorder which can occur at any age but is more common in school-age children and young adults. A prodrome of malaise, headache, and mild constitutional symptoms occasionally precedes the rash. In about half of the cases the eruption begins with the appearance of a "herald patch." This 3-cm to 5-cm isolated, oval, scaly, pink patch can appear anywhere on the body, although it occurs most commonly on the trunk and thighs (Fig. 3.38). Central clearing produces a lesion that often simulates tinea corporis. Within one to two weeks many smaller lesions appear on the body, usually concentrated on the trunk and proximal extremities. These begin as small, round papules which enlarge to form 1-cm to 2-cm oval patches with a dusky center and scaly border. The long axes of the patches often run parallel to the skin lines over the thorax and back, creating a "Christmas tree" pattern. Occasionally, PR spreads to involve much of the skin surface, including the face and distal extremities. Inflammation may be so intense

that some blistering and hemorrhage becomes clinically apparent. The rash reaches a peak in several weeks and slowly fades over six to 12 weeks.

Ultraviolet light may hasten the disappearance of the eruption. However, postinflammatory hyperpigmentation, particularly in dark-complexioned individuals, may persist for months. Although the cause is unknown, the peak incidence in late winter and low recurrence rate favor an infectious, probably viral, etiology.

Other eruptions that can resemble PR include guttate psoriasis, viral exanthems, drug rashes and secondary syphilis (Fig. 3.39). The herald patch may suggest tinea, but fungus can be excluded by a negative KOH prep and fungal culture.

Pityriasis Lichenoides

This includes a group of self-limited disorders with a spectrum of clinical presentations from the acute papulonecritic eruption of pitryiasis lichenoides et varioliformis acuta (PLEVA, Mucha–Habermann disease) to the chronic dermatitic papules of pityriasis lichenoides chronica (PLC). Although most common in older children and young adults, pityriasis lichenoides occasionally occurs in infants and young children, with a slight predominance in boys.

Acute forms usually begin with the sudden onset of 2-mm to 4-mm red macules and papules which evolve over several days into vesicular, necrotic, and eroded

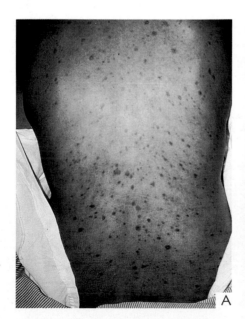 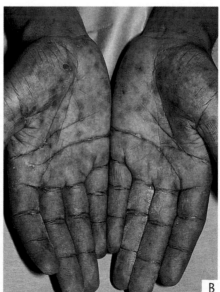 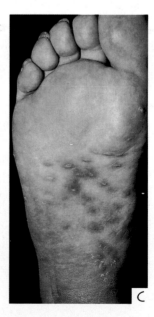

FIGURE 3.39 The rash of secondary syphilis may mimic pityriasis rosea. (**A**) A truncal rash in a Christmas tree pattern on this young adult resolved after treatment with intramuscular penicillin. Her VDRL titer was 1:2056. Hyperkeratotic "copper penny" papules, which are distinctive for syphilis, are seen on the palms of a black adolescent (**B**) and soles of a white adolescent (**C**). These also resolved quickly with antibiotics.

lesions (Fig. 3.40). Healing occurs within several weeks, with postinflammatory pigmentary changes and ocasionally chicken pox-like scars. Although the rash is usually asymptomatic and has a predilection for the trunk, pruritus may be intense and lesions may spread to involve the neck, face, and extremities, including the palms and soles. Fever and other mild constitutional symptoms may precede or accompany the acute phase. The eruption appears in successive crops, which settle down over weeks to months. Relapses and remissions occur episodically, but after several months most patients develop the more subtle lesions of PLC. In PLC, which may also appear de novo, the typical rash consists of round 2-mm to 10-mm reddish-brown papules which develop a shiny brown scale adherent at the center (Fig. 3.41). Episodic crops of papules heal over several weeks, with pigmentary changes but no evidence of scarring. In fact, postinflammatory pigmentary changes may be the first findings to bring attention to the rash (Fig. 3.42).

The histopathology of skin biopsies is distinctive but not diagnostic. In the mild form, minimal dermatitic changes are seen, with spongiosis and parakeratosis. A mild chronic perivascular infiltrate is found in the dermis associated with some hemorrhage and pigment incontinence. In acute disease the inflammation may be intense and can extend down into the deep dermis and up into the epidermis. Dyskeratosis is usually marked, and necrosis of the epidermis may occur with the formation of erosions. Endothelial cell swelling is marked, and vascular necrosis may occur. Hemorrhage is seen in the dermis and epidermis.

Although most children do well without treatment, phototherapy consisting of UVB, PUVA, or natural sunlight may be useful in persistently symptomatic patients. There may also be a role for oral antibiotics, such as erythromycin or tetracycline, in difficult patients. However, the use of systemic corticosteroids and methotrexate does not seem warranted.

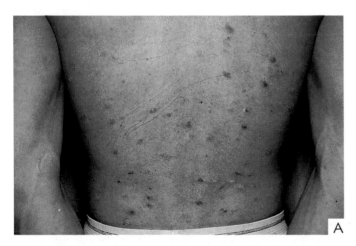

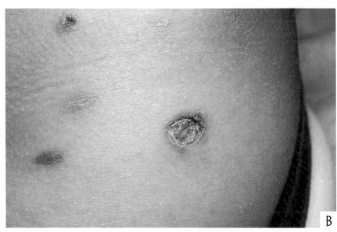

FIGURE 3.40 Pityriasis lichenoides et varioliformis acuta. **(A)** Asymptomatic hemorrhagic papules erupted in a pityriasis rosea-like pattern on the trunk and proximal extremities of this 15 year-old boy. **(B)** Recurrent papulonecrotic lesions continued to evolve on the trunk of this five-year-old for more than a year.

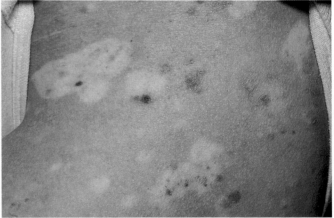

FIGURE 3.41 Pityriasis lichenoides chronica. A few diffusely scattered, shiny, hyperpigmented papules continued to appear for years in this 11 year-old boy. Note the central adherent scale.

FIGURE 3.42 Postinflammatory hyperpigmentation was severe in this child with generalized PLEVA. Fortunately, the pigmentary changes healed over several months as his disease evolved into the more indolent PLC.

Rare reports have suggested a relationship between pityriasis lichenoides and lymphoma. However, discussion of the generally innocent nature of this eruption and regular long-term follow-up should be reassuring to patients and their parents.

At the onset, PLEVA may be mistaken for varicella. However, the lack of symptoms or mucous membrane lesions and the subsequent chronic course will help to exclude chicken pox. Lymphomatoid papulosis is a benign, self-limited disorder which is clinically indistinguishable from PLEVA. However, the histopathology is characterized by an atypical lymphohistiocytic infiltrate suggestive of lymphoma. In adults a lymphomatoid papulosis-like eruption rarely occurs as a presenting picture for systemic lymphoma. Cutaneous vasculitis, impetigo, insect bites, and scabies should also be considered during the acute phase. PLC may be distinguishable from PR only by the extremely protracted course and the skin biopsy findings

LICHENOID DERMATOSES

Lichen Planus

Lichen planus (LP) is a distinctive dermatosis characterized by pruritic, purple, polygonal papules (the "4-p sign") which involve the flexures of the arms and legs, the mucous membranes, genitals, nails, and scalp (Fig. 3.43). The eruption in LP typically demonstrates the Koebner or isomorphic phenomenon in which cutaneous lesions appear or extend in areas of trauma (scratches, excoriations, burns, scars). Only 2 percent of cases present before the age of 20; however, patients with the familial variant develop LP in childhood. Although the cause of LP is unknown, complement and immunoglobulin deposition along the basement membrane zone suggests an immunologic mechanism.

Typically, itchy, violaceous 3-mm to 6-mm papules appear abruptly on the wrists, ankles, and/or genitals. Lesions may spread over the forearms, shins, and lower back. Rarely, a widespread rash covers much of the

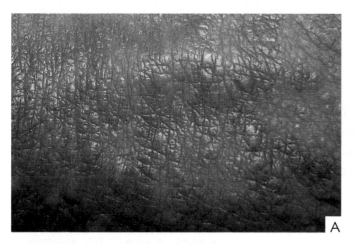

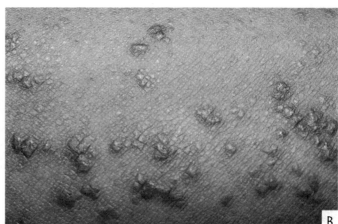

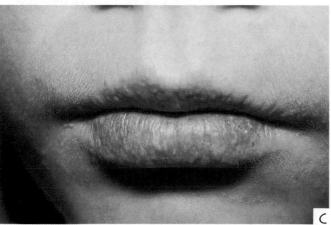

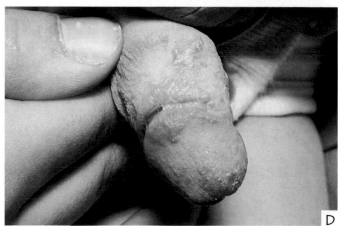

FIGURE 3.43 Lichen planus. (**A**) Violaceous polygonal papules almost to confluence appeared over several weeks on the dorsum of the hands and feet, ankles, and wrists of a 16 year-old boy. (**B**) Lesions are somewhat hyperpigmented on the forearm of this black adolescent. (**C,D**) White papules forming Wickham's striae were present on the lips of this child, who also had typical papules on the penis.

body. In areas of involvement, contiguous shiny-topped papules may form a white, lacy, reticulated network known as Wickham's striae. Their visibility may be enhanced by the application of a small quantity of mineral oil and examination with side lighting and a hand lens. Confluent lesions may form annular or linear plaques. Intense dermal inflammation may be associated with the development of vesiculobullous lesions, and hypertrophic, verrucous plaques may evolve, particularly on the shins, in chronic disease (Fig. 3.44).

Wickham's striae may also be present on the buccal mucosa, gingivae, lips, and tongue. Mucous membrane findings, which are present in two-thirds of patients with LP, also include erythema, white papules, resembling leukoplakia, vesicles, erosions, and deep, painful ulcerations.

LP may also present with follicular papules, particularly in the scalp where cicatricial alopecia may be progressive. Nail involvement, seen in about 10 percent of patients, includes brittleness, thinning, fragmentation, longitudinal ridging or striations, and partial or complete shedding of the nail (see Chapter 8). Pterygian formation, atrophy, subungual hyperkeratosis, and lifting of the distal nail plate may also occur. Rarely, nail disease appears without cutaneous involvement.

Skin biopsies characteristically demonstrate hyperkeratosis, focal thickening of the granular layer, irregular acanthosis, and a band-like infiltrate of lymphocytes and histiocytes in the dermis close to the epidermis and associated with damage to the basal cell layer.

Graft versus host disease and a number of medications have also been implicated in the development of a

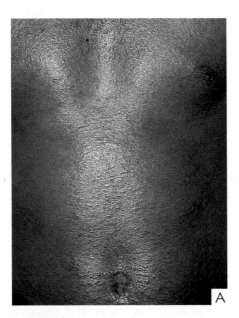
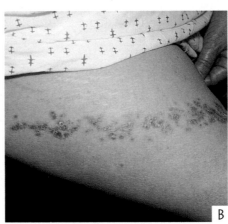
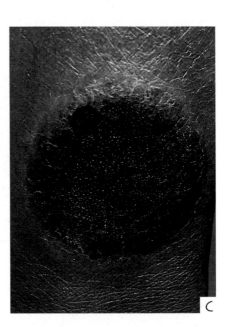

FIGURE 3.44 LP variants. (**A**) Diffuse eruptive LP responded to treatment with PUVA. Over 90 percent of this boy's body was involved with confluent papules on the trunk and extremities. (**B**) This asymptomatic linear plaque progressed slowly for over a year. (**C**) Extremely pruritic hypertrophic plaques were present on the shins of this 18 year-old girl.

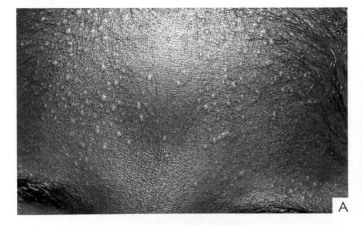
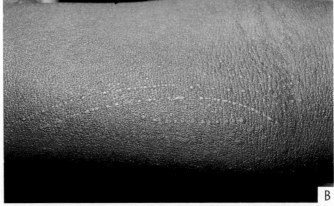

FIGURE 3.45 Lichen nitidus. (**A**) Asymptomatic, uniform, 2-mm to 3-mm shiny papules began on the face and spread to the trunk and extremities of this six-year-old boy. (**B**) Note the Koebner phenomenon on the arm, where papules developed in an incidental excoriation.

lichenoid rash indistinguishable from LP. The presence of eosinophils in the dermal infiltrate should suggest the possibility of a drug reaction. Prurigo nodules in eczema may be associated with other stigmata of atopic dermatitis, and the lesions of discoid lupus erythematosus usually demonstrate atrophy. Nail disease must be distinguished from other causes of nail dystrophy, and oral LP may mimic viral infection, primary blistering dermatoses, erythema multiforme, and leukoplakia.

Although many cases resolve within one to two years, some eruptions persist for 10 to 20 years. Localized lesions often respond well to topical steroids. Oral LP may be resistant to treatment, and some success has been achieved with topical retinoic acid, intralesional steroids, oral retinoids, oral steroids, and swish-and-spit cyclosporine. Although quite painful, intralesional injection of steroids is also useful in treating nail disease. Patients with generalized LP have been treated with systemic corticosteroids and retinoids. However, therapeutic benefits must be weighed against the long-term consequences of these medications. PUVA may, in fact, provide a relatively safe alternative for disseminated disease.

Lichen Nitidus
This uncommon, chronic, asymptomatic eruption is characterized by flat-topped, flesh-colored 2-mm to 3-mm papules which demonstrate the isomorphic phenomenon (Fig. 3.45). Although many practitioners

consider lichen niditus a variant of LP, the peak incidence in children between seven and 13 years, the uniformly tiny lesions which do not have a tendency to coalesce, and the lack of pruritus establish this disorder as a distinct entity. The rash progresses slowly over months to years, with a predilection for the arms, abdomen, and genitals. The majority of patients are male.

Skin biopsies demonstrate findings reminiscent of LP but are restricted to only one or a few papillae. The overlying horny layer exhibits parakeratosis, and at the lateral margin of the lesion the rete ridges extend downward to form a claw around the underlying infiltrate.

Papular or follicular eczema can be differentiated from lichen nitidus by the presence of pruritus and other markers of atopy. Keratosis pilaris appears in characteristic locations and is inherited as an autosomal dominant trait. Examination of flat warts with side lighting and magnification usually reveals a rough surface, unlike the smooth, shiny surface of papules in lichen nitidus. However, both lichen nitidus and flat warts koebnerize, and a skin biopsy may be necessary to distinguish them.

Lichen Striatus
This linear, lichenoid eruption appears most commonly in school-age children. Flat-topped papules arise suddenly in streaks and swirls, usually on the extremities, upper back, or neck (Fig. 3.46). However, any area, including the palms, soles, nails, genitals, and face, can

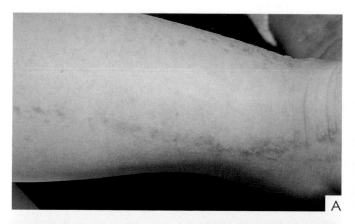

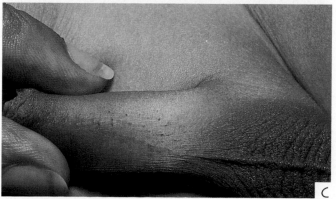

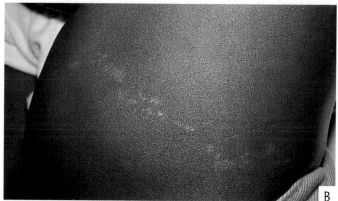

FIGURE 3.46 Lichen striatus. Asymptomatic linear scaly papules appeared on the (**A**) leg, (**B**) flank, and (**C**) penis of these young children. In each case histology demonstrated findings typical of lichen striatus. After a variable period of progression, from six to 24 months, these lesions resolved without treatment.

be involved. Lesions usually develop some overlying dusty scale and mild erythema. Hypopigmentation may bring attention to the eruption especially in dark-skinned children.

Lichen striatus usually fades without treatment in one to two years. Lubricants and topical corticosteroids may be useful to decrease scale and inflammation in cosmetically important areas.

This condition can be mistaken for linear epidermal nevi, linear lichen planus, linear porokeratosis, flat warts, linear psoriasis, and linear ichthyotic eruptions. When the clinical course is confusing, a skin biopsy is helpful in distinguishing these disorders. Lichen striatus usually demonstrates dermatitic changes in the epidermis, with a lymphocytic perivascular infiltrate in the superficial and mid-dermis that not infrequently extends into the deep dermis.

FUNGAL INFECTIONS

Tinea

Two types of fungal organisms, dermatophytes and yeasts, produce clinical cutaneous disease. Dermatophytes include tinea or ringworm fungi, which infect skin, nails, and hair (see Chapter 8). Mucous membranes are not usually involved.

Tinea Corporis This is a superficial fungal infection of nonhairy or glabrous skin. It has been called "ringworm" because of its characteristic configuration, which consists of pruritic annular plaques with central clearing or scale and an active indurated and/or vesiculopustular border (Fig. 3.47). Lesions, which can be single or multiple, typically begin as red papules or pustules which expand over days to weeks to form 1-cm to 5-cm plaques. Tinea corporis can occur in any age group and is usually acquired from an infected domestic animal (*Microsporum canis*)

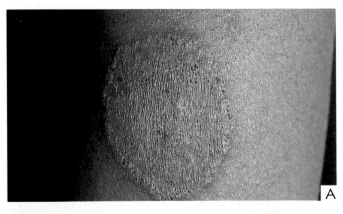
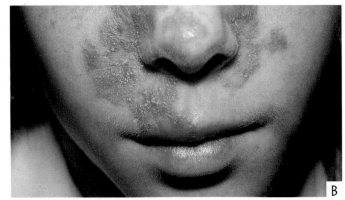
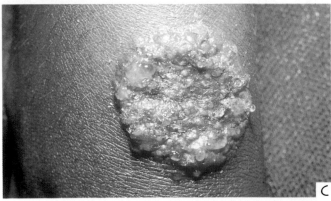
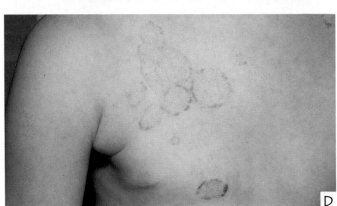

FIGURE 3.47 Tinea corporis. The characteristic annular lesions show many variations in appearance. (**A**) This lesion has a raised active border and shows some central clearing and scale. (**B**) Sharply circumscribed tinea faciale demonstrates erythema, scale, and pustule formation throughout the expanding patch. (**C**) An inflammatory tinea or kerion on the arm has marked edema and vesiculation. (**D**) Multiple expanding lesions spread quickly in a toddler who acquired infection from the family kitten.

or through direct human contact (*Trichophyton, Microsporum,* and *Epidermophyton*).

Clinically, tinea can be differentiated from atopic dermatitis by its propensity for autoinnoculation from the primary patches to other sites on the patient's skin, by spread to close contacts, and by the central clearing noted in many lesions. Moreover, the rash of atopic dermatitis tends to be symmetric, chronic, and recurrent in a flexural distribution. Unlike tinea, patches of nummular eczema are self-limited and do not clear centrally. The herald patch of pityriasis rosea is often mistaken for tinea. However, it is KOH-negative, and subsequent development of the generalized rash with its characteristic truncal distribution is distinctive. The clinical patterns, associated findings, and chronicity help differentiate psoriasis and seborrhea from tinea. Granuloma annulare produces a characteristic ringed plaque. However, on palpation the lesions are firm and do not exhibit epidermal changes (scales, vesicles, pustules). Granuloma annulare is also asymptomatic.

The diagnosis of tinea is confirmed by potassium hydroxide examination of the skin (Fig. 3.48). The first step is to obtain material by scraping the loose scales, vesicles, and pustules at the margin of a lesion. These should be mounted on the center of a glass slide and one or two drops of 20% KOH added. Next, a glass coverslip is applied and gently pressed down with a fingertip or the be heated gently, taking care not to boil the KOH solution, and again the coverslip is pressed down. The slide is then placed under a microscope, with the condenser and light at low levels to maximize contrast, and the objective at low power. On focusing up and down, true hyphae are seen as long, greenish, hyaline, branching, often septate rods of uniform width that cross the borders of epidermal cells (Fig. 3.49). Cotton fibers, cell borders or other artifacts may be falsely interpreted as positive findings.

Tinea infections on glabrous skin respond readily to topical antifungal creams (imidazoles such as clotrimazole, econazole, miconazole, ketoconazole; naftifine; cyclopirax; tolnoftate). When lesions are multiple and widespread, oral therapy with griseofulvin is indicated.

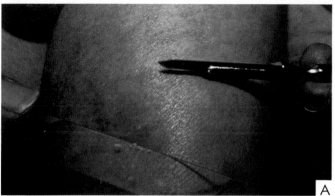

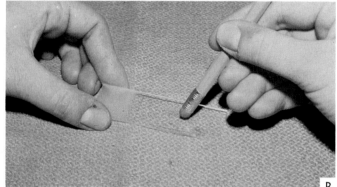

FIGURE 3.48 Potassium hydroxide (KOH) preparation. **(A)** Small scales should be scraped from the edge of the lesion onto a microscope slide. **(B)** Crush the scales to make a thin layer of cells in order to visualize the fungus easily.

FIGURE 3.49 Positive KOH preparation of skin scrapings. Fungal hyphae are seen as long septate branching rods at the margins and center of the scales.

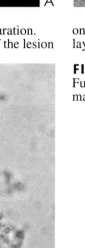

Tinea Pedis Commonly referred to as athlete's foot, tinea pedis is a fungal infection of the feet, with a predilection for web space involvement. It is common in adolescence, somewhat less so in prepubertal children. The infecting organisms are probably acquired from contaminated showers, bathrooms, and locker room and gym floors, and their growth is fostered by the warm, moist environment of shoes.

In some cases, scaling and fissuring predominate; in others, vesiculopustular lesions, erythema, and maceration are found (Fig. 3.50). The infection starts and may remain between and along the sides of the toes. However, lesions can extend over the dorsum of the foot and can involve the plantar surface as well, particularly the instep and the ball of the foot. Patients complain of burning and itching, which are frequently intense.

Diagnosis is suspected on clinical grounds and is confirmed by KOH preparation of skin scrapings. The mainstays of treatment include topical antifungal creams or powders and measures to reduce foot moisture. Many patients do better during the summer months while wearing sandals. For those with severe inflammatory lesions, oral antifungal agents may be required, and secondary bacterial infections (particularly with Gram-negative organisms) may be a problem.

Tinea pedis is distinguished from contact dermatitis of

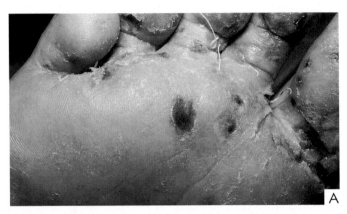

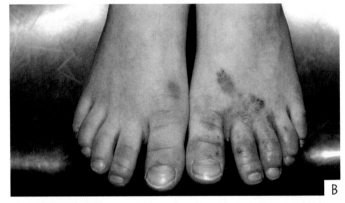

FIGURE 3.50 Tinea pedis. **(A)** Macerated, eroded, and crusted patches extend from the web spaces to the plantar surfaces of the toes and foot. **(B)** Dry, scaly, red patches extend from the web spaces to the top of the toes and foot. **(C)** The instep and medial surface of the foot is another commonly involved area. All of these children were under five years of age and had at least one parent with chronic or recurrent tinea pedis.

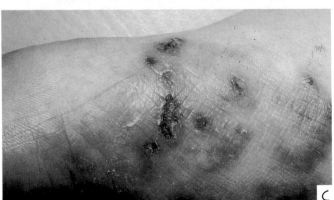

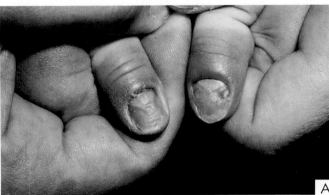

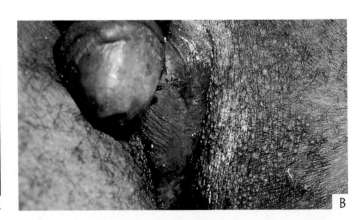

FIGURE 3.51 Candidiasis. **(A)** Chronic paronychia with erythema at the base of the nail, loss of the cuticle, and dystrophic changes of the nail developed in a two-year-old thumb sucker.

(B) A teenage diabetic on antibiotics developed a painful, red, macerated eruption dotted with pustules on the scrotum, penis, and groin. Scrapings from both patients grew *Candida* organisms.

the feet by the tendency of the latter to involve the dorsum of the feet and to spare the interdigital web spaces. In dyshidrotic eczema, KOH preparations and fungal cultures are negative. Psoriasis and PRP can be differentiated from tinea by their symmetric moccasin–glove distribution and other characteristic stigmata.

Yeasts

Candida and *Pityrosporum* account for the majority of yeast-related cutaneous disease.

Candidiasis *Candida* colonizes the gastrointestinal tract and skin shortly after birth and may produce both localized (thrush and diaper dermatitis) and disseminated cutaneous infection, as well as systemic infection, in the newborn. Recurrent and persistent infection in infancy may be associated with the use of antibiotics. However, it should also raise the suspicion of heritable or acquired immunodeficiency. *Candida* paronychia is also a common problem in otherwise healthy toddlers who suck on fingers and toes (Fig. 3.51). Yellowing, pit-

ting, and other signs of nail dystrophy associated with candida in this setting usually resolve without therapy; however, they may benefit from the application of topical antifungal creams. Perleche, manifested as erythema, maceration, and fissuring of the corners of the mouth, is common in diabetics and lip-lickers and can become secondarily infected by *Candida* (Fig. 3.52). Topical antifungals and aggressive use of lubricants may be necessary to eradicate the condition.

Tinea Versicolor This common dermatosis is characterized by multiple small, oval scaly patches measuring 1 to 3 cm in diameter, usually located in a guttate or raindrop pattern on the upper chest, back, and proximal portions of the upper extremities of adolescents and young adults (Fig. 3.53). However, all ages can be affected, including infants. Facial lesions are occasionally seen and may be the only area of involvement in breast-feeding infants who acquire the organism from their mothers. Some individuals may develop folliculitis on the chest, back, and occasionally the face.

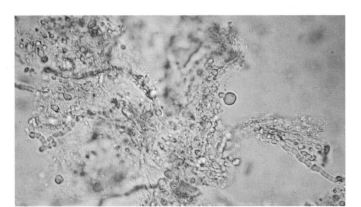

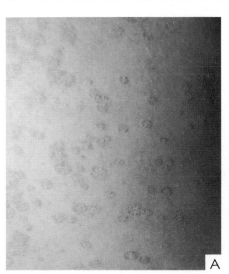 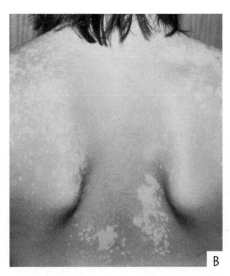 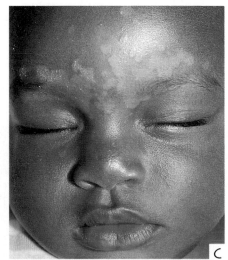

FIGURE 3.52 Positive KOH preparation for candidiasis. Note the stubby septate pseudohyphae and budding yeasts.

FIGURE 3.53 Tinea versicolor. (**A**) The well demarcated, scaly papules appear darker than surrounding skin on the back of a white adolescent. (**B**) Sun-exposed papules on the back of this child failed to tan, resulting in a hypopigmented rash. (**C**) A four-month-old black girl developed hypopigmented, scaly papules on her face. Her mother had widespread lesions on the chest and back.

When folliculitis does not respond to antibiotics, *Pityrosporum* should be considered. Tinea versicolor is caused by a dimorphous form of *Pityrosporum* which commonly colonizes the the skin by four to six months of age. Warm, moist climates, pregnancy, immunodeficiency states, and genetic factors predispose to the development of clinical lesions.

The rash is usually asymptomatic, although some patients complain of mild pruritus. Typically, the cosmetic appearance of the variably pigmented patches is more bothersome to them. Lesions may be light tan, reddish or white in color, giving rise to the term "versicolor." They are darker than surrounding skin in non-sun-exposed areas and lighter in areas that have tanned in response to sunlight. The diagnosis of tinea versicolor can usually be made on the basis of the clinical appearance of lesions and their distribution. It can be confirmed by a KOH preparation of the surface scale, which demonstrates short pseudohyphae and yeast forms that resemble spaghetti and meatballs (Fig. 3.54). Although the pathogenesis of the color change is not fully understood, the fungus is known to produce a substance that interferes with tyrosinase activity and subsequent melanin synthesis.

The differential diagnosis of tinea versicolor includes postinflammatory hypopigmentation and vitiligo. The history, distribution, and distinct borders help to distinguish tinea versicolor from postinflammatory hypopigmentation, and the presence of fine superficial scaling and some residual pigmentation helps to exclude vitiligo.

Confluent and reticulated papillomatosis of Gougerot and Carteud is an uncommon eruption characterized by brown or gray papules which aggregate on the seborrheic areas of the chest and back, particularly in black teenagers and young adults. Reticulated patches may extend over much of the back, shoulders, chest, and abdomen. Although the cause is not known, many investigators attribute the rash to *Pityrosporum* infection. Unfortunately, the rash is usually refractory to treatment. However, some patients improve spontaneously, and others respond to traditional therapy for tinea versicolor.

Topical desquamating agents, such as selenium sulfide and propylene glycol, produce rapid clearing of tinea versicolor. Localized lesions can be treated effectively with topical antifungal creams, and recalcitrant cases respond to oral ketocinazole. Patients must be counselled about the high risk of recurrence and reminded that pigmentary changes may take months to clear, even after eradication of the fungus.

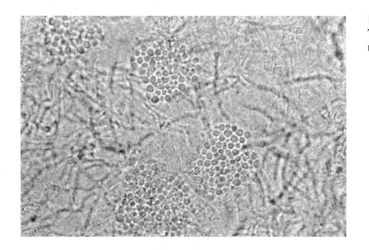

FIGURE 3.54 Positive KOH preparation for tinea versicolor. The combination of hyphal and yeast forms of the fungus simulates the appearance of spaghetti and meatballs.

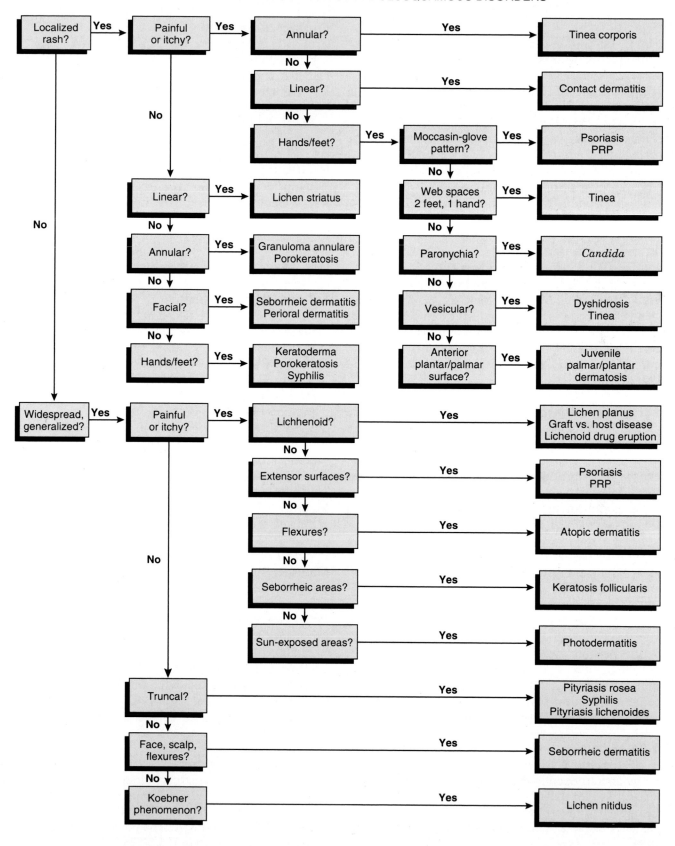

BIBLIOGRAPHY

Psoriasis

Beylot C, Puisant A, et al. Particular clinical features of psoriasis in infants and children. *Acta Dermatol Venereol* (suppl) 87:95, 1979.

Farber EM, Nall ML.The natural history of psoriasis in 5600 patients. *Dermatologica* 148:1, 1974.

Menter MA, Whiting DA, McWilliams J. Resistant childhood psoriasis: an analysis of patients seen in a day care center. *Pediatr Dermatol* 2:8–12, 1984.

National Psoriasis Foundation Bulletin, Suite 210, 6443 SW Beaverton Hwy, Portland, OR 97221.

Nyfors A, Lemholt K. Psoriasis in children. *Br J Dermatol* 92:437,1975.

Pityriasis rubra pilaris

Braun-Falco O, Ryckmanns F, Schmoeckel C, et al. Pityriasis rubra pilaris: a clinicopathological and therapeutic study. *Arch Dermatol Res* 275:287–295, 1983.

Cohen PR, Prystowsky JH. Pityriasis rubra pilaris. A review of diagnosis and treatment. *J Am Acad Dermatol* 20:801–807, 1989.

Huntley CC. Pityriasis rubra pilaris. *Am J Dis Child* 122:22, 1971.

Keratosis follicularis

Beck AL Jr, Finochio AF, White JP. Darier's disease: a kindred with a large number of cases. *Br J Dermatol* 97:335,1977.

Svendsen IB, Albrechtseb B. The prevalence of dyskeratosis follicularis (Darier's disease) in Denmark. An investigation of the hereditary in 22 families. *Acta Dermatol Venereol* 39:356, 1959.

Hyperkeratosis of the palms and soles

Baden HP. Keratoderma of palms and soles. In: Fitzpatrick TB, Eisen AZ, Freedberg IM, Austen KF, eds. *Dermatology in General Medicine.* New York: McGraw–Hill, 1987, p 529–533.

Ortega M, Quintana J, Camacho F. Keratosis punctata of the palmar creases. *J Am Acad Dermatol* 13: 381–382, 1985.

Poulin Y, Perry HO, Muller SA. Olmsted syndrome—congenital palmoplantar and periorificial keratoderma. *J Am Acad Dermatol* 10:600–610, 1984.

Porokeratosis

Cox GF, Jarratt M. Linear porokeratosis and other linear cutaneous exeptions of childhood. *Am J Dis Child* 133:1258–1259, 1979.

Madojana RM, Katz R, Rodman OG. Porokeratosis plantaris discreta. *J Am Acad Dermatol* 10:679–682, 1984.

Mikhail GR, Wertheimer FW. Clinical variants of porokeratosis (Mibelli). *Arch Dermatol* 98:124, 1968.

Contact dermatitis

Cronin E. *Contact dermatitis.* Edinburgh: Churchill Livingstone, 1980.

Fisher AA. *Contact dermatitis,* 2d ed. Philadelphia: Lea & Feibiger, 1973

Weston WL. Allergic contact dermatitis in children. *Am J Dis Child* 138:932, 1984.

Atopic dermatitis

Hanifin JM. Basic and clinical aspects of atopic dermatitis: a review. *Ann Allerg* 52:368–375, 1984.

Rajka G. *Atopic dermatitis.* London: WB Saunders, 1975.

Rajka G. Some aetiological data on atopic dermatitis. Paper presented at Second International Symposium on Atopic Dermatitis. Norway, 1984.

Seborrheic dermatitis

Ford GP, Farr PM, Ive FA, et al. The response of seborrheic dermatitis to ketoconazole. *Br J Dermatol* 111:603, 1984.

Skinner RB, Noah PW, Taylor RM, Zanolli MD, West S, Guin JD. Doubleblind treatment of seborrheic dermatitis with 2% ketoconazole cream. *J Am Acad Dermatol* 12:852–856, 1985.

Yates VM, Kerr RE, Frier K, et al. Early diagnosis of infantile seborrheic dermatitis and atopic dermatitis: clinical features. *Br J Dermatol* 108:633, 1983.

Juvenile palmar–plantar dermatosis

Moorthy TT, Rajan VS. Juvenile plantar dermatosis in Singapore. *Int J Dermatol* 23:476, 1984.

Perioral dermatitis

Marks R, Black MM. Perioral dermatitis. A histopathological study of 26 cases. *Br J Dermatol* 84:242, 1971.

Pityriasis rosea

Cavanaugh RM. Pityriasis rosea in children. *Clin Pediatr* 22:200, 1983.

Chuang Tsu-Yi, Ilstrup DM, Perry HO, Kurland LT. Pityriasis rosea in Rochester, Minnesota, 1969 to 1978. *J Am Acad Dermatol* 7:80, 1982.

Parsons. Pityriasis rosea update. *J Am Acad Dermatol* 15:159–167, 1986.

Pityriasus lichenoides

Hood AF, Mark EJ. Histopathologic diagnosis of pityriasis lichenoides et varioliformis acuta and its clinical correlation. *Arch Dermatol* 118:478, 1982.

Lambert WC, Everett MA. The nosology of parapsoriasis. *J Am Acad Dermatol* 5:373,1981.

Truhan AP, Hebert AA, Esterly NB. Pityriasis lichenoides in children: therapeutic response to erythromycin. *J Am Acad Dermatol* 15:66–70, 1986.

Lichen planus

Boyd AS, Neldner KH. Lichen planus (CME review). *J Am Acad Dermatol* 25:593–619, 1991.

Brice SL, Barr RJ, Rattet JP. Childhood lichen planus— a question of therapy. *J Am Acad Dermatol* 3:370, 1980.

Ragaz A, Ackerman AB. Evolution, maturation, and regression of lesions of lichen planus. *Am J Dermatopathol* 3:5–25, 1981.

Rivers JK, Jackson R, Orozaga M. Who was Wickham and what are his striae? *Int J Dermatol* 25:611–613, 1986.

Silverman RA, Rhodes AR. Twenty-nail dystrophy of childhood: a sign of localized lichen planus. *Pediatr Dermatol* 1:207, 1984.

Lichen nitidus

Lapins NA, Willoughby C, Helwid EB. Lichen nitidus: a study of 43 cases. *Cutis* 21:634, 1978.

Lichen striatus

Charles CR, Johnson BL, Robinson TA. Lichen striatus. *J Cutan Pathol* 1:265–274, 1974.

Taieb A, Youbi AE, Grosshaus E, Maleville J. Lichen striatus. A blachko linear acquired inflammatory skin eruption. *J Am Acad Dermatol* 25:637–642, 1991.

Fungal infections

Jacobs PH. Fungal infections in children. *Pediatr Clin North Am* 25:357–370, 1978.

McLean et al. Ecology of dermatophyte infections in South Bronx, New York, 1969 to 1981. *J Am Acad Dermatol* 16:336–340, 1987.

Confluent and reticulated papillomatosis of Gougerot and Carteud

Nordby CA, Mitchell AJ. Confluent and reticulated papilomatosis responsive to selenium sulfide. *Int J Dermatol* 25:194–199, 1986.

chapter four

VESICULOPUSTULAR ERUPTIONS

ANATOMY OF VESICULOPUSTULAR DERMATOSES

Cutaneous Anatomy	Site of Blister Formation	Disorder
	Upper Epidermis	Staphylococcal scalded skin syndrome
	Mid-Epidermis	Dermatitis Friction blister Pemphigus foliaceus
	Lower Epidermis	Herpes simplex Varicella-zoster Pemphigus vulgaris Epidermolytic epidermolysis bullosa
	Basement Membrane Zone	Bullous pemphigoid Chronic bullous disease of childhood Dermatitis herpetiformis Junctional epidermolysis bullosa
	Dermis	Epidermolysis bullosa acquisita Dermolytic epidermolysis bullosa Toxic epidermal necrolysis Burn

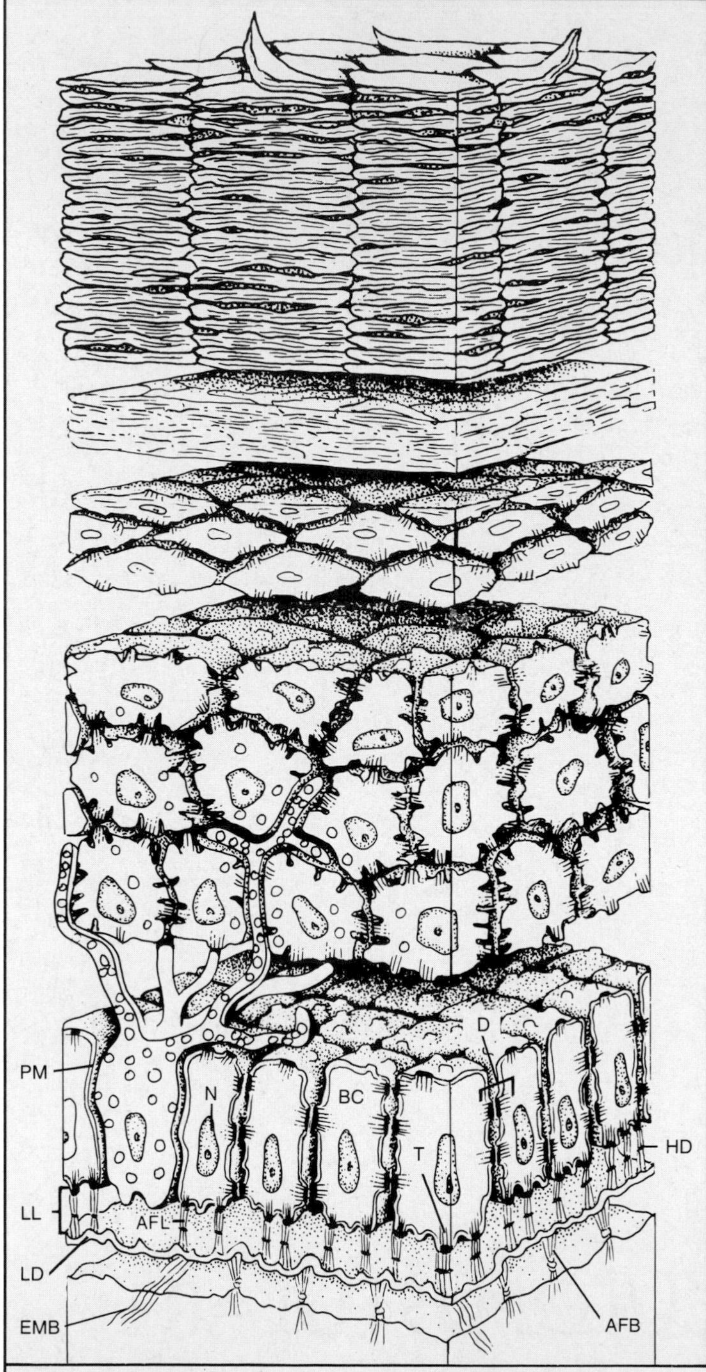

BC = Basal cell
N = Basal cell nucleus
T = Tonofilament
D = Desmosome
HD = Hemidesmosome
LL = Lamina lucida
LD = Lamina densa
PM = Plasma membrane of basal cell
EMB = Elastic microfibril bundle
AFL = Anchoring filament
AFB = Anchoring fibril

FIGURE 4.1 Anatomy of vesiculopustular dermatoses.

Vesiculopustular eruptions range from benign, self-limited conditions to life-threatening diseases. Early diagnosis, especially in the young or immunocompromised child, is mandatory.

An understanding of the structures that account for normal epidermal and basement membrane zone adhesion will provide clues to the clinical diagnosis and pathogenesis of blistering diseases (Fig. 4.1). Epidermal cells are held together by desmosome–tonofilament complexes. Electron-dense tonofilaments insert into desmosomes in the keratinocyte plasma membrane and project toward the nucleus. Intercellular bridges extend between keratinocytes and are associated with a sticky, glycoprotein-rich intercellular cement substance. In the basement membrane zone, tonofilaments insert into hemidesmosomes. These are attached to the lamina densa by anchoring filaments which traverse an electron-lucent layer known as the lamina lucida. The electron-dense lamina densa is, in turn, affixed to the dermis by anchoring fibrils. Elastic microfibril bundles that arise in the upper dermis also insert into the lamina densa.

A number of proteins that probably play a role in the structural integrity of the skin have been identified in the basement membrane zone. Bullous pemphigoid antigen appears on the bottom of the basal cell plasma membrane and within the lamina lucida. Laminin is present within the lamina lucida, and Type IV collagen has been isolated to the lamina densa. Epidermolysis bullosa acquisita antigen has recently been found in the dermis just beneath the lamina densa. Fluorescein-tagged antibodies directed against these proteins can be used to identify the site of blister formation in disorders that involve the dermal–epidermal junction.

In general, flaccid bullae arise within the epidermis and tense lesions involve the dermis. Specific diagnoses, however, rely on identification of clinical patterns, histopathology, and immunofluorescent findings. A few rapid diagnostic techniques will also aid in developing a differential diagnosis.

VIRAL INFECTIONS

Herpes simplex virus is a common cause of oral lesions in toddlers and school-age children. Primary herpetic gingivostomatitis begins with extensive perioral vesicles and pustules and intraoral vesicles and erosions (Fig. 4.2). The gingivae become edematous, red, and friable, and bleed easily. Epithelial debris and exudates may form a membrane on the mucosal surfaces. The eruption is usually accompanied by fever, irritability, and cervical adenopathy. Lesions may also be scattered on the face and upper trunk. In infants and toddlers, lesions are frequently autoinoculated onto the hands. Patients should be observed for dehydration as symptoms abate over seven to ten days.

Herpetic gingivostomatitis can be differentiated from enteroviral infections, which usually produce vesicles, ulcerations, and petechiae on the hard palate and spare the gingivae. Although aphthae may be very painful, they are usually isolated lesions that lack the diffuse inflammation associated with herpes.

Primary herpes simplex infections can involve any cutaneous or mucous membrane surface and usually result from direct inoculation of previously injured sites. Lesions consist of herpetiform or clustered red papules, which evolve into vesicles and sometimes into

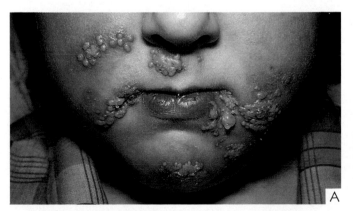
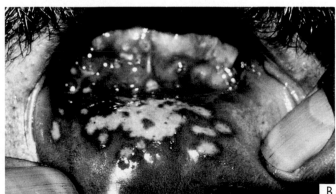

FIGURE 4.2 Herpetic gingivostomatitis. (**A**) This six-year-old boy developed extensive perioral vesicles and mucous membrane erosions with his first bout of herpes simplex. (**B**) A 19-year-old experienced severe pain from widespread gingival and buccal mucosal vesicles and erosions during the peak of his primary herpes infection.

pustules in 24 to 48 hours (Fig. 4.3A). During the following five to seven days the vesicles rupture and become encrusted. Desquamation and healing are complete in ten to 14 days. Primary herpes infections on the fingers are called herpetic whitlows (Fig. 4.3B). Just as in herpes gingivostomatitis, primary infections at other sites may be associated with painful local adenopathy and flu-like symptoms.

In children, most infections are caused by HSV Type 1. HSV Type 2 is most commonly found in genital infections in adolescents and adults (Fig. 4.4). However, it can also be found in nongenital areas, and Type 1 virus may be spread from mouth to hand to genital sites. Although the possibility of sexual contact should be considered in any child who develops genital herpes, nonvenereal sources are probably most common. Vesicles are usually restricted to the perineum and genital skin, and they quickly become ulcerated. Erythema and edema may lead to severe dysuria and urinary retention.

In immunocompromised children or patients with certain skin conditions, such as atopic dermatitis, seborrheic dermatitis, or immunologic blistering disorders, herpes simplex may disseminate over the entire skin surface (eczema herpeticum or Kaposi's varicelliform eruption) and to the lungs, viscera, and central nervous system. Herpes simplex may also produce life-threatening disease in the nursery environment.

After the initial episode, HSV enters a dormant state. A number of endogenous and environmental factors may trigger reactivation of the virus, such as a strep throat, an upper respiratory infection, sunburn, or surgery. Lesions usually occur near the site of the primary eruption, mucous membranes are rarely involved, systemic symptoms are absent, and the rash heals in less than a week. Although recurrences are unpredictable, disease-free periods tend to increase with time even in patients who initially experience frequent recurrences.

A clinical suspicion of herpes simplex can be confirmed quickly by performing a Tzanck smear in the emergency room or at the bedside. Viral cultures in reliable laboratories should turn positive within 12 to 36 hours. In some centers, immunofluorescent staining of blister fluid debris on glass slides or electron microscopy is used for rapid confirmation.

The Tzanck smear is obtained by removing the roof of a blister with a scalpel or scissors and scraping its base to obtain the moist, cloudy debris. This is then spread on a glass slide with the scalpel blade, dessicated with 95 percent ethanol, and stained with Giemsa or Wright's stain. The diagnostic finding in viral blisters is the multinucleated giant cell (see Fig. 2.40B). This is a syncytium of epidermal cells with multiple overlapping nuclei; hence, it is much larger than other inflammatory cells. Unfortunately, a positive Tzanck smear cannot be

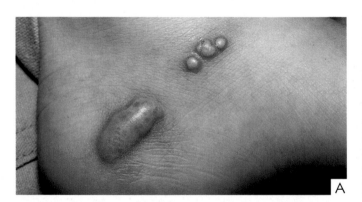

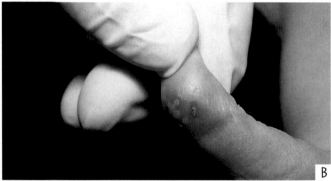

FIGURE 4.3 (A) Over 24 hours herpetic vesicles evolved into pustules on the foot of a five-year-old boy. In one area near the heel several vesicles fused to form a multiloculated bulla.

(B) A herpetic whitlow developed by autoinoculation from oral lesions in this four-year-old boy. Oral and finger lesions resolved without treatment in two weeks.

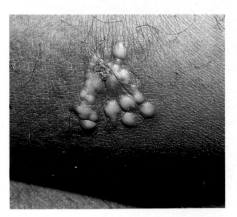

FIGURE 4.4 Clustered pustules appeared on the posterior thigh of a teenager with recurrent herpes simplex Type 2.

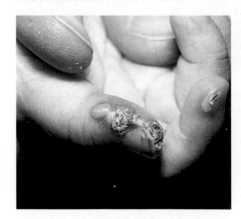

FIGURE 4.5 Blistering distal dactylitis developed on the right thumb and index finger of a five-year-old girl. Cultures from her throat and thumb grew Group A β-hemolytic *Streptococcus*. The infection responded quickly to oral amoxicillin.

used to differentiate one blistering viral eruption from another, and a viral culture should therefore be obtained when the clinical situation dictates.

In general, management of herpes infections is symptomatic, with cool compresses, lubricants, and oral analgesics. Topical acyclovir is of little use in the treatment of uncomplicated infections in normal hosts. Hospitalized patients with primary herpes gingivostomatitis or genital herpes may improve with parenteral acyclovir (5 mg/kg every eight hours). In recurrent disease, initiation of oral acyclovir at the time of prodromal tingling in the skin before the appearance of blisters may abort the episode. In selected children with frequent, multiple, widespread recurrent eruptions, long-term suppressive therapy may be necessary.

Herpes simplex infections can usually be distinguished from other blistering eruptions by the typical clustering of lesions, the clinical course, a positive Tzanck smear, and characteristic skin biopsy findings. Impetigo may mimic herpes. However, bullae tend to be relatively large with a central crust and peripheral extension, and a Gram-stain demonstrates Gram-positive cocci. Blistering distal dactylitis, which is caused by Group A β-hemolytic *Streptococcus*, may be mistaken for a herpetic whitlow (Fig. 4.5). In streptococcal infection the

lesions on the fingertips usually coalesce to form one or several 5-mm to 10-mm blisters, and Gram stains and cultures demonstrate the causative bacterium. Occasionally the eruption of herpes simplex forms a dermatomal pattern. In this situation a viral culture is required to exclude herpes zoster.

Varicella is a mild, self-limited infection in most children. However, disseminated disease is a problem in the neonate and in immunosuppressed children. Early administration of varicella-zoster immunoglobulin to immunocompromised children exposed to varicella may be preventative, and antiviral therapy in patients with disseminated lesions may be lifesaving. The recent availability of varicella vaccine for high-risk children may reduce the incidence of serious complications. Several studies are under way to assess the efficacy of immunization in normal children.

After exposure to varicella, the incubation period varies from seven to 21 days. Fever, sore throat, decreased appetite, and malaise precede the skin lesions by several days. Early cutaneous findings vary from a few scattered, pruritic red papules to generalized papules that evolve in 24 hours to vesicles on a bright-red base (dewdrops on a rose petal) (Fig. 4.6A–C). Central umbilication of blisters follows rapidly, and crusting and

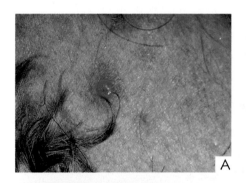 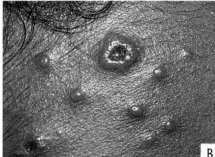 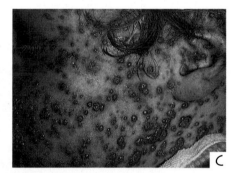

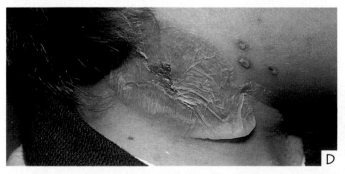 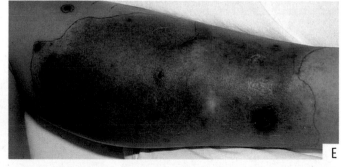

FIGURE 4.6 Chicken pox. (**A**) A dewdrop on a rose petal is the characteristic primary lesion in chicken pox. (**B**) Lesions in various stages of development including red papules, vesicles, umbilicated vesicles, and crusts developed in close proximity on the forehead of a toddler with varicella. (**C**) Severe varicella with blisters almost to confluence erupted within 24 hours over much of the skin surface of a six-year-old boy who was on high-dose systemic corticosteroids for inflammatory bowel disease. (**D**) Bullous impetigo spread quickly by scratching in a four-year-old boy with chicken pox. Bacterial cultures grew *Staphylococcus aureus* which was sensitive to erythromycin. (**E**) Purpura fulminans. A seven-year-old girl with resolving chicken pox developed expanding bruises on her legs. Laboratory studies were consistent with disseminated intravascular coagulation, which resolved on heparin therapy. Note the dark-purple crusted papules of healing chicken pox scattered on her leg.

desquamation occur within ten days. New papules and vesicles continue to appear for three to four days. Vesicles may also be identified on mucous membranes, particularly the buccal mucosa and gingivae. Although the blisters are intraepidermal and usually heal without scarring, some develop deep inflammation or become secondarily infected and heal with pitted or hypertrophic scars.

Pruritus may be intense and responds to cool compresses, calamine lotion, and antihistamines. Secondary infection is usually caused by *Staphylococcus* and should be treated with oral antibiotics such as erythromycin, dicloxacillin, or cephalexin (Fig. 4.6D). When cellulitis or other deep soft-tissue infection complicates chicken pox, hospitalization and parenteral therapy may be required. Rarely, progressive purpura and necrosis of large areas of skin heralds the onset of disseminated intravascular coagulation. This phenomenon, referred to as purpura fulminans, occurs in less than one in 20,000 cases of varicella (Fig. 4.6E).

Administration of systemic corticosteroids, even in normal children, is contraindicated during varicella infection and may result in severe blistering, disseminated viral infection, and increased risk of complications. As a consequence, it is important to differentiate chicken pox from contact dermatitis, insect bites, and mononucleosis or other viral infections. The Tzanck smear may be particularly useful early in the course of disease when only a few skin lesions are present.

Herpes zoster, or *shingles,* represents a reactivation of the dormant varicella virus from the sensory root ganglia. The most commonly involved sites include the distribution of the head and neck and the thoracic sensory nerves (Fig. 4.7). After a variable prodrome, which may include mild constitutional symptoms and localized itching and burning, clustered red papulovesicles appear in a unilateral, linear pattern in one or several dermatomes. In some children the eruption may be completely asymptomatic. Over three to five days the rash reaches its full extent, and during the ensuing one to two weeks vesicles and erosions develop umbilicated crusts and desquamate, similar to the course in chicken pox.

Although six to ten lesions may appear outside the primary dermatomes in normal individuals, the development of widespread cutaneous lesions suggests the possibility of an immunodeficiency state and an increased risk of visceral involvement. Children with lymphoreticular malignancies are more than 100 times as likely to develop zoster as healthy children. However, most cases of childhood zoster occur in normal hosts.

Normal children who develop chicken pox during the first two months of life may also be prone to zoster. In these patients, protective antibody titers tend to be low and skin-test reactions are diminished, suggesting a blunted immunologic response to varicella in early infancy. This phenomenon may result from transient maternal antibody protection which wanes during the first four months of life.

The presence of a dermatomal bullous eruption is virtually diagnostic for herpes zoster. However, herpes simplex occasionally presents in a dermatomal pattern. Moreover, zoster may be confused with herpes simplex early in the course when only a few clustered vesicles are present and the dermatomal organization is not yet apparent.

Management of shingles is usually limited to supportive measures, similar to the case with chicken pox. In disseminated disease administration of parenteral acyclovir may be lifesaving. Normal individuals who develop eye involvement will also benefit from antiviral therapy and should be followed closely by an ophthalmologist. Because of the high risk of zoster in children undergoing bone marrow transplantation or other elective immunosuppression, antiviral prophylaxis should be considered in these patients.

Although systemic corticosteroids can be administered to reduce the risk of post-herpetic neuralgia in adults over the age of 60, this treatment has not been shown to be beneficial in young adults or children. Moreover, the incidence of this problem in childhood is extremely low. Children with shingles should be isolated from individuals who are susceptible to chicken pox because of the risk of acquiring infection from direct contact with skin lesions.

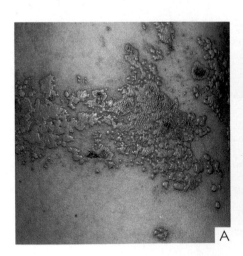 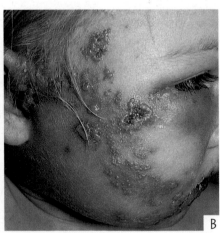

FIGURE 4.7 (**A**) Herpes zoster involved the right midthoracic dermatomes in an otherwise healthy ten-year-old girl with a history of chicken pox at age two. (**B**) Periorbital cellulitis was initially considered in this toddler with impressive edema and erythema of the right eye. The diagnosis of shingles became apparent one day later when the characteristic dermatomal vesiculopustular rash appeared. Both children had uneventful recoveries without treatment.

Hand, foot, and mouth syndrome is a distinctive, self-limited viral eruption caused most frequently by Coxsackie A16. The disease is highly infectious and, like other enteroviruses, peak incidence occurs in the late summer and fall. After exposure, the incubation period ranges from four to six days. A one- to two-day prodrome of fever, anorexia, and sore throat is followed by the development of 3-mm to 6-mm elongated, gray, thin-walled vesicles on a red or noninflamed base. As the name sugests, lesions appear most commonly on the palms, soles, and sides of the hands and feet, but red papules and vesicles may also erupt on the buttocks, trunk, face, arms, and legs (Fig. 4.8A and B). The enanthem is characterized by vesicles which rapidly ulcerate, leaving sharply marginated erosions on a red base on the tongue, buccal mucosa, and posterior pharynx (Fig. 4.8C). Although cutaneous and mucosal lesions may be completely asymptomatic, pruritus and burning are occasionally severe. Systemic symptoms including fever, diarrhea, sore throat, and cervical adenopathy may be absent or mild, and treatment is supportive. The eruption usually clears in less than a week.

BACTERIAL INFECTIONS

Expanding honey-colored, crusted patches or bullae with a central crust should suggest the diagnosis of *impetigo* (see Chapter 2) (Fig. 4.9). In older children, lesions appear most commonly on exposed skin during

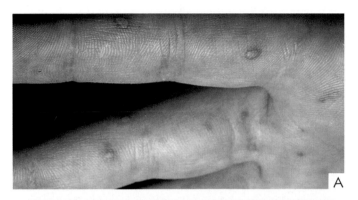

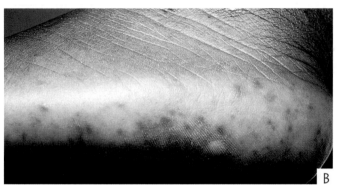

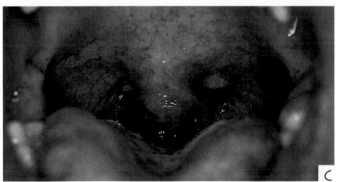

FIGURE 4.8 **(A,B)** Characteristic elongated vesicles on a red base are shown on the palmar surface of the fingers and plantar surface of the foot of a child with Coxsackie hand, foot, and mouth syndrome. **(C)** The enanthem, consisting of shallow yellow ulcers surrounded by red halos, may be found on the labial or buccal mucosa, the tongue, soft palate, uvula, and anterior tonsilar pillars. When the enanthem occurs in the absence of a rash, the disorder is known as herpangina.

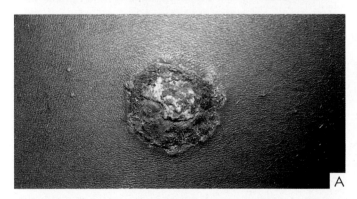

FIGURE 4.9 **(A)** A large doughnut-shaped blister with a central crust and smaller satellite lesions suggests the diagnosis of bullous impetigo. Widespread blisters in this toddler responded quickly to oral cephalexin. **(B)** Painful impetiginized pustules obscured the primary diagnosis of scabies in this teenager. A careful examination, however, revealed burrows under her breasts and in the genital area, and she was treated with oral cephalexin and topical 5 percent permethrin cream.

the summer months. Although Group A β-hemolytic *Streptococcus* was the predominant organism 20 to 30 years ago, *Staphylococcus aureus,* alone or in combination with streptococci, is now recovered from a majority of cultures. As a consequence, antistaphylococcal antibiotics are now the drugs of choice for treatment.

Impetigo is often a self-limited process. However, complications, including cellulitis and disseminated infection, as well as spread to family members and classmates, can be limited by antibiotic therapy. Topical antibiotics such as bacitracin, polymyxin B, neomycin, and mupirocin can be used in localized disease. Widespread lesions should be treated with oral agents including dicloxacillin, cephalexin, amoxicillin–clavulinate, and erythromycin. Unfortunately, up to 40 percent of staphylococcal isolates have been reported to be resistant to erythromycin in a number of studies around the country. Consequently, practitioners should select antibiotic coverage based on the resistance patterns in their respective communities.

Staphylococcal scalded skin syndrome (SSSS) occurs almost exclusively in infants and toddlers (see Chapter 2). However, it has been reported with increasing frequency in older children and adults, particularly in debilitated patients with decreased renal function (Fig. 4.10). This process should be considered in any child who develops a generalized, tender erythema associated with a Nikolsky sign. When a Nikolsky sign is present, minimal shearing force produced by finger pressure will induce a skin slough or blister formation.

Although SSSS is usually self-limited in healthy children, immunocompromised patients may develop complications related to their primary staphylococcal infection. Most SSSS is associated with a primary cutaneous infection. However, the soluble toxin that causes the rash may be produced by an occult infection such as osteomyelitis, septic arthritis, pneumonia, or meningitis. Healthy children respond to oral antistaphylococcal antibiotics. Infants, severely ill older children, and patients with occult infection require appropriate culturing and parenteral therapy. Parents should also be counseled about the generalized desquamation that develops ten to 14 days after the acute infection.

Staphylococcal folliculitis is a common problem in older children and adults. Red papules and pustules on an inflamed base erupt in a follicular pattern, most frequently on the buttocks, thighs, back, and upper arms (Fig. 4.11). Occasionally, superficial follicular pustules evolve into painful, deep-seated furuncles or spread to neighboring follicles and soft tissue, creating an abscess or carbuncle. Abscesses and resulting cellulitis may be associated with fever, malaise, and sepsis.

Localized folliculitis may improve with topical antibiotics. However, widespread lesions respond best to systemic therapy. In addition, abscesses should be incised and drained, and cellulitis may require parenteral antibiotics.

Children with chronic folliculitis often have predisposing dermatoses such as keratosis pilaris. Children with Down's syndrome are particularly prone to folliculitis on the trunk and proximal extremities. Long-term use of antiseptic soaps, topical antibiotics (e.g., clindamycin, tetracycline, erythromycin) and peeling agents (e.g., benzoyl peroxide, retinoic acid, salicylic acid) may reduce the risk of recurrent infection. Certain hydrating lotions and creams which are also designed to remove scale (e.g., Carmol and Aquacare with urea, Lacticare and LacHydrin with lactic acid) may be beneficial. Patients should also be instructed to avoid tight clothing and occlusive moisturizers. In toddlers, folliculitis may improve after toilet training. Older children with enuresis should also be encouraged to remove wet clothing as soon as possible.

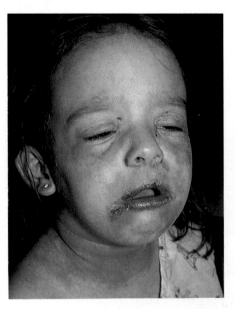

FIGURE 4.10
Staphylococcal scalded skin syndrome. A healthy four-year old boy developed fever, periorificial crusting, and generalized tender red skin. A Nikolsky sign was present, and *Staphylococcus aureus* was cultured from his nares.

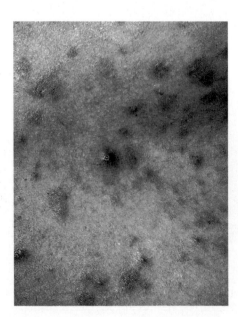

FIGURE 4.11
Staphylococcal folliculitis recurred chronically on the buttocks of a 13-year-old with Down's syndrome. Note the red papules and pustules around the gluteal cleft. He improved considerably with the use of topical benzoyl peroxide and mupriocin ointment, but he still required intermittent oral antibiotic therapy.

IMMUNOBULLOUS DERMATOSES

Although there is clinical overlap among the various immunologically mediated vesiculobullous dermatoses, they can be distinguished on the basis of specific clinical patterns, histopathology, immunopathology, and response to therapy. In pemphigus, blisters form within the epidermis. Chronic bullous dermatosis of childhood or linear IgA dermatosis, bullous pemphigoid, dermatitis herpetiformis, and epidermolysis bullosa acquisita are characterized by subepidermal blisters.

Intraepidermal Disorders

Childhood pemphigus refers to a group of rare, chronic, and potentially life-threatening immunobullous disorders characterized by flaccid intraepidermal bullae which erupt on normal-appearing or erythematous skin. Clinically and histologically, pemphigus can be divided into two types: pemphigus vulgaris (PV) and pemphigus foliaceous (PF).

In half of patients with PV, intraoral erosions or scalp blisters precede more widespread lesions for months. Eventually, vesicles and bullae develop on the trunk, scalp, face, and extremities in a seborrheic distribution (Fig. 4.12). By progressive extension, large areas of the body surface may become involved. Blisters heal insidiously without scarring unless they become secondarily infected. Ninety-five percent of patients have intraoral involvement, which may extend into the posterior pharynx and larynx. Pruritus, pain, and burning of the skin and mucous membranes may be severe, resulting in decreased oral intake and marked weight loss. A Nikolsky sign is usually present, and downward pressure on previously formed blisters may cause extension at the periphery (Asbaugh–Hansen sign). Pemphigus may also occur transiently in the newborn as a result of transplacental passage of the pemphigus antibody from the mother to the baby.

Although the pathogenesis of PV has not been completely determined, an IgG antibody directed against epidermal intercellular cement substance has been identified in the skin, serum, and blister fluid of these patients. When the purified IgG obtained from blister fluid is injected into the peritoneal cavity of neonatal nude mice, it produces widespread blistering which demonstrates acantholysis. Complement, IgA, and IgM have also been identified in blister fluid, but their roles in the development of bullae are not clear.

Biopsies of fresh, intact vesicles with perilesional skin demonstrate intercellular edema and disappearance of intercellular bridges in the lower portion of the epidermis at the periphery. Separation of epidermal cells from one another leads to the formation of suprabasilar clefts and then to frank blister formation, with the basal rounded-up acantholytic keratinocytes may be found within the bullae and are easily demonstrated on Tzanck smears.

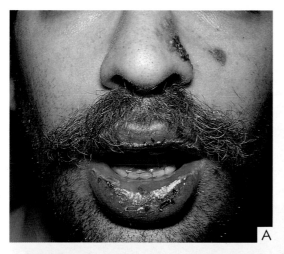

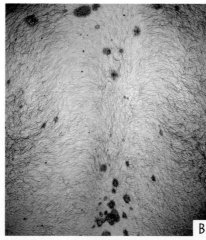

FIGURE 4.12 Pemphigus vulgaris. (**A,B**) A 20-year-old developed superficial hemorrhagic blisters on his face, lips, and trunk in a seborrheic distribution. Histopathology and immunofluorescence demonstrated findings typical of pemphigus vulgaris. (**C**) Note these flaccid blisters on a minimally inflamed base. (**D**) Anti-IgG antibody marks the epidermal intercellular cement substance on direct immunofluorescence.

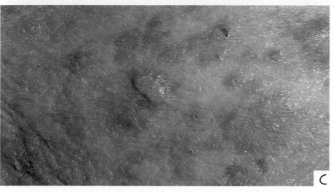

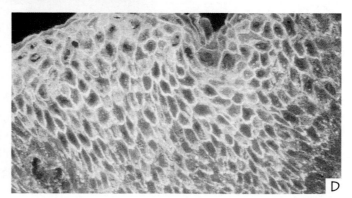

In virtually 100 percent of patients, fluorescein-labeled IgG can be demonstrated to bind to the epidermal intercellular space in the patient's normal-appearing and perilesional skin (see Fig. 4.12D). This finding is referred to as positive direct immunofluorescence (DIF). Deposits of C3, IgA, or IgM are also identified in almost half of these patients. For study of indirect immunofluorescence (IIF), unfixed frozen sections of various epithelia, such as monkey esophagus or normal human skin, are used. The patient's serum is applied to the specimen, followed by fluorescein-labeled antihuman IgG at various dilutions. When the study is positive, fluorescence is seen in the intercellular spaces of the test specimen. The antibody titer refers to the highest dilution at which fluorescence is still noted. Although DIF is very sensitive, even early in the course of disease, IIF is less useful, particularly before lesions become widespread.

Early PV restricted to the mouth must be differentiated histologically from other disorders that involve the oral mucosa, such as erosive lichen planus and aphthosis. Once cutaneous lesions appear, the typical clinical pattern, histology, and immunofluorescence will distinguish PV from other immunobullous disorders.

Before the introduction of corticosteroids, patients often succumbed to sepsis. Management of fluid and electrolyte losses and supportive skin care may require admission to a burn unit. High-dose prednisone (2–5 mg/kg/day) may be lifesaving. After the eruption comes under control, steroids can usually be tapered over nine to 12 months to acceptable maintenance levels. Some patients may require steroid-sparing immunosuppressive agents such as methotrexate, cyclophosphamide, or azathioprine, depending on their response to the steroid taper.

Pemphigus foliaceus (PF) is a more superficial and

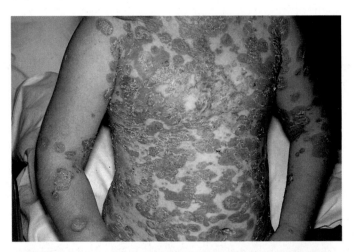

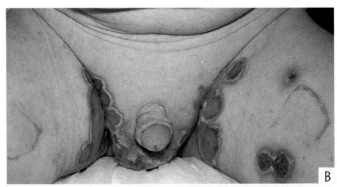

FIGURE 4.13 Pemphigus foliaceus. A ten-year-old girl with generalized, slightly itchy, scaly, and crusted patches was referred for evaluation of possible pemphigus foliaceus. Although a skin biopsy was suggestive of pemphigus, a skin culture grew *Staphyloccus aureus,* and the rash resolved after seven days of oral dicloxacillin. Widespread bullous impetigo, staphyloccal scalded skin syndrome, drug reactions, and other disorders that produce erythroderma should be considered in the differential diagnosis of pemphigus foliaceus.

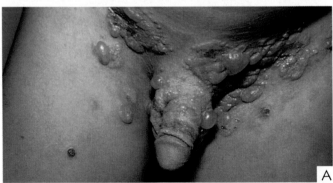

FIGURE 4.14 Chronic bullous dermatosis of childhood. Two three-year-old boys presented with chronic, recurrent blisters in the diaper area. (**A**) Fresh, tense bullae have spread along the inguinal creases onto the thighs and penis. (**B**) Ruptured bullae have left annular and scalloped erosions.

less aggressive immunobullous disorder. Although it occurs most commonly in middle age, this variant is more common than pemphigus vulgaris in children. Although PF tends to be sporadic and most cases have been reported in North America and Europe, an endemic variant known as fogo selvagem occurs primarily in children and adolescents in Brazil. Clinically and histologically, PF is indistinguishable from Brazilian pemphigus. Some medications, such as penecillamine, have also been reported to trigger a PF-like eruption.

Like PV, PF begins with crops of vesicles, flaccid bullae, and erosions on an erythematous base in a seborrheic distribution. However, because the blisters arise high in the epidermis, they quickly crust over. The Nikolsky sign is usually positive, but mucous membranes are invariably spared. When lesions become generalized, vesicles may be obscured by crust and scale, giving the patient the appearance of an exfoliative erythroderma (Fig. 4.13). Even with widespread rash, patients tend to appear clinically well, and the course is often self-limited.

Histopathology demonstrates acantholysis and bullae formation, much as in PV. However, the action occurs in the upper half of the epidermis, sometimes restricted to the area immediately beneath the stratum corneum. Direct immunofluorescence shows IgG staining of the intercellular space in the upper half of the epidermis, and indirect immunofluorescence is also usually positive. Chronic lesions typically show acanthosis, eosinophilic spongiosis, and eosinophilic dermal inflammation.

Patients with mild disease may respond to moderate- or high-potency topical steroids. In many cases, systemic corticosteroids may be required for a while, and some investigators have reported success with antimalarials (hydroxychloroquine and chloroquine) and sulfonamides (sulfapyradine and avlusulfone).

Subepidermal Disorders

Chronic bullous dermatosis of childhood (CBDC) is probably the most common subepidermal immunobullous disease in children. It is also known as linear IgA dermatosis, which describes the characteristic immunofluorescent finding in perilesional skin.

Although tense, 1-cm to 2-cm bullae typically appear in preschoolers on the lower trunk, buttocks, legs, and top of the feet, children of any age can be affected (Fig. 4.14). Widespread lesions may involve any site on the body surface, including the face, scalp, upper trunk, hands, and arms (Fig. 4.15). Lesions erupt on red as well as normal-appearing skin and often form rings of sausage-shaped bullae around a central crust or healing blister. Linear vesicles on an inflamed base may suggest a "string of pearls." Mucous membranes are not usually involved, the Nikolsky sign is not present, and burning and pruritus are variable. Some children are completely asymptomatic.

Histopathology is indistinguishable from bullous pemphigoid, which demonstrates a subepidermal blister with a dermal infiltrate of neutrophils and eosinophils. Occasionally, eosinophils form microabscesses at the tips

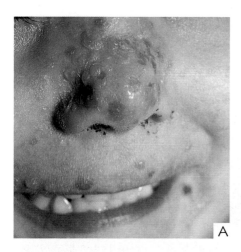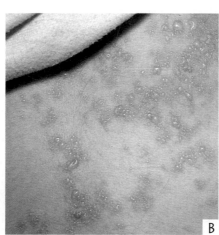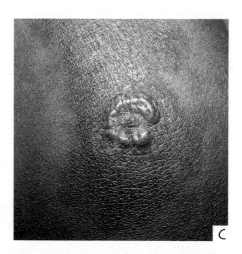

FIGURE 4.15 **(A,B)** Widespread vesicles erupted over several days in a five-year-old girl with chronic bullous dermatosis of childhood. Blisters were densest on the face and trunk. **(C)** Characteristic annular blisters spread over the trunk and extremities of this four-year-old boy. The bullous dermatosis in both children responded quickly to 25 mg/day of Dapsone.

of the dermal papillae, reminiscent of dermatitis herpetiformis. However, direct immunofluorescence showing linear deposits of IgA at the dermal–epidermal junction is diagnostic (Fig. 4.16). Investigators have also shown that the site of deposition is within the lamina lucida, with accentuation near the basal cell membrane around hemidesmosomes. Circulating IgA antibodies are present in 50 percent to 75 percent of patients.

Although CBDC is often self-limited, with spontaneous resolution over three to five years, occasional cases persist after adolescence. Many children are exquisitely sensitive to small doses of Dapsone (0.5–1.0 mg/kg/day). Blisters often respond within one to three days of initiating therapy and can be tapered to low maintenance doses (12.5–25 mg/day or less). Resistant cases may require systemic corticosteroids, at least until the eruption comes under control. All patients on Dapsone must be monitored for clinical and laboratory signs of hemolysis, methemoglobinemia, and neurologic complications.

CBDC must be distinguished from a less common immunobullous dermatosis, *juvenile bullous pemphigoid (BP)*, in which the bullae are often large (>2 cm) and mucous membranes are frequently involved (Fig. 4.17). Skin biopsies in BP also demonstrate subepidermal bullae with an eosinophilic dermal infiltrate. However, linear deposition of IgG and C3 at the dermal–epidermal junction in the lamina lucida is diagnostic for BP. An unusual cicatricial variant of BP involves primarily the mucous membranes and occurs only rarely in childhood. *Dermatitis herpetiformis (DH)* is suggested by symmetric, extremely pruritic, clustered 3-mm to 4-mm vesicles on extensor surfaces of the extremities, lower trunk, and buttocks (Fig. 4.18). In DH the lesions arise on both red and normal-appearing skin and may occasionally exceed 1 cm. Biopsy of perilesional skin reveals characteristic granular IgA deposits in the basement membrane zone and prominent neutrophilic microabscesses at the dermal papillary tips. DH is also defined by the high incidence of HLA B8 antigens, a gluten-sensitive enteropathy, and rapid response to Dapsone.

The target lesions of erythema multiforme (EM), particularly when blistering is present, may be confused with CBDC. However, the acute clinical course, histopathology, and negative immunofluorescence will readily distinguish EM. Early in its course CBDC is often misdiagnosed as bullous impetigo. Moreover, bullae of CBDC that are secondarily infected will respond to antibiotic therapy. However, the persistence of blistering despite antibiotic therapy, the widespread distribution of the eruption, and negative Gram stains and cultures should suggest a noninfectious etiology.

MECHANOBULLOUS DISORDERS

Friction blisters occur frequently on the soles, palms, and palmar surfaces of the fingers after vigorous exercise or other repetitive activities that cause shearing of thick areas of epidermis that are firmly attached to

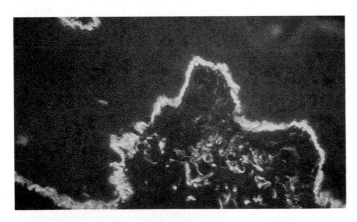

FIGURE 4.16 Direct immunofluorescence in bullous dermatosis of childhood shows diagnostic linear IgA deposition along the dermal–epidermal junction.

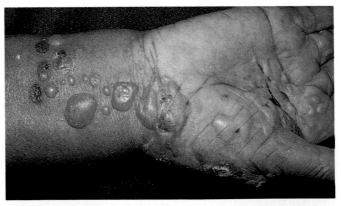

FIGURE 4.17 Tense, large blisters developed insidiously on the extremities and trunk of a patient with bullous pemphigoid.

underlying tissue. In patients with chronic localized or generalized edema, particularly in the setting of malnutrition, minor trauma may lead to blister formation (Fig. 4.19). Histologically, these lesions can be identified as noninflammatory intraepidermal blisters which are usually located just beneath the granular layer. Although blisters heal quickly in healthy individuals, impetiginization and cellulitis are frequent complications in compromised hosts.

Epidermolysis bullosa is a heterogeneous group of mechanobullous disorders differentiated by clinical findings, depth of blister formation, biochemical markers, and inheritance patterns (see Chapter 2). In most of these conditions, vesiculobullous lesions appear at birth or in early infancy. Several variants, however, do not present until adolescence or adult life.

In *recurrent epidermolysis bullosa of the hands and feet* or *Weber–Cockayne syndrome,* an autosomal dominant epidermolytic variant, blisters may first appear on the soles during rigorous physical activity, such as track and field sports or military boot camp. Vesicles and bullae are usually restricted to the distal extremities and particularly to the palms and soles. Healing occurs without scar formation, and the nails and mucous membranes are not affected. Histopathology demonstrates a suprabasilar split in the epidermis, and electron microscopy shows cytolysis within the basal cell layer. Although these findings are also typical of friction blisters in normal individuals, clumping of tonofilaments in basal cell keratinocytes is specific for Weber–Cockayne.

Recurrent blistering of the palms and soles, particularly during warm weather when blistering is more common, suggests the disorder. A positive family history will clinch the diagnosis. Blistering can be reduced by using extra cushioning in shoes and avoiding unnecessary trauma to the hands and feet, particularly during warm weather. Cool tapwater compresses may be helpful acutely, and topical antibiotics will reduce the risk of secondary infection. The use of topical antiperspirants 10–20 percent aluminum hydroxide, 10 percent formaldehyde, or 10 percent glutaraldehyde may decrease the blistering as well as the associated hyperhidrosis of the palms and soles. Some patients have also benefitted from applications of tincture of benzoin or Mastisol.

Epidermolysis bullosa acquisita (EBA), an acquired mechanobullous dermatosis, may clinically resemble hereditary EB. However, onset of skin fragility and blister formation is widespread and does not usually occur until adolescence. EBA is actually an immunobullous dermatosis and is frequently associated with an underlying systemic disorder, such as inflammatory bowel disease. Although skin biopsies show a subepidermal blister indistinguishable from CBDC and BP, immunoelectron microscopy reveals characteristic deposition of IgG and complement in the upper dermis, beneath or contiguous with the lamina densa. Patients usually respond to systemic corticosteroids. However, in patients with bowel disease, cutaneous lesions may improve in conjunction with aggressive management of gastrointestinal symptoms.

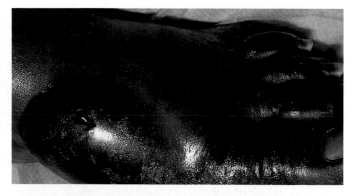

FIGURE 4.18 Excoriated, eroded vesicles are all that remain of the primary lesions of dermatitis herpetiformis in this teenager. Similar lesions were symmetrically distributed on the anterior thighs, knees, buttocks, back, and abdomen. Intact vesicles are only occasionally seen in DH because of the intense pruritus and resultant scratching.

FIGURE 4.19 Friction blisters. Large, hemorrhagic blisters developed in areas of minor trauma on the trunk and extremities of a cachectic, chronically ill child during an episode of acute renal failure. Blistering healed as renal function returned to normal and cutaneous edema resolved. A skin biopsy demonstrated intraepidermal blisters without inflammation.

DERMATITIS

In acute *dermatitides* inflammation and associated edema may be so intense that vesiculation occurs. Blisters erupt frequently in acute contact irritant and allergic dermatitis, as well as atopic dermatitis, seborrhea, and insect bite reactions (Fig. 4.20). When blistering develops in this setting, secondary infection with *Staphylococcus* or herpes simplex virus should also be considered.

A Tzanck smear and Gram stain will exclude bacterial and viral infection. Skin biopsies demonstrate variable acanthosis or thickening of the epidermis, exocytosis or an influx of lymphocytes into the epidermis, and spon-

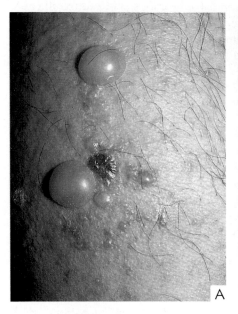
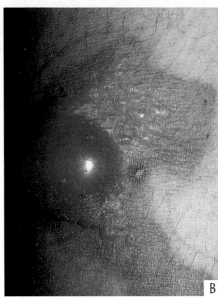
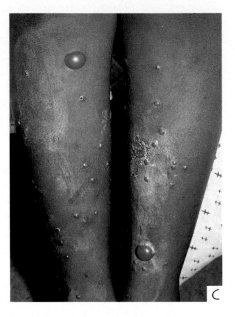

FIGURE 4.20 Dermatitic blisters. **(A)** Acute poison ivy dermatitis resulted in blisters on the arm of a nine-year-old boy. Note the surrounding erythema, edema, and papules typical of an allergic contact dermatitis. **(B)** Vesicles and a large bulla erupted on an extremely well-demarcated red base on the arm of a teenager who admitted to applying acid to create the lesions. **(C)** This child's lower legs are studded with many thick-walled vesicles and bullae which formed in response to flea bites.

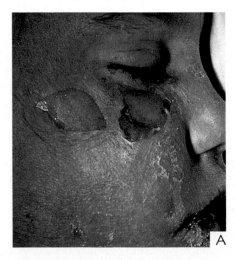
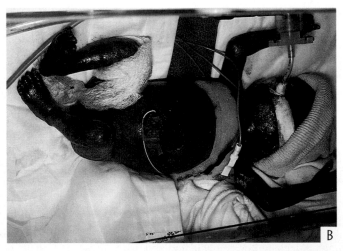

FIGURE 4.21 Toxic epidermal necrolysis. **(A)** Seven days into a course of oral trimethoprin/sulfamethorisole (Bactrim) for otitis media, this eight-year-old girl developed high fever and generalized erythema and edema, followed by sloughing of large sheets of skin. Mucous membranes were severely involved. Note the Nikolsky sign on her upper cheek induced by accidental minor trauma. **(B)** At ten days of age this tiny premature infant developed TEN while on multiple antibiotics. Denuded areas of skin occurred over bony prominences and around tape and monitor sites.

giosis or intercellular edema. It is the intense edema that eventually breaks apart desmosomal attachments and results in spongiotic blister formation. Immunofluorescent studies should be negative.

Blistering from dermatitic reactions can usually be distinguished clinically from thermal burns, cold injury, and ischemic insults to the skin that result in subepidermal blisters.

TOXIC EPIDERMAL NECROLYSIS

Although originally reported in adults, *toxic epidermal necrolysis (TEN)* has been recently described in children, particularly in association with drug hypersensitivity reactions. One or two days of flu-like symptoms are followed abruptly by the development of generalized painful erythema, blistering, and sloughing of large areas of skin (Fig. 4.21A). A Nikolsky sign is present, and skin biopsies demonstrate full-thickness epidermal

necrosis (Fig. 4.21B). Mucous membrane involvement is usually severe, and lesions may extend to the gastrointestinal tract and tracheobronchial tree. Intensive supportive measures are required to avoid massive fluid and electrolyte disturbances and bacterial superinfection. Transfer to a regional burn unit should be considered. Unfortunately, re-epithelialization may not be complete for over a month, and mortality may exceed 40 percent.

Allopurinol, anticonvulsants, and sulfonamides have often been associated with the development of TEN. However, bacterial and viral infections, connective tissue disorders, and malignancies have also been implicated as triggering factors.

TEN must be distinguished from staphylocccal scalded skin syndrome (SSSS), in which a circulating staphylococcal exotoxin produces a superficial epidermal injury. SSSS is usually self-limited, and treatment is directed against the causative organism. Frozen sections of skin biopsies or sheets of sloughed skin can be examined quickly to determine the level of epidermal injury.

ALGORITHM FOR EVALUATION OF VESICULOPUSTULAR DERMATOSES

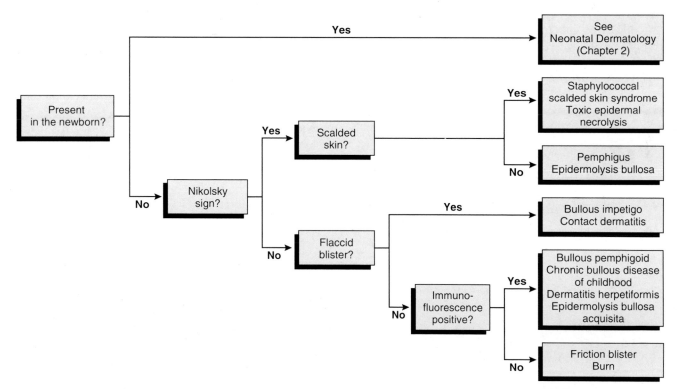

BIBLIOGRAPHY

Herpes simplex infection

Corey L, Spear PG. Infections with herpes simplex viruses. *N Engl J Med* 314:686–691, 1986.

Douglas JM, Critchlow C, Benedetti J, et al. A double-blind study of oral acyclovir for suppression of recurrences of genital herpes simplex virus infecton. *N Engl J Med* 310:1551–1556, 1984.

Symposium on antiviral drugs and vaccines for herpes simplex and herpes zoster. *J Am Acad Dermatol* 18: 161–238, 1988.

Varicella-zoster infection

Baba K, Yabuuchi H, Takahashi M, Ogra P. Immunologic and epidemiologic aspects of varicella infection acquired during infancy and early childhood. *J Pediatr* 100:881–885, 1982.

Dunkle LM, Arvin AM, Whitley RJ, et al. A controlled trial of acyclovir for chickenpox in normal children. *N Engl J Med* 325:1539–1544, 1991.

Preblud SR, Orenstein WA, Bart KJ. Varicella: clinical manifestations, epidemiology and health impact in children. *Pediatr Infect Dis* 3:505, 1984.

Weibel RE, Neff BJ, Kuter BJ, et al. Live attenuated varicella virus vaccine: efficacy trial in healthy children. *N Engl J Med* 310:1409–1415, 1984.

Hand, foot, and mouth syndrome

Cherry JD. Viral exanthems. *Current Probl Pediatr* 13: 1, 1983.

Esterly NB. Viral exanthems: diagnosis and management. *Semin Dermatol* 3:140, 1984.

Bacterial infections (see Chapter 2)

Pemphigus

Anhalt GJ, Labib RS, Vorhees JJ, Beals TF, Diaz LA. Induction of pemphigus in neonatal mice by passive transfer of IgG from patients with the disease. *N Engl J Med* 306:1189–1196, 1982.

Smitt JH. Pemphigus vulgaris in childhood: clinical features, treatment and prognosis. *Pediatr Dermatol* 2:185, 1985.

Bullous pemphigoid and chronic bullous dermatosis of childhood

Korman N. Bullous pemphigoid. *J Am Acad Dermatol* 16:907–924, 1987.

Sweren RJ, Burnett JW. Benign chronic bullous dermatosis of childhood: a review. *Cutis* 29:350–357, 1982.

Wojnarowska F, Marsden RA, Bhogal B, Black MM. Chronic bullous dermatosis of childhood, childhood cicatricial pemphigoid and linear IgA disease of adults. *J Am Acad Dermatol* 19:792–805, 1988.

Mechanobullous disorders

Borok M, Heng MCY, Ahmed AR. Epidermolysis bullosa acquisita in an 8-year-old girl. *Pediatr Dermatol* 3:315–322, 1986.

Toxic epidermal necrolysis

Amon RB, Dimond RL. Toxic epidermal necrolysis: rapid differentiation between staphylococcal and drug-induced disease. *Arch Dermatol* 111:1433–1437, 1975.

Hawk RJ, Storer JS, Danon RS. Toxic epidermal necrolysis in a 6-week-old infant. *Pediatr Dermatol* 2:197–200, 1985.

chapter five

LUMPS AND BUMPS

Lumps and bumps in the skin often raise fears of skin cancer. Fortunately, primary skin cancer is extremely rare in childhood, and most infiltrated plaques and tumors are benign (Fig. 5.1). Hemangiomas, congenital nevi, and tumors of the newborn are reviewed in Chapter 2, "Neonatal Dermatology." This chapter focuses on disorders of childhood and adolescence.

Several clinical clues, including the depth and color of lesions, will aid in developing a differential diagnosis. Superficial growths are readily moved back and forth over the underlying dermis, whereas the overlying epidermis and superficial dermis may slide over deep-seated tumors. Some dermal and subcutaneous lesions characteristically produce tethering of the overlying skin. Epidermal tumors include warts, molluscum, and seborrheic keratoses. Milia, neurofibromas, granuloma annulare, mastocytomas, scars, keloids, xanthomas, xanthogranulomas, nevocellular nevi, and adnexal tumors involve the superficial and mid-dermis. Leukemia, lymphoma, melanoma, lipomas, and metastatic solid tumors involve the dermis and/or fat and may extend deep into subcutaneous structures.

Color may suggest the specific cell type in various cutaneous lumps and bumps. For example, yellow tumors might include large quantities of fat in a lipoma or lipid-laden histiocytes in xanthomas or xanthogranulomas. Nevocellular nevi, epidermal nevi, mastocytomas, and seborrheic keratosis contain variable amounts of the brown pigment melanin in nevus cells or keratinocytes. Vascular tumors are usually red or blue, and primary or metastatic nodules may appear in various shades of red, purple, and blue, depending on their depth and degree of vascularity.

The diagnosis of certain genodermatoses associated with cutaneous and/or internal malignancies enables the clinician to develop strategies for close monitoring. Early recognition of malignancy in this setting may be lifesaving (Fig. 5.2).

Figure 5.1 Histologic Diagnosis of 775 Superficial Lumps Excised in Children

Type	Number
Epidermal inclusion cysts	459 (59%)
Congenital malformations (pilomatrixoma, lymphangioma, brachial cleft cyst)	117 (15%)
Benign neoplasms (neural tumors, lipoma, adnexal tumors)	56 (7%)
Benign lesions of undetermined origin (xanthomas, xanthogranulomas, fibromatosis, fibromas)	50 (6%)
Self-limiting processes (granuloma annulare, urticaria pigmentosa, insect bite reaction)	47 (6%)
Malignant tumors	11 (1.4%)
Miscellaneous	35 (4%)

Modified from Knight and Reiner, 1983.

Figure 5.2 Cancer-associated Genodermatoses

Disease	Associated Cancer	Clinical Manifestations	Mode of Inheritance
Basal cell nevus syndrome	Many basal cell carcinomas (mean age of onset 15 years) on sun-exposed and non-sun-exposed areas; medulloblastoma, astrocytoma	Many basal cell nevi, palmar and plantar pits, jaw cysts, calcification of the falx cerebri, ovarian fibromas, fused ribs	Autosomal dominant
Hidrotic ectodermal dysplasia	Squamous cell cancer of palms, soles, and nailbed	Normal sweating, total alopecia, severe nail dystrophy, palmar and plantar hyperkeratosis	Autosomal dominant
Bazex syndrome	Basal cell carcinomas of the face (second to third decade)	Follicular atrophoderma; localized anhidrosis and/or generalized hypohidrosis	Autosomal dominant
Dysplastic nevus syndrome; familial atypical multiple-mole syndrome	Cutaneous and intraocular melanoma, lymphoreticular malignancy, and sarcomas	Multiple large reddish-brown moles with irregular borders and nonuniform colors, usually on trunk and arms; familial occurrence of melanoma	Autosomal dominant
Multiple hamartoma syndrome (Cowden's disease)	Carcinoma of the breast, colon, and thyroid	Coexistence of multiple ectodermal, mesodermal, and endodermal nevoid neoplasms, punctate keratoderma of the palms, multiple angiomas and lipomas	Autosomal dominant
Neurofibromatosis (von Recklinghausen's disease)	Malignant degeneration of the neurofibromas in 3–15% of cases; optic and acoustic neuromas, meningiomas, gliomas, pheochromocytoma, nonlymphocytic leukemia	Cafe-au-lait spots, multiple skeletal anomalies, fibromatous skin tumors	Autosomal dominant
Multiple mucosal neuroma syndrome	Pheochromocytoma, medullary thyroid carcinoma	Pedunculated nodules on eyelid margins, lip; tongue with true neuromas	Autosomal dominant
Intestinal polyposis II (Peutz–Jeghers syndrome)	Adenocarcinoma of the colon, duodenum; granulosa cell ovarian tumors	Pigmented macules on oral mucosa and lips, conjunctivae, and digits; intestinal polyps	Autosomal dominant
Intestinal polyposis III (Gardner's syndrome)	Malignant degeneration of colon, adenomatous polyps, sarcomas, thyroid cancer	Polyps of the colon and small intestine, globoid osteotoma of mandible with overlying fibromata, epidermoid cysts, desmoids	Autosomal dominant

continued on next page

Figure 5.2 *continued*

Disease	Associated Cancer	Clinical Manifestations	Mode of Inheritance
Tuberous sclerosis	Rhabdomyoma of myocardium, gliomas, mixed tumor of kidney	Triad of angiofibroma, epilepsy, and mental retardation; ash-leaf macules; shagreen patches; subungual fibromas; intracranial calcification in 50%	Autosomal dominant
Epidermolysis bullosa dystrophica	Squamous cell carcinoma in chronic lesions	Lifelong history of bullae; phenotype not as severe as autosomal-recessive forms	Autosomal dominant
Albinism	Increased incidence of cutaneous malignancies	Lack of skin pigment, incomplete hypopigmentation of ocular fundi, horizontal congenital mystagmus, myopia	Autosomal recessive
Bloom's syndrome	High incidence of leukemia and lymphoma; squamous cell cancers of esophagus and adenocarcinoma of the colon; often by age 20	Small stature; cutaneous photosensitivity presenting as telangiectatic facial (malar) erythema	Autosomal recessive
Chediak–Higashi syndrome	Malignant lymphoma	Decreased pigmentation of hair and eyes; photophobia; nystagmus; abnormal susceptability to infection	Autosomal recessive
Epidermolysis bullosa dystrophica	Basal and squamous cell carcinoma developing in skin and cancer of mucous membranes (esp. esophagus)	Bullae develop at sites of trauma; present at birth or early infancy; may involve mucous membranes, esophagus, conjunctivae, cornea	Autosomal recessive
Rothmund–Thomson syndrome (poikiloderma congenitale	Cutaneous malignancies	Poikiloderma, short stature, cataracts, photosensitivity, nail defects, alopecia, bony defects	Autosomal recessive
Xeroderma pigmentosum	Basal and squamous cell carcinomas of skin, malignant melanoma	Marked photosensitivity, early freckling, telangiectasia, keratoses, papillomas, photophobia, keratitis, corneal opacities	Autosomal recessive
Wiskott–Aldrich syndrome	Lymphoreticular malignancies, malignant lymphoma, myelogenous leukemia, astrocytoma	Eczema, thrombocytopenia, bleeding problems (i.e., melena, purpura, epistaxis), increased susceptibility to skin infections, otitis, pneumonia, meningitis	X-linked recessive
Dyskeratosis congenita	Squamous cell carcinoma, oral cavity, esophagus, nasopharynx, skin, anus	Reticulated hypo- and hyperpigmentation of the skin, nail dystrophy, leukoplakia of oral mucosa, thrombocytopenia, anemia, testicular atrophy	X-linked recessive

From Edwards et al., 1988.

SUPERFICIAL LUMPS AND BUMPS

Warts

Warts are benign epidermal tumors produced by human papillomavirus (HPV) infection of the skin and mucous membranes. In children they most commonly occur on the fingers, hands, and feet (Figs. 5.3–5.5). The incubation period for warts varies from one to three months and possibly up to several years, and most lesions disappear within three to five years. Local trauma promotes inoculation of the virus. Therefore, periungual warts are common in children who bite their nails or pick at hangnails.

Investigators have identified more than 50 HPV types capable of causing warts, and many of these organisms produce characteristic lesions in specific locations. For instance, the discrete, round, skin-colored papillomatous papules typical of *verruca vulgaris* (common warts) are produced by HPV types 2 and 4. The subtle, minimally hyperpigmented flat warts (verruca plana) caused by

HPV 3 are frequently spread by deliberate or accidental scratching, shaving, or picking, and may become widespread on the face, arms, and legs (Fig. 5.6).

Plantar warts are most commonly caused by HPV 1. Although not proven, the transmission of the virus is probably by contact with contaminated, desquamated skin in showers, pool decks, and bathrooms. Although their surface appearance is often subtle, their large size may be hidden by a collarette of apparently normal skin, and they often cause pain when the patient walks. Although plantar warts can be confused with corns, calluses, or scars, they can be distinguished by their disruption of the normal dermatoglyphics. Characteristic black dots in the warts are thrombosed capillaries.

Warts can also be found on the trunk, oral mucosa, and conjunctivae. *Condyloma acuminatum* and flat warts in the anogenital area are usually caused by HPV types 6 and 11 (Fig. 5.7). Although sexual abuse should

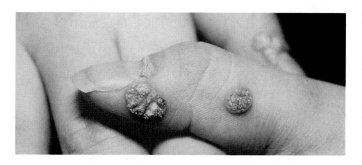

FIGURE 5.3 Verruca vulgaris. Dry, rough, and crusty, these common warts usually involve the hands. The periungual distribution in this girl was due, in part, to her habit of picking at her cuticles.

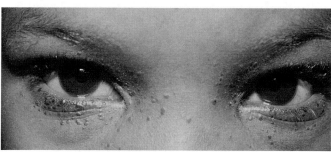

FIGURE 5.4 Flat warts or verruca plana. These tiny, light-brown warts are spread by scratching.

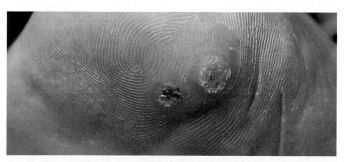

FIGURE 5.5 Plantar warts. Two painful lesions are seen over the ball of the foot. Note how they interrupt the normal skin lines.

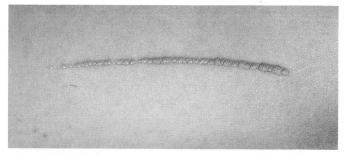

FIGURE 5.6 Flat warts spread in a line on the flank of a five-year-old girl after scratching.

FIGURE 5.7 Anogenital warts developed at eight months of age in this toddler whose mother had extensive vaginal and cervical HPV infection. These lesions resolved after several treatments with podophyllin.

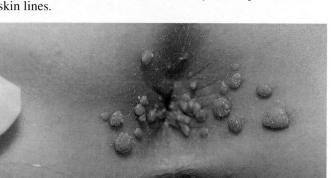

be considered in any child with anogenital warts, most are transmitted in a nonvenereal manner.

Although warts are self-limited in most children (Fig. 5.8A and B), persistent, widespread lesions should suggest the possibility of congenital or acquired immunodeficiency (Fig. 5.9A and B). In fact, warts may present a serious management problem in oncology and transplant patients who are chronically immunosuppressed.

Topical irritants, including salicylic acid and lactic acid, in occlusive vehicles such as collodion or under tape occlusion, are safe, effective, and relatively painless preparations for treating warts that are not in sensitive areas, such as the eyelids and perineum. Recalcitrant lesions may respond to destructive measures, including liquid nitrogen, electrocautery, and carbon dioxide laser surgery. However, patients and parents should be cautioned about the risk of recurrence and scarring (Fig. 5.10). Immunotherapy with topical contact sensitizers, such as dinitrochlorobenzene, diphencyclopropenone, and *Rhus* extract, is still considered experimental, and

parents should be counseled accordingly, with emphasis on the fact that most warts will resolve without treatment in three to five years.

Large warts in the diaper area may cause itching, burning, bleeding, and secondary bacterial infection. Although not yet approved for use in children, topical application of podophyllin and podophylotoxin is safe and effective in severe, symptomatic cases. Scissor excision with electrocautery and carbon dioxide laser ablation may be effective in recalcitrant cases.

Several innocent epidermal growths are often confused with warts. *Dermatosis papulosa nigra (DPN)* is a variant of seborrheic keratosis which appears in about a third of black individuals (Fig. 5.11). Although seborrheic keratoses usually do not erupt until middle age, small, brown, warty DPN typically begin to develop during adolescence in a symmetric malar distribution on the face. The neck and upper trunk may also be involved. Although DPN are of no medical consequence, irritated or unsightly lesions can be snipped, frozen, or

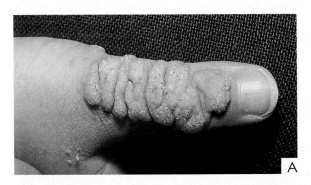
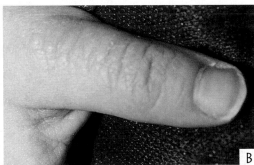

FIGURE 5.8
(A) Multiple common warts grew to confluence on the thumb of a four-year-old boy.
(B) Shortly before surgery was scheduled, the lesions began to regress without treatment.

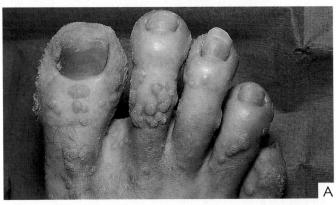
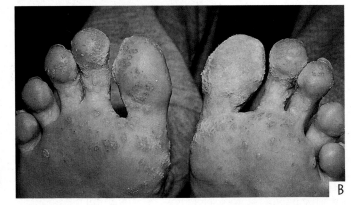

FIGURE 5.9 (A,B) Extensive, recalcitrant warts spread over the feet of a teenager with severe combined immunodeficiency.

cauterized. Patients should be warned about the risk of postinflamatory pigmentary changes after treatment. Pearly penile papules, often diagnosed as warts, are also innocent. These uniform, 1-mm to 3-mm papules ring the corona at the base of the glans penis. They are asymptomatic and probably represent a normal variant. No treatment is required.

Molluscum Contagiosum

Molluscum contagiosum, caused by a large poxvirus, is characterized by sharply circumscribed single or multiple superficial, pearly, dome-shaped papules (Fig. 5.12A–D). They usually start as grouped pinpoint papules and increase in size to 3 to 5 mm. Many lesions have umbilicated centers which are best seen with a hand

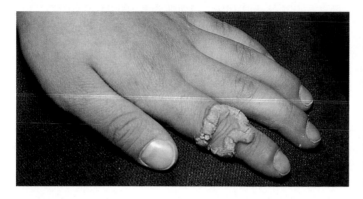

FIGURE 5.10 A 10-year-old boy developed a recurrent ring wart around a scar after treatment of a large common wart on the index finger.

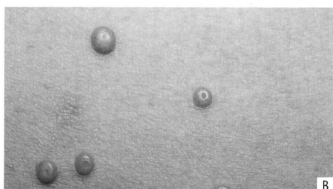

FIGURE 5.11 Small brown papules typical of dermatosis papulosa nigra slowly increase in number and size on the face of this black adolescent. Her parents had similar lesions which began to appear in late childhood.

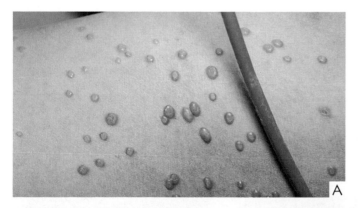

A

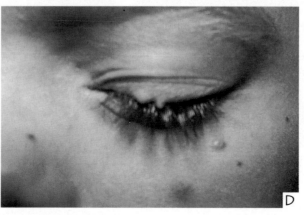

FIGURE 5.12 Molluscum contagiosum. **(A)** Multiple pearly papules dot the arm of this eight-year-old girl with widespread molluscum. **(B)** A close-up view demonstrates the central umbilication present on mature molluscum lesions. **(C)** Note the linear spread of papules on the neck of this child, which followed scratching. **(D)** Molluscum lesions on the eyelid margin and conjunctive are particularly irritating and difficult to treat.

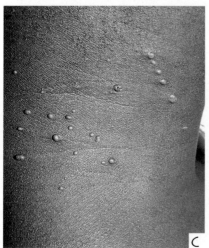

C

D

lens. Molluscum is endemic in young children, in whom involvement of the trunk, axillae, face, and diaper area is common. Lesions are spread by scratching and often appear in a linear arrangement. In teenagers and adults, molluscum frequently occurs as a sexually transmitted disease affecting the genital area.

A white, cheesy core can be expressed from the center of the papule for microscopic examination, which reveals the typical molluscum bodies. Destruction of lesions by curetting their cores or by application of a blistering agent (cantharidin) and plastic tape which is peeled off after one to three days is curative of individual lesions. However, recurrences and the development of new papules are common, although most cases undergo spontaneous remission. Consequently, treatment should be directed against symptomatic lesions only. Bacterial superinfection can be treated with appropriate topical or oral antibiotics. The development of scaly, red rings around old papules may herald the onset of a delayed hypersensitivity reaction and resolution of the infection. As in children with warts, patients with widespread, recalcitrant molluscum should be screened for congenital and acquired immunodeficiency disease.

Basal Cell Carcinoma

Basal cell carcinoma (BCC) presents as a nonhealing, pearly, reddish-gray to brown papule or plaque with a central dell or crust and peripheral telangiectasias (Fig. 5.13). Although BCC occurs primarily in the middle aged and the elderly, the tumor is being recognized with increasing frequency in adolescents and young adults,

particularly fair-skinned individuals in sunny climates. The risk of developing BCC has been clearly linked to ultraviolet light exposure, and most lesions appear on sun-exposed sites such as the face, ears, neck, and upper trunk. BCC is an indolent, superficial malignancy which responds readily to electrodessication and curettage or simple excision. However, neglected lesions may become locally destructive and invade deep soft tissues, bone, and dura. Protection from excessive sun exposure, aggressive use of sunscreens, and careful skin surveillance should reduce the risk from BCC.

When BCC is diagnosed in sun-protected areas or in childen, the practitioner should search for predisposing factors such as radiation or arsenic exposure, a preexisting nevus sebaceus or scar, or a hereditary condition such as basal cell nevus syndrome (Fig. 5.14). In this autosomal dominant disorder, many basal cell nevi appear on the trunk, scalp, face, and extremities during the first decade. Over time, many of these lesions enlarge and develop into progressive BCCs. Other stigmata include palmar and plantar pits, jaw cysts, calcification of the falx cerebri, ovarian fibromas, and fused ribs. Early diagnosis and removal of enlarging BCCs will reduce the need for more extensive and disfiguring surgery.

In children BCC may be confused with warts, molluscum contagiosum, seborrheic keratoses, pigmented nevi, and other epidermal and superficial dermal growths. BCC should be considered in any slowly progressive, crusted or ulcerated plaque, particularly when risk factors are present.

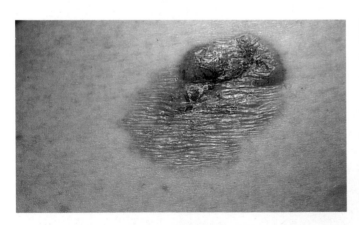

FIGURE 5.13 A slowly enlarging, reddish-tan plaque on the upper chest of an 18-year-old boy developed a nodular component with overlying telangiectasias. A skin biopsy demonstrated basaloid budding typical of basal cell carcinoma. The child had red hair, blue eyes, light complection, and a history of frequent sunburns since early childhood.

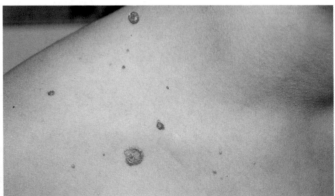

FIGURE 5.14 Basal cell nevus syndrome. Many 1-mm to 3-mm papules composed of proliferating basaloid cells and two larger nodules which demonstrated changes typical of basal cell carcinoma are seen on the shoulder and neck of a 15-year-old girl with basal cell nevus syndrome. In addition to the widespread cutaneous tumors, she had subtle palmar and plantar pits and a history of jaw cysts. Her father, uncle, and grandmother had similar cutaneous lesions.

DERMAL LUMPS AND BUMPS

Granuloma Annulare

When fully evolved, *granuloma annulare* is an annular eruption histologically characterized by dermal infiltration of lymphocytes and histiocytes around altered collagen (Fig. 5.15A–E). The lesion begins as a papule or nodule which gradually expands peripherally to form a ring 1 to 4 cm in diameter. Multiple rings may overlap to form large annular plaques. In some cases the rings are broken up into segments. The overlying epidermis is usually intact and is the same color as adjacent skin, but may sometimes be slightly red or hyperpigmented. Most lesions are asymptomatic, although a few are reported to be mildly pruritic. Granuloma annulare most commonly erupts on the extensor surfaces of the lower legs, feet, fingers, and hands, but other areas can be involved.

Over months to years, old plaques and papules regress while new lesions appear. Granuloma annulare eventually resolves without treatment. The origin is unclear, but some lesions may be associated with insect bite reactions or other antecedent trauma. In adults, granuloma annulare, especially multiple eruptive lesions, has appeared in association with diabetes mellitus (see Fig. 5.15E). This is not the case in children.

Granuloma annulare is most commonly confused with tinea corporis or ringworm. However, the thickened indurated character of the ring and the lack of epidermal changes such as scale, vesicles, or pustules enable clinical distinction. A deep dermal or subcutaneous variant of granuloma annulare can be mistaken for the rheumatoid nodules characteristic of rheumatic fever and other connective tissue disorders. These lesions are referred to as subcutaneous granuloma annulare and

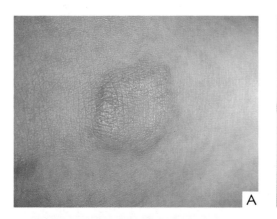
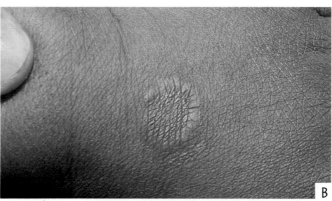
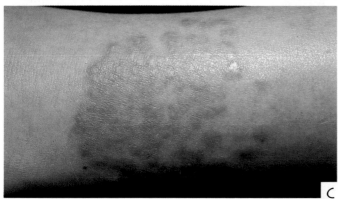
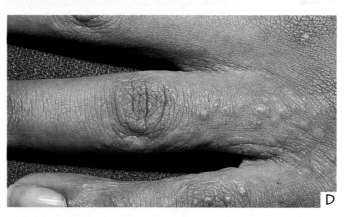

FIGURE 5.15 Granuloma annulare. Characteristic doughnut-shaped dermal plaques are seen on the foot of a white boy (**A**) and the hand of a black girl (**B**). In both children the epidermal markings are intact. (**C**) A large confluent plaque is developing from merging papules on the arm of a nine-year-old boy. (**D**) Multiple asymptomatic 2-mm to 4-mm papules erupted on the hand of a teenager. (**E**) Disseminated granuloma annulare developed in an adult with insulin-dependent diabetes mellitus.

pseudo-rheumatoid nodules. However, practitioners should avoid the latter term because the subcutaneous variant is not associated with local symptoms or systemic disease. Subcutaneous nodules usually appear on the extremities and scalp, where they are often fixed to the underlying periosteum. The diagnosis is often suggested by the presence of typical annular dermal plaques. When skin biopsy is necessary, pathologic examination reveals changes similar to the more superficial lesions.

Adnexal Tumors

Neoplasms can arise from any structure in the skin. Although many tumors of the adnexal structures can be distinguished only by specific histopathology, some lesions demonstrate distinctive clinical patterns.

Epidermal inclusion cysts (EICs) are slow-growing dermal or subcutaneous tumors that usually reach a size of 1 to 3 cm and occur most commonly on the face, scalp, neck, and trunk. Occasionally they develop on the palms and soles. These cysts account for most cutaneous nodules in children. They can be present at birth or can appear at any time during childhood. Although they are usually associated with hair follicles, EICs can also arise from the epithelium of any adnexal structure. Primary lesions probably represent a keratinizing type of benign tumor. Other cysts occur as a response to trauma or inflammation, such as in nodulocystic acne. Histologically, EICs consist of epidermis-lined sacs usually arising from the infundibular portion of the hair follicle. Rupture of the cyst and spillage of the epithelial debris contained within results in acute and chronic dermal inflammation. These lesions may become red and painful. Noninflamed cysts can be readily excised. Inflamed lesions may respond to intralesional injections of corticosteroids and oral antibiotics before surgery is attempted.

Most EICs are solitary. When multiple lesions are present, the preceding injury or inflammatory process is usually apparent. In other cases, the development of multiple cysts should suggest the diagnosis of *Gardner's syndrome,* or *intestinal polyposis type III*. In this syndrome, increasing numbers of cysts, especially on the face and scalp, are associated with large-bowel polyposis and a 50 percent risk of malignant transformation,

osteomatosis involving the bones of the head, and desmoid tumors, particularly of the abdominal wall.

Milia are miniature EICs ranging from 1 to 3 mm in diameter (see Fig. 2.16). Although they are usually seen in the newborn, they can also be acquired after acute and chronic cutaneous injury such as abrasions, surgery, and recurrent blistering in epidermolysis bullosa (see Fig. 2.48). Milia often resolve without treatment, but some may remain indefinitely. Curettage or gentle puncture and expression with a comedone extractor is usually curative.

A number of other cystic tumors in the skin, including trichilemmal cysts, pilomatrixomas, vellus hair cysts, steatocystomas, and dermoid cysts, may be confused clinically with EICs.

Trichilemmal cysts are clinically indistinguishable fron epidermal cysts. However, they are less common than EICs, occur almost exclusively on the scalp, and appear as multiple lesions in a majority of patients. Trichilemmal cysts tend to be inherited in an autosomal dominant pattern. Histologically, these lesions can be distinguished from epidermal cysts by the absence of a granular layer and the presence of a palisading arrangement of the peripheral cells in the cyst wall. The cyst cavity contains homogeneous keratinous material, unlike the laminated horny material seen in EICs.

Pilomatrixoma, or calcifying epithelioma of Malherbe, presents as a sharply demarcated, firm, deep-seated nodule covered by normal or tethered overlying skin (Fig. 5.16). Superficial tumors develop a bluish-gray hue, and occasionally protuberant red nodules are present. Lesions range in size from less than 1 cm to more than 3 cm. Although pilomatrixomas can arise at any age, 40 percent appear before age 10, and over 50 percent by adolescence. These tumors often come to the attention of anxious patients or parents when rapid enlargement follows hematoma formation after trauma.

Pilomatrixomas most commonly affect the face, scalp, and upper trunk. They are usually solitary, but occasionally multiple lesions develop. Although most pilomatrixomas do not appear to be inherited, there are several reports of familial cases.

Histologically, this well-demarcated, encapsulated tumor demonstrates a distinctive pattern, with islands of

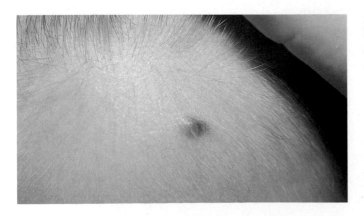

FIGURE 5.16 A pilomatrixoma was removed from the forehead of a seven-year-old boy. Note the characteristic bluish-gray dermal papule.

basophilic and shadow epithelial cells. Eosinophilic foci of keratinization and basophilic deposits of calcification are scattered throughout.

Although pilomatrixomas are usually asymptomatic, rapid enlargement or gradual progression to a large size may prompt surgical removal. They can usually be excised easily with local anesthesia.

Vellus hair cysts erupt as multiple 1-mm to 2-mm follicular papules on the chest, abdomen, and arm flexures of children and young adults (Fig. 5.17). Some of the papules have an umbilicated center suggestive of molluscum contagiosum, and impacted, lightly pigmented vellus hairs may be seen poking out of the center. These asymptomatic lesions resolve over months to years without treatment. Familial cases with autosomal dominant inheritance have been described.

Steatocystoma appears either sporadically as a solitary tumor or in an autosomal dominant pattern with many nontender, 1-cm to 3-cm, firm, rounded cystic nodules tethered to the overlying skin (Fig. 5.18). Cysts usually begin to develop on the chest, arms, and face in childhood or adolescence. Ruptured cysts exude an oily or milky fluid and in some cases small hairs. The walls of the cyst characteristically contain flattened sebaceous gland lobules or aborted hair follicles. Electron microscopic findings suggest that steatocystoma arises either from se-

baceous ductal epithelium or from the hair outer root sheath. A few bothersome cysts can be removed by simple excision. In some patients with hundreds of lesions, 13-*cis*-retinoic acid has been shown to shrink existing tumors and suppress the development of new ones.

Dermoid cysts are congenital subcutaneous cysts from 1 to 4 cm in diameter which are found most commonly around the eyes and on the head and neck (see Fig. 2.71). Most dermoids on the head are immobile because they are fixed to the periosteum. Dermoid cysts grow slowly and may cause thinning of the underlying bone. Unlike epidermal cysts, the epithelial lining of dermoid cysts contains multiple adnexal structures including hair follicles, eccrine glands, sebaceous glands, and apocrine glands.

Multiple facial papules and nodules should suggest the diagnosis of *syringoma, angiofibroma,* or *trichoepithelioma.* Differentiation can be made on the basis of clinical and histologic findings.

Syringomas appear as multiple 1-mm to 2-mm, skin-colored to yellow-brown papules on the lower eyelids and cheeks (Fig. 5.19). Occasionally they occur as isolated lesions or in a widely disseminated eruptive form with hundreds of papules on the face, axillae, chest, abdomen, and genitals. Although they are most common in adolescent girls and young women, they can

FIGURE 5.17
Multiple, asymptomatic 1-mm to 3-mm vellus hair cysts erupted on the chest of this nine-year-old boy.

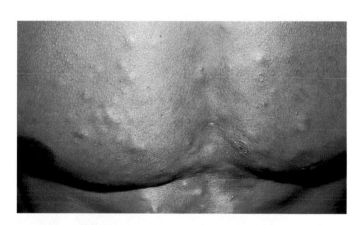

FIGURE 5.18 Many steatocystomas began to appear on the chest, neck, and face of this adolescent at age eight. His father and brother had similar nodulocystic lesions.

FIGURE 5.19 Syringomas dot the eyelids of this adolescent. The papules responded quickly to gentle carbon dioxide laser vaporization.

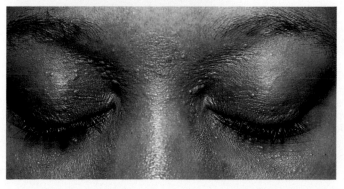

appear at any age in both sexes, and are also common in children with Down's syndrome.

Histologic examination reveals characteristic multiple small ducts lined with two rows of flattened epithelial cells in the superficial dermis. The lumina of the ducts contain amorphous debris, and some ducts possess comma-like tails, giving the appearance of tadpoles.

Although occasionally disfiguring, these lesions are usually asymptomatic. Syringomas can be effectively removed by a number of methods, including carbon dioxide laser, electrocautery, cryosurgery, and surgical excision.

Angiofibromas first appear in the early school years as subtle 1-mm 2-mm red or brownish-red papules on the cheeks, chin, and nasolabial folds. Papules increase in size and number, particularly as the child approaches puberty. Multiple lesions are the hallmark of tuberous sclerosis (see Chapter 6), and should prompt a search for other stigmata of this autosomal dominant disorder.

The typical histology of angiofibromas shows concentric rings of fibrosis around atrophic sebaceous glands and capillary dilation. Fibrous papules of the nose are solitary 2-mm to 3-mm shiny dome-shaped papules with similar histologic appearance. However, they are innocent solitary lesions which probably represent involuting nevi and should not be confused with the multiple angiofibromas of tuberous sclerosis.

In adolescents and adult, angiofibromas may become pedunculated and friable, and bleeding and infection may develop after minor trauma. Fortunately, these lesions respond readily to carbon dioxide laser ablation as well as to dermabrasion.

Trichoepitheliomas occur most commonly as solitary skin-colored tumors less than 2 cm in diameter on the faces of children or young adults (Fig. 5.20A and B). Multiple lesions are inherited as an autosomal dominant

trait. In this setting, trichoepitheliomas first appear in childhood and increase slowly in number and size. Many papules and nodules between 2 and 8 mm in diameter are scattered over the cheeks, nasolabial folds, nose, and upper lip. Histopathology shows a typical dermal tumor consisting of horn cysts of various sizes and formations resembling basal cell carcinomas. Histologic differentiation from basal cell tumors is occasionally difficult.

Unfortunately, a continuing increase in the number and size of tumors may lead to severe disfigurement. Surgical excision, electrocautery, and laser ablation have been used to deal with the most recalcitrant lesions.

Xanthomas

Xanthomas are yellow dermal tumors composed of lipid-laden histiocytes (Fig. 5.21A–C). They are usually associated with an abnormality of lipid metabolism, and their presence may point to an underlying systemic disease.

Poorly soluble lipids are transported in serum by lipoproteins. Abnormalities in lipid transport and metabolism may cause elevations of serum triglycerides and/or cholesterol. The deposition of these lipids in skin and soft tissue leads to the development of xanthomas. Although conditions such as poorly controlled diabetes mellitus and fulminant hepatic necrosis associated with serum hepatitis can trigger hyperlipidemia, a number of primary inherited dyslipoproteinemias have been defined.

The recognition of a number of clinical variants may help in the identification of a particular systemic disorder. Planar xanthomas present as soft, slightly infiltrated yellow plaques at any site, but with a predilection for previously injured skin such as old lacerations and acne scars. Xanthelasma, an example of planar lesions on the eyelids, is associated with hypercholesteremia in about half of the cases. Diffuse lesions may involve the

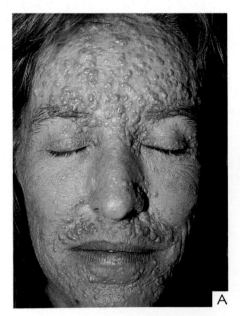

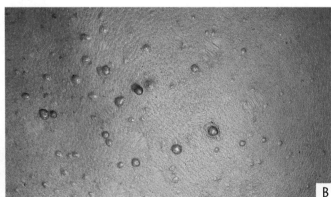

FIGURE 5.20 Trichoepitheliomas slowly increased in size and number on the face (**A**) and the chest and back (**B**) of this 17-year-old boy. Note the involvement of the nasolabial folds and the upper lip. At least five individuals in three generations of his family were affected.

extremities, trunk, face, and neck. In childhood, planar xanthomas occur in diabetes mellitus, liver disease, and histiocytosis syndromes.

Tuberous xanthomas arise as reddish-yellow nodules on the extensor surfaces of the extremities and buttocks. Although they may coalesce to cover a large area, tuberous lesions do not become adherent to the underlying soft-tissue structures as tendinous xanthomas do. They may be associated with elevations of cholesterol or triglycerides.

Tendinous xanthomas present as smooth, asymptomatic nodules on ligaments, tendons, and other deep soft-tissue structures. They are usually several centimeters in size and are most common on the ankles, knees, and elbows.

Eruptive xanthomas develop suddenly as 1-mm to 4-mm yellowish-red papules over the extensor surfaces of the extremities, buttocks, and bony prominences. Their appearance is usually associated with marked elevation in triglycerides, especially in poorly controlled diabetics or in patients with types I, III, IV, and V hyperlipidemia.

Xanthomas must be distinguished from xanthogran-ulomas because the latter are not usually associated with systemic disease (see Chapter 2). Xanthogranulomas rarely appear in large numbers; they are single in about 50 percent of cases, and less than five nodules are present in most of the rest. Moreover, serum lipids are normal.

Fibrous Tumors

A number of benign dermal tumors are caused by proliferation of fibroblasts in the dermis. During the healing process that follows an injury to the skin, loss of normal structures and the laying down of collagen by fibroblasts may lead to the formation of a *scar.* In certain predisposed individuals the collagen may become particularly thick, resulting in a *hypertrophic scar.* Over the ensuing six to nine months many of these scars will flatten. However, some may persist or develop into *keloids,* which continue to thicken and extend beyond the margins of the initial injury (Fig. 5.22A and B). These rubbery nodules or plaques can be pruritic or tender, especially during the active phase of growth. Keloids may arise sporadically or occur in a familial form. They are

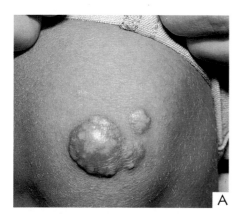
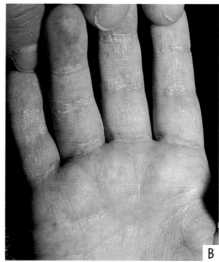
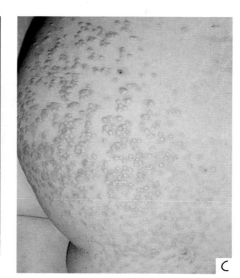

FIGURE 5.21 Xanthomas erupted in two children (**A,B**) with congenital biliary atresia and chronic liver failure. The infiltrated nodules and plaques resolved after liver transplantation. (**C**) Widespread xanthomas also appeared in this young adult with primary biliary cirrhosis.

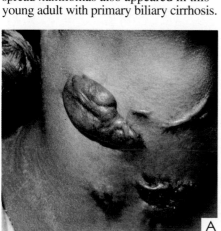
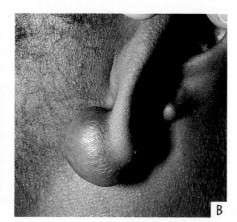

FIGURE 5.22 Keloids. (**A**) An abnormal reparative reaction to skin injury, keloids are characterized by proliferation of fibroblasts and collagen beyond the margins of the original wound. (**B**) A large keloid developed on the ear of this teenage girl after ear piercing.

most common in blacks, and have a predilection for the earlobes, upper trunk, and shoulders. Fortunately, they are rare on the midface. If treated early, hypertrophic scars and keloids may regress with intralesional steroid injections alone or in combination with surgery. However, recurrences are common.

Dermatofibromas present as firm, indolent, 0.3-cm to 1.0-cm, reddish-brown dermal nodules (Fig. 5.23). Although they are most common in adults, about 20 percent occur before age 20, and they account for 2 percent of all cutaneous nodules in children. Tumors may arise as single or multiple lesions (usually less than five) at any site, including the palms and soles. However, they usually appear on the arms and legs. Although the cause is unknown, many lesions are believed to follow minor trauma, such as insect bites or folliculitis.

On examination, dermatofibromas often demonstrate dimpling with lateral pressure because of attachment of the dermal nodule to an overlying thickened and hyperpigmented epidermis. Dermatofibromas may come to the attention of the patient after sudden enlargement following trauma and resultant hemorrhage. Histologic examination, which reveals proliferating fibroblasts and histiocytes, permits easy differentiation from melanocytic tumors such as nevi and melanomas.

Although *angiofibromas* may develop as isolated papules, their presence should alert the clinician to the diagnosis of tuberous sclerosis (see Chapter 2). These dermal tumors usually increase gradually in size and number during childhood, involving the scalp, cheeks, and nasolabial folds but sparing the upper lip (Fig. 5.24A and B). Subtle angiofibromas may be mistaken for flat warts, comedones, or seborrheic keratoses. Histopathology demonstrates a fibrous tumor with increased numbers of fibroblasts and collagen as well as capillary dilatation. The presence of acne-like papules beginning well before puberty should suggest the diagnosis even in otherwise healthy children of normal intelligence.

Pyogenic Granuloma

Pyogenic granuloma, also known as lobular capillary hemangioma, is a common, acquired, benign vascular tumor that resembles a small capillary hemangioma (Fig. 5.25A and B). Although it is usually thought to represent an overgrowth of granulation tissue after trauma or a reaction to a foreign body, such as a thorn or splinter, most pyogenic granulomas probably arise de novo. Lesions are usually solitary, bright-red, soft papules which are often pedunculated and range in size from 2 mm to 2 cm. Two-thirds arise on the head and

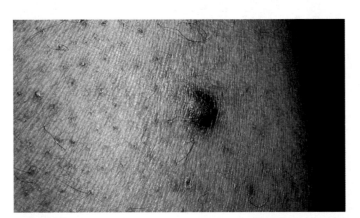

FIGURE 5.23 Dermatofibroma. An indolent 5-mm firm brown nodule appeared two years ago on the leg of this 17-year-old girl. The overlying epidermis was thickened and hyperpigmented.

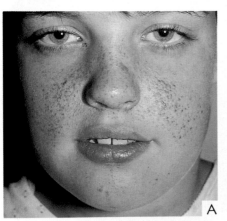
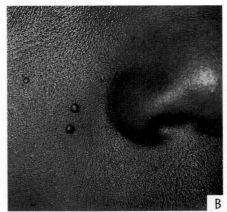
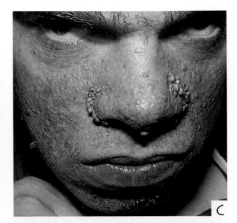

FIGURE 5.24 Angiofibromas. (**A**) Small red facial papules were initially dismissed as acne. (**B**) Subtle brown papules were diagnosed as moles. Both children were of normal intelligence and had no history of seizures. Skin biopsies demonstrated find- ings typical of angiofibromas. (**C**) This profoundly retarded boy with tuberous sclerosis developed progressive angiofibromas over much of his face. Note the involvement of the nasolabial folds and sparing of the upper lip.

neck, followed in frequency by the trunk, upper extremities, and lower extremities. Although they are most common in children and young adults, they can appear at any age.

The term "pyogenic granuloma" is misleading because the tumor is neither an infectious pyoderma nor a granuloma. Skin biopsy demonstrates proliferating capillaries in a loose, edematous fibrous matrix. The surface may become friable and secondarily infected. Minimal trauma then results in profuse bleeding, which prompts a visit to the practitioner. Treatment consists of surgical excision, laser ablation, or shave excision with electrodessication of the base. Care must be taken to destroy residual vessels or the lesion will recur. Occasionally surgical removal of pyogenic granulomas is followed by the eruption of multiple satellite lesions. Although these may regress spontaneously, further surgery is sometimes required. Laser surgery is sometimes particularly useful in the management of recurrent or multiple lesions.

Neural Tumors

Neurofibromas are the most common tumors of neural ori-
gin for which a patient might seek dermatologic consultation (Fig. 5.26). These soft, compressible, skin-colored, 0.5-cm to 3-cm tumors arise in the dermis and occasionally in the subcutaneous fat. Neurofibromas occur sporadically as solitary lesions or progressively in large numbers in patients with neurofibromatosis (see Chapter 6).

Neuromas arise in three settings. Traumatic neuromas are solitary, painful nodules that develop in scars after surgery or trauma. Pain usually resolves quickly after surgical excision. Traumatic neuromas also include amputation neuromas and rudimentary supernumerary digits which occur most commonly on the ulnar side of the base of the fifth finger (see Fig. 2.21). *Idiopathic neuromas* are rare lesions that develop at any time from early childhood through adult life as solitary or multiple 0.2-cm to 1-cm dermal nodules on the skin and oral mucosa (Fig. 5.27). They are not associated with multiple endocrine neoplasia (MEN). Finally, *multiple mucosal neuromas* are part of an autosomal dominant syndrome (MEN type IIB), in which many small tumors appear on the lips, oral mucosa, and face in early childhood. Recognition of this syndrome is important because of its association with

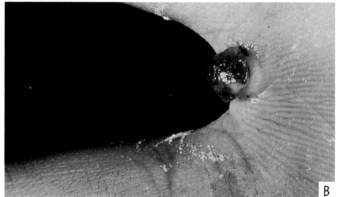

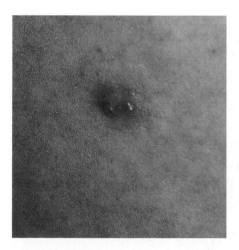

FIGURE 5.25 Pyogenic granuloma. **(A)** A raised hemorrhagic papule developed on this infant's cheek. **(B)** Another rapidly growing, friable lesion is present between his fingers.

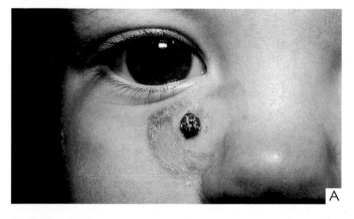

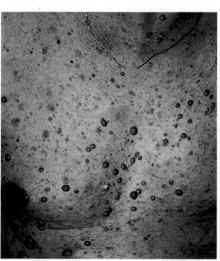

FIGURE 5.26 Neurofibromas. Widespread compressible tumors developed over much of the body surface of this young man with neurofibromatosis type I (von Recklinghausen's disease). He had a four-year-old son with multiple cafe-au-lait spots but no cutaneous tumors.

FIGURE 5.27 Idiopathic neuromas. More than 50 small, yellow, dermal nodules erupted on the face, neck, trunk, and extremities of a three-year-old girl. She has no signs of MEN, and the family history is negative.

medullary thyroid carcinoma in young children and adults and with pheochromocytoma in adolescents and adults.

In multiple mucosal neuroma syndrome, facial lesions may be confused with angiofibromas, trichoepitheliomas, multiple trichilemmomas in Cowden's disease, and extensive papillomavirus infection. However, the large numbers of nerve bundles histologically indentified in skin biopsy specimens are distinctive. Nodules on the trunk and extremities cannot be distinguished from other dermal tumors without a biopsy.

Lymphocytoma Cutis

Lymphocytoma cutis presents as asymptomatic nodules and plaques, usually affecting the face, although any site can be involved (Fig. 5.28). Although multiple lesions may erupt, solitary nodules ranging from under 1 cm to several centimeters in diameter are the rule. Most tumors develop in adolescents and young adults.

The distinction from a non-Hodgkin's lymphoma, which also presents as a single nodule, may be impossible. Histologic study demonstrates a mixed dermal

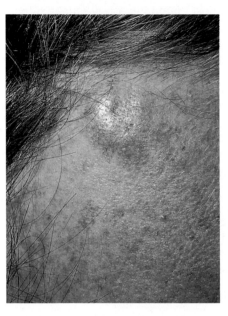 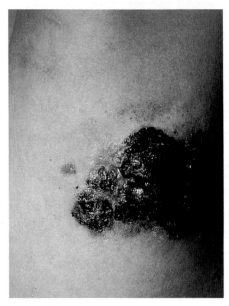 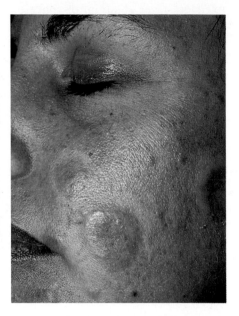

FIGURE 5.28 Lymphocytoma cutis. A 1-cm painless nodule persisted for over a year on the forehead of a teenage boy. A skin biopsy from the center of the lesion demonstrated a lymphocytic infiltrate in the dermis, forming lymphoid follicle-like structures. Intralesional steroids produced some improvement.

FIGURE 5.29 Lymphoma. An indolent nodule on the thigh of a seven-year-old boy was initially diagnosed as a persistent insect bite reaction. During the following year several new nodules appeared on his legs and buttocks and regressed without treatment. Biopsy of the initial lesion shown here, which persisted throughout the period, demonstrated a Ki-1 marker-positive lymphoma.

FIGURE 5.30 Follicular (alopecia) mucinosis. Multiple nodules and indurated plaques appeared on the face and neck of an 18-year-old girl. Histopathology of a skin biopsy showed intracellular edema, formation of cystic spaces, and accumulation of mucin in the external root sheaths of involved hair follicles and sebaceous glands. Several plaques were treated successfully with intralesional injections of corticosteroids. The remainder resolved over several years without treatment.

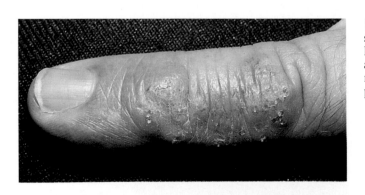

FIGURE 5.31 Sporotrichosis. A teenage boy developed a slowly expanding, painless, violaceous, indurated plaque on his left fifth finger. Sporotrichosis was diagnosed on a skin biopsy and confirmed by fungal culture. The lesion healed in three months with oral administration of a saturated solution of potassium iodide.

infiltrate of large and small lymphocytes, separated from the epidermis by a small band of normal collagen. The infiltrate may become organized into structures resembling lymph follicles. The frequent presence of an admixture of plasma cells and/or eosinophils speaks against malignancy. Unfortunately, the histology is not specific, and the usual innocent nature of the eruption in children is defined by the clinical course. Nodules heal without treatment over months to years. Some patients may benefit from intralesional corticosteroids.

Clinically, lymphocytoma cutis is indistinguishable from lymphoma (Fig. 5.29), and all children deserve a careful history and complete physical examination to exclude signs and symptoms of systemic disease. Other infiltrative processes, such as histiocytosis X, follicular mucinosis (Fig. 5.30), and mastocytomas, as well as insect bite reactions, sarcoidosis, deep fungal infections (Fig. 5.31), and dermatofibromas, may resemble lymphocytoma cutis. The clinical course and histologic findings help to define these entities. Rarely, other malignancies such as leukemia, rhabdomyosarcoma, neuroblastoma, and renal carcinoma present initially with cutaneous nodules. Their rapid growth and their histologic pattern distinguish these malignancies from benign lymphocytoma cutis.

ALGORITHM FOR EVALUATION OF LUMPS AND BUMPS

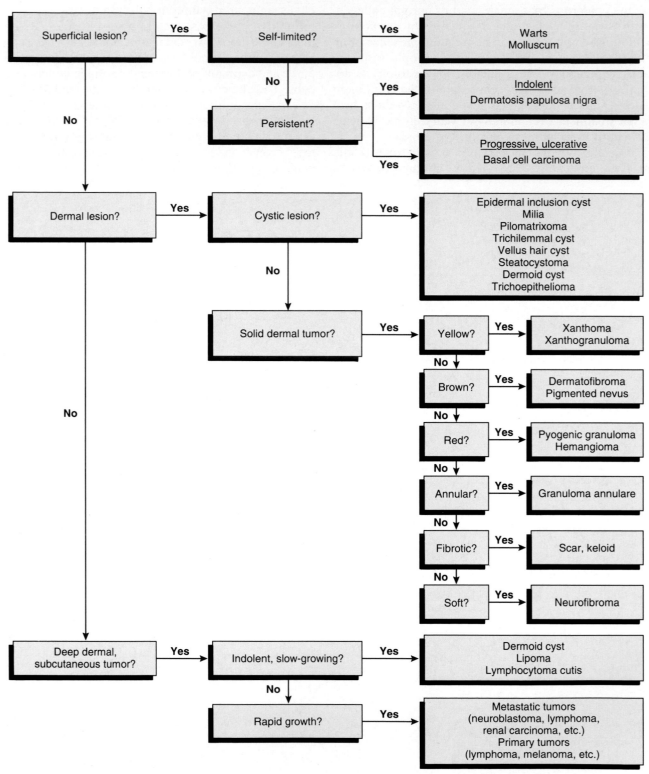

BIBLIOGRAPHY

Warts

Androphy EJ. Human papillomavirus: current concepts. *Arch Dermatol* 135:683–685, 1989.

Barnett N, Mark H, Winkelstein JA. Extensive verrucosis in primary immunodeficiency diseases. *Arch Dermatol* 119:5–7, 1983.

Cohen BA, Honig PG, Androphy E. Anogenital warts in children. *Arch Dermatol* 126:1575–1580, 1990.

Ingelfinger JR, Grupe WE, Topor M, et al. Warts in a pediatric renal transplant population. *Dermatologica* 155:7–12, 1977.

Lutzner MA. The human papillomaviruses. A review *Arch Dermatol* 119:631–635, 1983.

Silva PD, Micha JP, Silva DG. Management of condyloma acuminatum. *J Am Acad Dermatol* 13:457–463, 1985.

Zur Hausen H. Papillomaviruses in human cancer. *Cancer* 59:1692–1696, 1987.

Molluscum contagiosum

Pauly CR, Artis WM, Jones HE. Atopic dermatitis, impaired cellular immunity, and molluscum contagiosum. *Arch Dermatol* 114:391–393, 1978.

Pierard-Franchimont C, Legrain A, Pierard GE. Growth and regression of molluscum contagiosum. *J Am Acad Dermatol* 9:669–672, 1983.

Steffen C, Markman JA. Spontaneous disappearance of molluscum contagiosum. *Arch Dermatol* 116:923, 1980.

Weston WL, Lane AT. Should molluscum be treated? *Pediatrics* 65:865–866, 1980.

Basal cell carcinoma

Edwards L, Bangert JL, Goldberg GN, Hansen RC. Benign neoplasms, premalignant conditions, and malignancy. In: Schachner LA, Hansen RC, eds. *Pediatric Dermatology*. New York: Churchill Livingstone, 1988.

Mallory SB. Genodermatoses with malignant potential. In: Alper JC, ed. *Genetic Disorders of the Skin*. St. Louis: Mosby Year Book, 1991:256–261.

Milstone E, Helwig E. Basal cell carcinoma in children. *Arch Dermatol* 108:523–527, 1978.

Granuloma annulare

Beatty JR. Rheumatic-like nodule occurring in nonrheumatic children. *Arch Pathol* 68:154–159, 1959.

Dicken CH, Carrington SG, Winkelmann RK. Generalized granuloma annulare. *Arch Dermatol* 99:556–563, 1969.

Mulhbauer JE. Granuloma annulare. *J Am Acad Dermatol* 3:217, 1980.

Wells RS, Smith MA. The natural history of granuloma annulare. *Br J Dermatol* 75:199–206, 1963.

Adnexal tumors

Brownstein MH, Helwig EB. Subcutaneous dermoid cysts. *Arch Dermatol* 107:237–239, 1973.

Esterly NB, Fretxin DF, Pinkus H. Eruptive vellus hair cysts. *Arch Dermatol* 1113:500–503, 1977.

Friedman SJ, Buttler DF. Syringoma presenting as milia. *J Am Acad Dermatol* 16:310–314, 1987.

Kligman AM, Kirschbaum JD. Steatocystoma multiplex: a dermoid tumor. *J Invest Dermatol* 42:383–387, 1964.

Knight PJ, Reiner CB. Superficial lumps in children. What, when, and why. *Pediatrics* 72:147, 1983.

Mallory SB. Genodermatoses with malignant potential. In: Alper JC, ed. *Genetic Disorders of the Skin*. St. Louis: Mosby Year Book, 1991:247–250.

Pariser RJ. Multiple hereditary trichoepitheliomas and basal cell carcinoma. *J Cutan Pathol* 13:111–117, 1986.

Pollard ZF, Robinson HD, Calhoun J. Dermoid cysts in children. *Pediatrics* 57:379–382, 1976.

Xanthomas

Parker F. Xanthomas and hyperlipidemias. *J Am Acad Dermatol* 13:1–30, 1985.

Fibrous tumors

Murray JC, Pollack SV, Pinnell SR. Keloids: a review. *J Am Acad Dermatol* 4:461–470, 1981.

Noemi KM. The benign fibrocystic tumors of the skin. *Acta Dermatol Venereol (Stockh)* 50 (suppl):63, 1970.

Pyogenic granuloma

Amerigo J, Gonzales-Camara R, Galera H, et al. Recurrent pyogenic granuloma with multiple satellites. *Dermatologica* 166:117–121, 1983.

Patrice SJ, Wiss K, Mulliken JB. Pyogenic granuloma (lobular capillary hemangioma): a clinicopathologic study of 178 cases. *Pediatric Dermatol* 8:267, 1991.

Neural tumors

Holm TW, Prawer SE, Sahl WJ Jr, et al. Multiple cutaneous neuromas. *Arch Dermatol* 107:608–610, 1973.

Khairi MRA, Dexter RN, Burzynski NJ, et al. Mucosal neuroma, pheochromocytoma and medullary thyroid carcinoma: multiple endocrine neoplasia type 3 (review). *Medicine (Baltimore)* 54:89–112, 1975.

Lymphocytoma cutis

Burg G, Kerl H, Schmoekel C. Differentiation between malignant B-cell lymphomas and pseudolymphomas of the skin. *J Dermatol Surg Oncol* 10:271–2735, 1984.

VanHale HM, Winkelmann RK. Nodular lymphoid disease of the head and neck: lymphocytoma cutis, benign lymphocytic infiltrate of Jessner, and their distinction from malignant lymphoma. *J Am Acad Dermatol* 12:455–461, 1985.

chapter six

DISORDERS
OF PIGMENTATION

Although most disorders of pigmentation in infancy and childhood are of cosmetic importance only, some lesions provide clues to the diagnosis of multisystem disease. Disorders of pigmentation may be differentiated clinically by the presence of increased or decreased pigmentation in a localized or diffuse distribution.

HYPERPIGMENTATION

Localized areas of hyperpigmentation are frequently developmental or hereditary in origin and appear early in childhood. However, pigmented lesions may also be acquired later in childhood following inflammatory rashes in the skin or environmental exposure to sunlight or after other traumatic, chemical, and thermal injury. *Epidermal melanosis* occurs when increased numbers of epidermal melanocytes are present in the basal cell layer or increased quantities of melanin are present in epidermal keratinocytes. *Dermal melanosis* results from increased melanin in dermal melanocytes or melanophages. Although epidermal melanosis may result in the development of dark-brown or black macules and papules, most lesions appear tan or light brown in color. Dermal melanosis tends to produce slate-gray, dark-brown, and bluish-green lesions.

Epidermal melanosis

Cafe-au-lait spots are discrete tan macules that appear at birth or during childhood in 10 percent to 20 percent of normal individuals. Lesions vary from the size of freckles to 20 cm or more in diameter and may involve any site on the skin surface (Fig. 6.1A).

Although most affected children are normal, cafe-au-lait spots, particularly six or more lesions over 1.5 cm in diameter, provide a marker for classic neurofibromatosis (von Recklinghausen disease or National Institutes of Health classification NF-1). Conversely, 90 percent of individuals with neurofibromatosis have at least one lesion. Although cafe-au-lait spots are often present at birth, they usually increase in size and number throughout childhood, particularly during the first few years of life in children with neurofibromatosis. Other stigmata including neurofibromas and Lisch nodules may not appear until later childhood or adolescence (Fig. 6.1B and C). Axillary freckling is also a characteristic sign of neurofibromatosis (see Fig. 6.1A).

Histologic findings include increased numbers of melanocytes and melanin in melanocytes and keratinocytes. Giant pigment granules have been identified in the cafe-au-lait spots of neurofibromatosis, but they may also be seen in sporadic cafe-au-lait spots, nevi, freckles, and lentigines.

Cafe-au-lait spots are not specific for neurofibromatosis and have also been associated with tuberous sclerosis, Albright's syndrome, leopard syndrome, epidermal nevus syndrome, Bloom's syndrome, ataxia-telangiectasia, and Russell–Silver syndrome (Fig. 6.2).

Freckles, or *ephelides*, are 2-mm to 3-mm reddish-tan and brown macules that appear on sun-exposed surfaces,

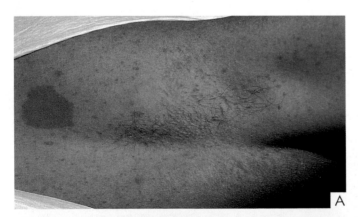

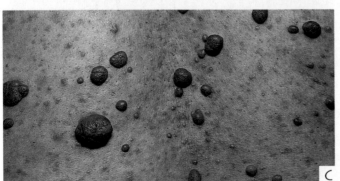

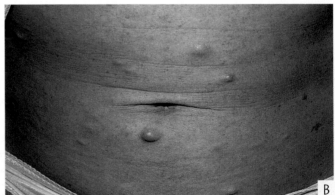

FIGURE 6.1 Neurofibromatosis. This 16-year-old girl had multiple cafe-au-lait spots since early childhood. (**A**) Her axilla demonstrates a single 4-cm cafe-au-lait spot and diffuse freckling. (**B**) At puberty she began to develop widespread neurofibromas. Note the variable size of the subcutaneous tumors. (**C**) A 19-year-old boy with NFI has mushroom-shaped neurofibromas dotting his entire skin surface as demonstrated on his back.

particularly the face, neck, upper chest, and forearms (Fig. 6.3). They typically arise in early childhood on lightly pigmented individuals. Lesions tend to fade in the winter and increase in number and pigmentation during the spring and summer months. Photoprotection with clothing, sunblocks, and sunscreens may decrease the summer exacerbation of freckles which are generally of cosmetic importance only. The development of progressive widespread freckling in sun-exposed sites may suggest an underlying disorder of photosensitivity (see Chapter 7).

Figure 6.2 Cafe-au-lait Spots

Disorder	Other Skin Findings	Systemic Involvement
Neurofibromatosis	Axillary freckling, Lisch nodules (iris) neurofibromas	Skeletal abnormalities, neurologic involvement
McCune–Albright syndrome	Few large cafe-au-lait spots	Precocious puberty in girls, polyostotic fibrous dysplasia
Watson's syndrome	Axillary freckling	Pulmonary stenosis, mental retardation
Russell–Silver dwarfism	Hypohidrosis in infancy	Small stature, skeletal asymmetry, clinodactyly of fifth finger
Ataxia-telangiectasia	Telangiectasia in bulbar conjunctivae and on face, sclerodermatous changes	Growth retardation, ataxia mental retardation, lymphopenia, IgA, IgE, lymphoid tissue, respiratory infections
Tuberous sclerosis	Hypopigmented macules, shagreen patch, adenoma sebaceum, subungual fibromas	Central nervous system, kidneys, heart, lungs
Turner's syndrome	Loose skin especially around neck, lymphedema in infancy, hemangiomas	Small stature, gonadal dysgenesis, skeletal anomalies, renal anomalies, cardiac defects
Bloom's syndrome	Telangiectatic erythema of cheeks, photosensitivity, ichthyosis	Short stature, malar hypoplasia, risk of malignancy
Multiple lentigines (leopard syndrome)	Lentigenes, axillary freckling	EKG abnormalities, ocular hypertelorism, pulmonic stenosis, genital abnormalities, growth retardation, sensorineural deafness
Westerhof's syndrome	Hypopigmented macules	Growth and mental retardation

Histologically, freckles demonstrate hyperpigmentation of the basal cell layer of the epidermis. The number of melanocytes may actually be decreased, but those that are present are larger and show more numerous and prominent dendritic processes.

Freckles must be distinguished from *lentigines* which are more uniform and darker in color, fewer in number, and do not demonstrate seasonal variation. Lentigines vary from 2 mm to 5 mm in diameter and may involve any site on the skin or mucous membranes.

Lentigo simplex arises most commonly during childhood and does not show a predilection for sun-exposed surfaces. The lentigines are scattered, 2-mm to 3-mm uniformly pigmented macules that range from brown to black in color and may be indistinguishable clinically from junctional pigmented nevi.

Microscopically, lentigo simplex shows elongation of the rete ridges, an increase in concentration of melanocytes in the basal layer, an increase in melanin in both melanocytes and basal keratinocytes, and melanophages in the upper dermis.

Several special variants of lentigo simplex are recognized, including *lentiginosis profusa, multiple lentigines syndrome*, and *speckled lentiginous nevus.*

Lentiginosis profusa is characterized by the presence of diffuse, multiple, small, darkly pigmented macules from birth or infancy. They are not usually familial, and children are otherwise healthy and develop normally. This entity should be distinguished from *multiple lentigines syndrome*, or *leopard syndrome*, in which diffuse lentigines are associated with multisystem disease.

In *leopard* (or *LEOPARD*) *syndrome* the lentigines are tan or brown in color, begin to appear in early infancy, and increase in number throughout childhood (Fig. 6.4). Axillary freckling and cafe-au-lait spots appear frequently. Other anomalies suggested by the leopard mnemonic and variably occur include electrocardiographic conduction abnormalities (E), ocular hypertelorism (O), pulmonic stenosis (P), abnormal genitalia (A), growth retardation (R), and neural deafness (D). This disorder is inherited as an autosomal dominant trait. In both lentiginosis profusa and leopard syndrome the mucous membranes are spared.

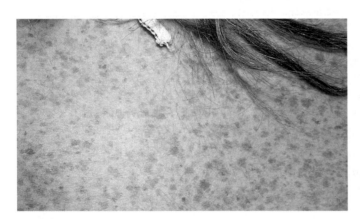

FIGURE 6.3 Ephiledes. Freckles cover sun-exposed areas of this red-haired, blue-eyed girl. The pigmented macules darken and increase in number during the summer.

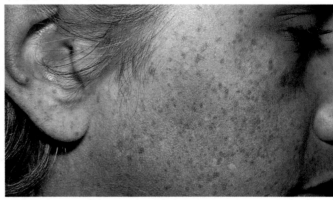

FIGURE 6.4 Lentigo. Multiple lentigines persisted year 'round on the face, upper trunk, and extremities of this 13-year-old boy with leopard syndrome. His sister, father, and grandfather had similar cutaneous findings.

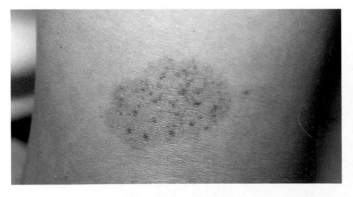

FIGURE 6.5 Nevus spilus. This speckled nevus was unchanged since it was noted shortly after birth.

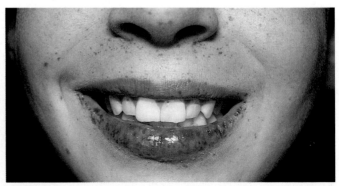

FIGURE 6.6 Peutz–Jeghers syndrome. This smiling 12-year-old girl developed progressive lentigines on her face, particularly her lips, in early childhood. She also has involvement of the extremities, trunk, and mucous membranes.

In a related disorder, *lamb* (or *LAMB*) *syndrome*, multiple lentigines are associated with atrial myxoma (A), cutaneous papular myxomas (M), and blue nevi (B).

Speckled lentiginous nevus or *nevus spilus* presents at birth as a discrete tan or brown macule that becomes dotted with darker pigmented macules during childhood (Fig. 6.5). The light-brown patch demonstrates histologic changes typical of lentigo simplex, while the dark pigmented macules show nests of nevus cells at the dermal-epidermal junction. The risk of malignant change is unknown but may be increased as in small congenital pigmented nevi.

Peutz–Jeghers syndrome is distinguished by the presence of diffuse, small, slate-gray to black macules on the skin and mucous membranes at birth or during early childhood. Lesions increase in number throughout childhood. The face is most commonly involved, particularly the vermilion border of the lips and buccal mucosa, but macules may appear on the hands, arms, trunk, and perianal and genital skin (Fig. 6.6). Axillary freckling may also occur in this autosomal dominant disorder. Cutaneous lesions occasionally occur alone. However, they are characteristically associated with intestinal polyposis which is usually restricted to the small bowel. Although the risk of malignant change in the gastrointestinal tract is low, polyps may act as the lead point for intussusception and result in bleeding or obstruction.

Although the clinical lesions in Peutz–Jeghers syndrome are clinically indistinguishable from lentigines, the histology reveals only increased pigmentation in the basal cell layer. Some investigators have found increased numbers of melanocytes, suggesting that this disorder may represent a distinct form of epidermal melanosis.

Cutaneous macules may become disfiguring and respond well to destructive measures such as gentle liquid nitrogen and carbon dioxide laser ablation. The new pigmented lesion lasers (Candela, Metalaser) may also provide a safe, effective, relatively painless therapeutic alternative.

Solar lentigines usually do not become apparent until the fourth and fifth decades of life. However, these irregularly shaped, darkly pigmented macules, which range from a few millimeters to a few centimeters in diameter on sun-exposed skin, may begin to appear in later childhood or adolescence, particularly in lightly pigmented individuals who spend long hours outdoors. Although the risk of malignant degeneration is minimal, they provide a marker of significant sun exposure. Children and parents should be counseled regarding the cumulative risk of actinic damage and use of protective clothing and sunscreens.

Becker's nevus, or *hairy epidermal nevus*, typically develops as a unilateral patch of hyperpigmentation on the trunk of an older child or adolescent (Fig. 6.7). This common lesion is usually followed by the appearance of hypertrichosis within two years. Although it occurs most frequently in boys on the shoulder, chest, or back, girls occasionally develop lesions, and any skin site may be involved. Pigmentation is usually uniform and well demarcated, but reticulated patches may be present. The coarse, long hairs may extend beyond the area of hyperpigmentation.

Histologically, the epidermis demonstrates acanthosis and rete ridge elongation in association with increased pigment in the basal cell layer and melanophages in the upper dermis. Smooth muscle bundles may be increased in some cases, reminiscent of the changes seen in congenital smooth muscle hamartomas.

As in other epidermal melanoses, gentle destructive measures and the new pigmented lesion lasers may result in improvement of hyperpigmentation. Use of photoprotection will decrease darkening from sun exposure during the summer months. Bleaching agents with hydroquinone (e.g., Solaquin Forte, Melanex) may also be effective. However, patients should be aware that inadvertent contact by the drug with normal contiguous skin may result in hypopigmentation. Shaving, depilatories, and electrolysis may be helpful for nevi with prominent hair.

Acanthosis nigricans is marked by distinctive velvety, warty hyperpigmentation in intertriginous areas. Four types are recognized. The inherited type usually

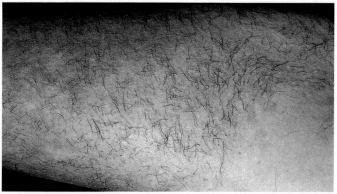

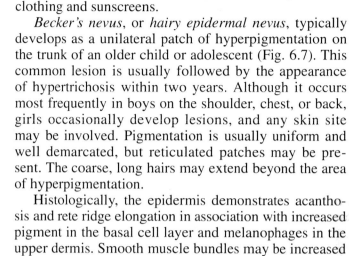

FIGURE 6.7 Becker's nevus. Progressive mottled hyperpigmentation beginning at age 13 years was followed by the development of dark, coarse hair on the shoulder of this 15-year-old boy.

erupts during infancy or childhood but occasionally at puberty (Fig. 6.8A). Lesions tend to intensify in adolescence and may fade somewhat during adulthood. There is no association with underlying medical disorders, and the inheritance is autosomal dominant. The endocrine type is usually associated with a pituitary tumor or polycystic ovary syndrome and insulin resistance. Obesity is a variable feature. Malignant acanthosis nigricans can usually be distinguished from the other types by its extensive and more florid lesions, progressiveness, and onset in middle age. The malignant type is only rarely seen in childhood. Associated tumors include gastric carcinoma, lymphoma, Hodgkin's disease, and osteogenic sarcoma. Idiopathic acanthosis nigricans is the most common type (Fig. 6.8B–D). There is no associated endocrine disorder, malignancy, or genetic predisposition. Idiopathic lesions occur most commonly in healthy, obese adolescents. Pigmentation may decrease after puberty, particularly in patients who experience a weight reduction.

Although brown to black pigmentation and thickening of the skin is most intense in skin creases of the neck, axillae, and groin, skin over bony prominences including the knuckles, elbows, knees, and ankles may be affected. In cases of malignant acanthosis nigricans, mucous membranes are occasionally involved.

Histopathology demonstrates hyperkeratosis, minimal acanthosis, and marked papillomatosis. Although there may be a slight increase in melanin in the basal cell layer, hyperpigmentation probably results from compact hyperkeratosis.

Melasma occurs primarily in pubertal girls and women but also occasionally in adolescent boys (Fig. 6.9). Although this symmetric, patchy, facial melanosis may be idiopathic, it is often associated with pregnancy or the ingestion of oral contraceptives. Lesions tend to increase after sun exposure.

Histologically, epidermal and dermal types of melanization are recognized, but many patients demonstrate pigment in both sites. There are increased numbers of epidermal melanocytes and increased pigment in epidermal keratinocytes and dermal melanophages.

Clinically, melasma must be differentiated from postinflammatory hyperpigmentation and phytophotocontact (berloque) dermatitis. Berloque dermatitis frequently appears after inadvertent application of a photosensitizer such as musk ambrette, a common component of perfumes, and sun exposure.

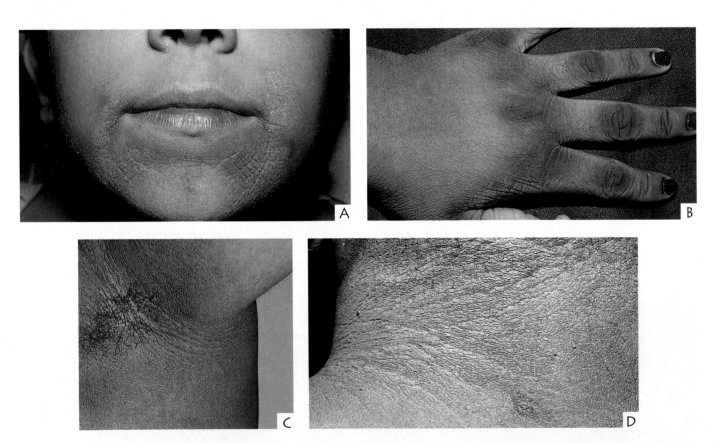

FIGURE 6.8 Acanthosis nigricans. **(A)** Progressive, leathery thickening of the skin and hyperpigmentation developed on the face, neck, chest, back, and flexures of this healthy nine-year-old boy with familial acanthosis nigricans. Note the symmetric patches on his chin and cheeks. **(B–D)** Symmetric, velvety patches appeared over the bony prominences and flexures of this obese black adolescent with benign acanthosis nigricans. Lesions were most prominent over the knuckles **(B)**, axillae **(C)**, and neck **(D)**.

Pigmentation often wanes after pregnancy or the discontinuation of oral contraceptives. However, treatment with potent topical sunscreens and bleaching agents (hydroquinone) may be helpful.

Dermal melanosis

Mongolian spots are poorly circumscribed slate-gray to blue-green congenital macules (Fig. 6.10A and B). Lesions range from a few millimeters to over 20 centimeters and are found on the trunk and proximal extremities of 80 percent to 90 percent of black infants, 75 percent of Orientals, and 10 percent of whites. Nearly 75 percent of lesions appear on the lumbosacral region. Mongolian spots do not require therapy and usually fade or are camouflaged by normal pigment by three to five years of age. When lesions are clinically confused with a pigmented nevus, a skin biopsy will reveal characteristic melanocytes in the dermis in a mongolian spot.

Special variants of the mongolian spot, the *nevus of Ota* and *nevus of Ito,* tend to persist into adult life. *Nevus of Ota (nevus fuscoceruleus ophthalmomaxillaris)* represents a unilateral patchy dermal melanosis of the skin of the face in the distribution of the trigeminal nerve. Although most cases are sporadic, rare family clusters have been reported. Lesions tend to be slate-gray to brown in color, with a "powder blast burn" appearance. The forehead, temple, periorbital area, cheek, and nose are commonly involved. Rarely pigmentation is bilateral, and large areas of the face and oral mucous membranes are affected. Melanin pigment involves the eye in about half the cases. About 50 percent of lesions are present at birth, and the remainder appear during puberty. Although lesions are most common on Orientals and blacks, all races are affected, and the majority of patients are female.

Nevus of Ito (nevus fuscoceruleus acromiodeltoideus) is a similar pathologic process in which unilateral pigmentation is located over the supraclavicular, deltoid, and scapular regions. Although it usually occurs as an isolated lesion, nevus of Ota may also be present.

Nevus of Ito and nevus of Ota are benign dermal melanoses. However, there are rare reports of malignant degeneration. Extensive lesions are amenable to corrective cosmetic camouflage. There is no effective, safe, definitive therapy available at this time, but some of the new pigmented lesion lasers may prove to be useful.

Incontinentia pigmenti (IP) is an inherited multisystem disorder which is defined by its splashy, reticulated

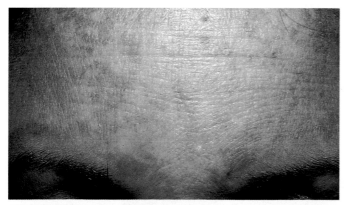

FIGURE 6.9 Melasma. Diffuse, mottled, tan pigmentation developed on the forehead and cheeks of this young woman shortly after she began taking oral birth control pills.

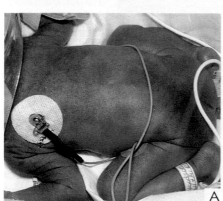
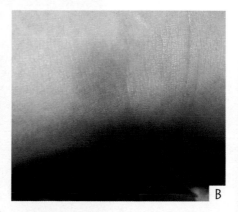
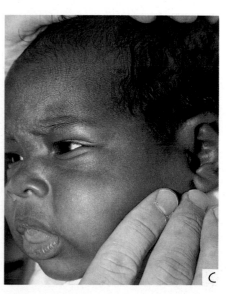

FIGURE 6.10 Mongolian spot. (**A**) Widespread and confluent mongolian spots were noted at birth on this premature black infant. The pigment was slate gray in color. (**B**) Note the solitary blue mongolian spot on the shin of a white newborn. (**C**) A nevus of Ota involved the forehead, cheek, and contiguous scalp of an otherwise healthy black infant. The lids and conjunctivae were spared.

hyperpigmentation (see Chapter 2). An inflammatory phase in the newborn precedes the pigmentary change in over 90 percent of affected children. However, 5 percent to 10 percent of patients demonstrate diffuse, whorled pigmentation at birth without antecedent inflammation (Fig. 6.11). These children may represent a distinct neurocutaneous syndrome and require the same close neurodevelopmental monitoring as those with classic IP. Inheritance may vary from the typical X-linked dominant pattern of IP.

The most common cause of increased pigmentation is *postinflammatory hyperpigmentation* (Fig. 6.12). This alteration in normal pigmentation follows many inflammatory processes in the skin such as a diaper dermatitis, insect bites, drug reactions, or traumatic injury. Lesions are usually localized and typically follow the distribution of the resolving disorder. Although epidermal melanocytes appear normal, aberrant delivery of melanin to surrounding keratinocytes results in deposition of pigment in the dermal melanophages. Areas of hyperpigmentation are more marked in darkly pigmented children. No therapy is necessary, and lesions usually fade over several months.

A special subset of drug reactions known as a *fixed drug eruption* produces peculiar, persistent hyperpigmentation, particularly on the face and genitals, and scattered on the trunk and extremities (see Chapter 7). After exposure to certain medications such as tetracycline, ibuprofen, phenobarbital, and phenolphthalein, patients develop acutely inflamed, dusky-red, edematous, round to oval, 1-cm to 3-cm plaques that may become frankly bullous in the center. When the drug is discontinued, the reaction subsides, leaving residual postinflammatory pigmentation. On re-exposure to the inciting agent, new lesions may appear, but the old lesions recur in the same "fixed" spots. The reactivity of the skin seems to reside in the dermis because normal epidermis grafted over affected dermis becomes reactive, whereas involved epidermis grafted onto normal dermis loses its sensitivity.

Acquired *nevomelanocytic nevi,* also referred to as *pigmented nevi* and *pigmented moles* begin to develop in early childhood as small, pigmented macules 1 mm to 2 mm in diameter (Fig. 6.13). In these early, flat nevi, nevus cells are located at the dermal-epidermal junction and are called junctional nevi. They then enlarge slowly and become papular. In such elevated lesions, the nevus cells have spread into the dermis to become compound nevi. Many nevi over a period of years become fleshy or pedunculated, particularly on the upper trunk, head, and neck. Histopathology of these nevi demonstrates nevus cells restricted to the dermis resulting in the so-called intradermal nevus.

During puberty nevi show an increase in darkening, size, and number. However, most normal acquired nevomelanocytic nevi do not exceed 0.5 cm in diameter, and they retain their regularity in color, contour, texture, and symmetry. The majority of nevi appear on sun-exposed areas, but lesions may involve the palms, soles, buttocks, genitals, scalp, mucous membranes, and eyes. Generally, nevi change slowly over months to years and warrant observation only.

Sudden enlargement of a nevus with redness and tenderness may occur because of an irritant reaction or folliculitis. Trauma from clothing or scratching may produce hemorrhage or crust formation that heals uneventfully. Another more gradual change causing concern in patients and parents is the appearance of a hypopigmented ring and mild local pruritus around a benign nevus (Fig. 6.14). This is called a halo nevus and is caused by a cytotoxic T-lymphocyte reaction

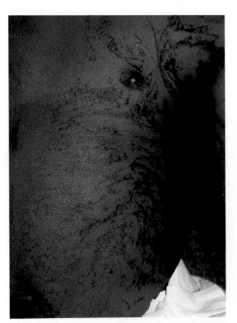

FIGURE 6.11
Incontinentia pigmenti. A toddler with developmental delay and seizures was noted to have swirled hyperpigmentation at birth. There was no history of an antecedent inflammatory eruption.

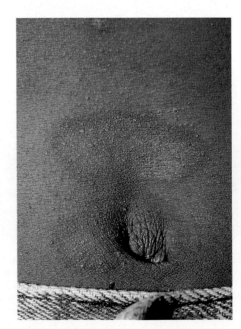

FIGURE 6.12
Postinflammatory hyperpigmentation. Dark-brown rings developed after a contact dermatitis from nickel in a belt buckle. The postinflammatory hyperpigmentation faded without treatment in four months.

against both the nevus cells and the innocent melanocytic bystanders. As a result, the nevus tends first to lighten and then to disappear completely, and the halo eventually repigments. Occasionally, halo nevi are associated with vitiligo or the loss of pigmentation in areas of normal skin without nevi.

As long as the clinical appearance of a nevus is innocent, excision is unnecessary. However, a number of changes in pigmented lesions may portend the development of melanoma. These include:

1. A change in size, shape, or contours with scalloped irregular borders;
2. A change in the surface characteristics, such as development of a small, dark, elevated papule or nodule within an otherwise flat plaque and flaking, scaling, ulceration, or bleeding;
3. A change in color, with the appearance of black, brown, or an admixture of red, white, or blue;

4. Burning, itching, or tenderness, which may be an indication of the body's immune reaction to malignancy.

Fortunately, melanomas are still rare in children. However, the incidence is increasing, and curative treatment is contingent on early diagnosis and prompt excision. A keen awareness of diagnostic features is important.

Melanomas in children may occur de novo or within acquired or congenital nevi (Fig. 6.15) (see Chapter 2). Family history of malignant melanoma—particularly if other family members have multiple, unusually large, and irregularly pigmented, bordered, and textured nevi—carries a high lifetime risk of melanoma which may approach 100 percent. Malignant melanoma in this hereditary setting is referred to as *familial dysplastic nevus syndrome*. During early childhood children in these families may develop only innocent-looking nevi.

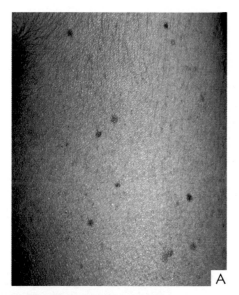

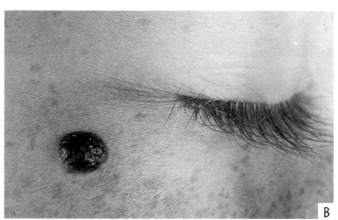

FIGURE 6.13 Pigmented nevi. Acquired nevomelanocytic nevi. **(A)** Junctional nevi. These brown macules are flat on palpation. **(B)** This typical compound nevus is raised, with a regular border and uniform pigmentation.

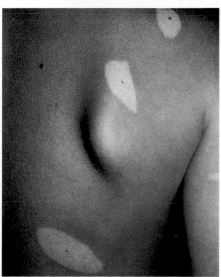

FIGURE 6.14 Large, hypopigmented halos surround these relatively small nevi on the back of this boy.

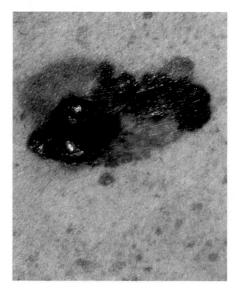

FIGURE 6.15 Melanoma. This lesion shows the irregularity of outline, color, and thickness typical of a melanoma.

However, the predisposition for the development of malignant melanoma is autosomal dominant, imparting a 50 percent risk to children of affected parents. The presence of a large number of nevi, particularly on the scalp and sun-protected sites in prepubertal children, may be an early marker for dysplastic nevus syndrome. Children in these high-risk families should be observed carefully for the development of dysplastic nevi at least through their adolescent years. Unusual appearance of nevi or changes in existing nevi should be biopsied to exclude malignant degeneration.

Another cause of melanoma in the pediatric age group is transplacental spread of maternal melanoma. Neonates born to mothers with a history of melanoma should be examined and followed carefully. Conversely, mothers of infants born with melanoma should be examined thoroughly for signs of the malignancy.

Differential diagnosis of childhood melanoma includes congenital and acquired nevomelanocytic nevi, the *blue nevus* (Fig. 6.16) (a small firm, blue papule consisting of deep nevus cells), traumatic hemorrhage, especially under the nails, on the heels, or in the mucous membranes, and a number of innocent vascular lesions such as pyogenic granuloma or hemangioma.

Spindle and epithelial cell nevus, also known generally as *Spitz nevus* after the author who first described it in 1948, is an innocent nevomelanocytic nevus that may be clinically and histologically confused with malignant melanoma (Fig. 6.17). Initially Spitz nevus was also referred to as *benign juvenile melanoma*. However, this term should be discarded because *melanoma* is misleading, and these lesions have recently been described in adults. Spitz nevi frequently appear as rapidly growing, dome-shaped, red papules or nodules on the face or extremities. Occasionally they contain large quantities of melanin and may appear brown or black. In most histopathologic specimens, malignant melanoma can be readily excluded. Consequently simple excision is usually adequate.

Diffuse hyperpigmentation has rarely been reported as progressive familial hyperpigmentation. Affected infants are born with splotches of macular hyperpigmentation that slowly increase in size and number to involve much of the skin surface. This can usually be differentiated from the normal pigmentary darkening that occurs during the first year of life in many infants, particularly those of dark races. Generalized bronze pigmentation may develop after phototherapy for hyperbilirubinemia, particularly in infants with a high direct bilirubin component. Most cases have resolved uneventfully after discontinuation of phototherapy, but occasional hepatic abnormalities and deaths have been reported.

Generalized hyperpigmentation may also occur after exposure to certain drugs (e.g., heavy metals, phenothiazines, antimalarials) and in association with a number of systemic endocrine and inflammatory disorders. In adrenocortical insufficiency, Cushing's syndrome, and acromegaly, melanotropin-stimulating hormone or other hormones with similar pigment-production-stimulating properties trigger generalized hyperpigmentation. Pigmentation may be particularly marked in skin creases on the palms and soles and mucous membranes in general. Increased epidermal and dermal melanin also occurs in hemochromatosis, chronic renal and hepatic disease, and extensive cutaneous fibrosis associated with dermatomyositis and scleroderma.

HYPOPIGMENTATION AND DEPIGMENTATION

Partial or complete pigmentary loss may be congenital or acquired in a localized or diffuse pattern. Localized disorders of pigmentation include hypopigmented macules of the newborn, incontinentia pigmenti achromians, piebaldism, postinflammatory hypopigmentation, and vitiligo. Generalized pigmentary disturbances occur in albinism and progressive vitiligo.

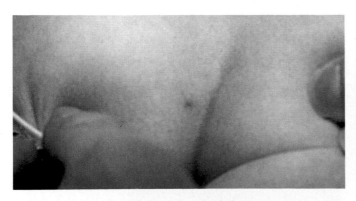

FIGURE 6.16 Blue nevus. This blue nodule was made up of deep nevus cells; it was firm on palpation.

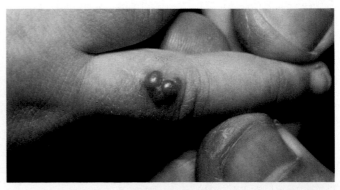

FIGURE 6.17 Spindle and epithelial cell nevus. This raised, red Spitz nevus grew rapidly.

Localized Hypopigmentation

Localized hypopigmentation is characteristic of several nevoid phenomena including hypopigmented macules, incontinentia pigmenti achromians, and piebaldism. Although 0.1 percent of normal newborns have *hypopigmented macules (ash leaf macules),* they may be a marker for tuberous sclerosis (Fig. 6.18). These macules appear at birth as 2-mm to 3-cm lesions on the trunk of 70 percent to 90 percent of individuals with tuberous sclerosis. Although macules are typically lancet-shaped, small confetti spots and oval, round, and irregularly shaped patches may appear on any body site.

The identification of hypopigmented macules may be enhanced in lightly pigmented children by the use of a Wood's light examination. The visible purple light emitted by the Wood's light is absorbed by melanin. In a darkened room subtle areas of depigmentation or hypopigmentation will appear bright violet; normal pigmented skin will absorb light and be dull purple or black.

Children with hypopigmented macules require close neurodevelopmental observation. Onset of other cutaneous findings, such as adenoma sebaceum (Fig. 6.19) or angiofibromas and subungual fibromas, and systemic symptoms of tuberous sclerosis, such as seizures and intracranial tumors, may be delayed for years. Tuberous sclerosis is transmitted as an autosomal dominant trait, but 25 percent to 50 percent of children represent new mutations. A careful family history and cutaneous exam-

ination of other family members may demonstrate subtle findings of tuberous sclerosis. The presence of asymptomatic rhabdomyomas, calcified intracranial tubers, renal angiolipomas, and cystic lesions in the kidneys and lungs will also support the diagnosis.

The term *nevus depigmentosus,* or *nevus achromicus,* should probably be used for the majority of children with one or two hypopigmented macules and no other signs of neurocutaneous disease (Fig. 6.20). However, nevus depigmentosus has rarely been reported in association with hemihypertrophy and mental retardation without findings of tuberous sclerosis. Hypopigmented macules on cosmetically important areas are readily camouflaged by rehabilitative cosmetics such as Dermablend and Covermark.

Nevus anemicus is often misdiagnosed as an ash leaf macule. This congenital patch, usually located on the trunk, appears pale compared to surrounding normal skin. However, a Wood's lamp examination demonstrates the presence of normal pigment. Rubbing the area results in erythema from vasodilitation in surrounding normal skin while the lesion remains unchanged. A persistent increase in vascular tone which results in maximal vasoconstriction in the nevus seems to account for this phenomenon.

Incontinentia pigmenti achromians, also known as *hypomelanosis of Ito* after the physician who first described the disorder in 1952, is characterized by con-

FIGURE 6.18 Ash leaf macules. A four-month-old boy was admitted to the pediatric neurology service for evaluation of seizures. Several ash-leaf-shaped hypopigmented macules were discovered on the back. A CT scan of the head demonstrated tumors typical of tuberous sclerosis.

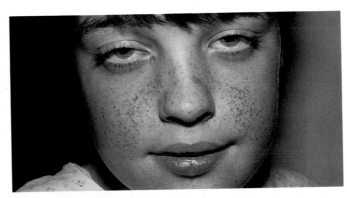

FIGURE 6.19 Adenoma sebaceum. Symmetric, red papules on the cheeks of this 12-year-old boy with a seizure disorder were initially dismissed as acne. A skin biopsy, however, demonstrated changes typical of an angiofibroma, and a CT scan of the head confirmed the diagnosis of tuberous sclerosis.

FIGURE 6.20 Nevus depigmentosus. An otherwise healthy infant was noted to have a congenital depigmented patch on the leg.

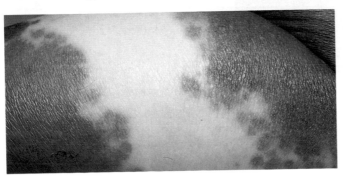

In oculocutaneous albinism (OCA) both sexes and all races are equally involved. OCA may be divided into a number of variants based on clinical findings and biochemical markers (Fig. 6.25). Tyrosinase-negative and tyrosinase-positive forms have been established based on the ability of plucked hairs incubated in tyrosine to produce pigment. In classic tyrosinase-negative OCA, children are born without any trace of pigment. Affected individuals have snow-white hair, pinkish-white skin, and blue eyes. Nystagmus is common as well as moderate to severe strabismus and poor visual acuity. Although children with tyrosinase-positive OCA may be clinically indistinguishable at birth from their tyrosinase-negative counterparts, they usually develop variable amounts of pigment with increasing age. Eye color may vary from gray to light brown, and hair may change to blond or light brown. Most black patients will acquire as much pigment as light-skinned whites.

In tyrosinase-negative albinism the enzyme tyrosinase is either absent or nonfunctional. Tyrosinase-positive albinism probably results from a number of different defects in pigment synthesis and transport.

In both tyrosinase-positive and -negative variants of albinism, "clear cells" are noted in the basal cell layer of the epidermis. However, epidermal melanocytes form pigment when incubated with dopa only in the tyrosinase-positive variants. Electron microscopy demonstrates the presence of small amounts of melanin and mature

Figure 6.25 Albinism		
Disorder	**Incidence**	**Inheritance**
Oculocutaneous (OCA)		
Tyrosinase-negative	1:30,000	Autosomal recessive
Tyrosinase-positive	1:37,000 whites 1:15,000 blacks	Autosomal recessive (rarely autosomal dominant)
Yellow mutant	Rare (described in Amish)	Autosomal recessive
Albinoidism	Uncommon	Autosomal dominant
Hermansky–Pudlak syndrome	Rare	Autosomal recessive
Chediak–Higashi syndrome	Rare	Autosomal recessive
Cross syndrome	Rare	Autosomal recessive
Ocular albinism		
Classic	Uncommon	X-linked recessive
Autosomal recessive	Rare	Autosomal recessive

melanosomes in tyrosinase-positive disease but no melanin and only early stages of melanosome development in tyrosinase-negative patients.

Patients with OCA require aggressive sun protection to prevent actinic damage and early development of basal cell and squamous cell skin cancers (see Fig. 6.24B). Strabismus and macular degeneration may also be associated with a progressive decrease in visual acuity. Consequently, ongoing ophthalmology input is also important for these patients.

Although the skin and hair appear clinically normal in ocular albinism, characteristic macromelanosomes have been demonstrated by electron microscopy. This finding is a reliable marker and may be used to confirm the diagnosis and identify asymptomatic female carriers.

Diffuse hypopigmentation may also suggest a number of other systemic disorders associated with defects in melanin synthesis in the skin, hair, and eyes. Children with inborn errors of amino acid metabolism (e.g., phenoketonuria, histidinemia, and homocystinuria) often demonstrate widespread pigment dilution. Hypopigmentation of skin and hair in Menke's kinky hair syndrome results from a defect in copper metabolism which interferes with the normal activity of copper-dependent tyrosinase. Hypohidrotic ectodermal dysplasia and deletion of the short arm of chromosome 18 are also associated with diffuse hypopigmentation and light hair color. Finally, children with malnutrition, particularly kwashiorkor, may develop hypopigmentation that resolves when adequate calorie and protein intake resume.

Figure 6.25 *continued*	
System Involved	**Comments**
Skin, hair, eyes	No pigment present, poor visual acuity
Skin, hair, eyes	Pigment with age, variable visual acuity
Skin, hair, eyes	Vision usually normal
Skin, hair, eyes	Vision usually normal
Light pigment generally, bleeding diathesis (platelet dysfunction), inflammatory bowel disease, pulmonary fibrosis	Tyrosinase-positive, ceroid-like material in system (variable visual acuity)
Pigment dilation generally, seizures, bone marrow failure, recurrent infection	Incidence of lymphomas
Skin, eyes, mental retardation, spasticity	Blind
Eye severely involved, skin appears normal	Macromelanosomes in skin of affected males and carrier females
Eye severely involved, freckling of generally lightly pigmented skin, light hair darkens with age	May have mild cutaneous pigment dilution

ALGORITHM FOR EVALUATION OF DISORDERS OF PIGMENTATION

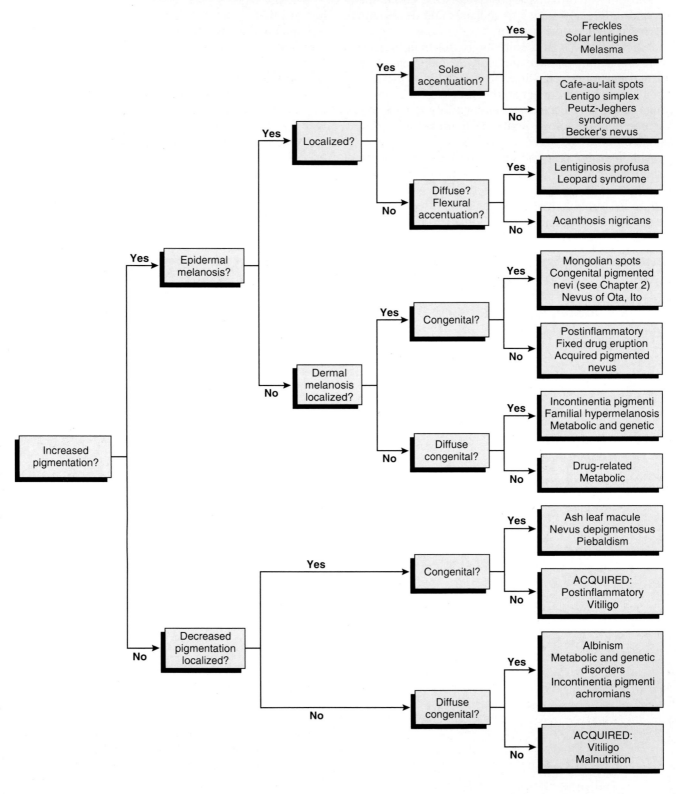

BIBLIOGRAPHY

Cafe-au-lait spot

Johnson BL, Charneco DR. Cafe-au-lait spot in neurofi-bromatosis and in normal individuals. *Arch Dermatol* 102:442–446, 1970.

Riccardi VM. Von Recklinghausen neurofibromatosis (review). *N Engl J Med* 305:1617–1627, 1981.

Riccardi VM. Neurofibromatosis and Albright's syndrome. In: Alper JA, ed. *Genetic Disorders of the Skin.* St Louis: Mosby Year Book, 1991:163–169.

Lentigo

Kaufmann J, Eichman A, Neves C, et al. Lentiginosa profusa. *Dermatologica* 153:116, 1976.

Voron DA, Hatfield HH, Kalkhoff RK. Multiple lentigines syndrome, case report and review of the literature. *Am J Med* 60:447–456, 1976.

Atherton DJA, Pitcher DW, Wells RS, et al. A syndrome of various cutaneous pigmented lesions, myxoid neu-rofibromata and atrial myxoma; The NAME syndrome. *Br J Dermatol* 103:421–429, 1980.

Cohen HJ, Minkin W, Frank SB. Nevus spilus. *Arch Dermatol* 102:433–437, 1970.

Tovar JA, Eizaguirre I, Albert A, et al. Peutz–Jeghers in children: report of two cases and review of the literature. *J Pediatr Surg* 18:1–6, 1983.

Becker's nevus

Becker SW. Concurrent melanosis and hypertrichosis in distribution of nevus unius lateris. *Arch Dermatol Syph* 60:155–160, 1949.

Urbanek RW, Johnson WC. Smooth muscle hamartoma associated with Becker's nevus. *Arch Dermatol* 114: 98–99, 1978.

Acanthosis nigricans and melasma

Sanchez NP, Pathak MA, Sato S, et al. Melasma: a clinical, light microscopic, ultrastructural, and immunoflu-orescence study. *J Am Acad Dermatol* 4:698–710, 1981.

Sanchez JL, Vasquez M. A hydroquinone solution in the treatment of melasma. *Int J Dermatol* 21:55–58, 1982.

Mongolian spot

Mevorah B, Frenk E, Delacretaz J. Dermal melanocyto-sis. *Dermatologica* 154:107–114, 1977.

Smalek JE. Significance of mongolian spots. *J Pediatr* 97:504–505, 1980.

Cordova A. The mongolian spot. *Clin Pediatr* 20:714–722, 1981.

Kopf AW, Weidman AJ. Nevus of Ota. *Arch Dermatol* 85:195–208, 1962.

Hidano A, Kajima H, Ikeda S, et al. Natural history of nevus of Ota. *Arch Dermatol* 95:187–195, 1967.

Fixed drug eruption

Korkij W, Soltani K. Fixed drug eruption. A brief review. *Arch Dermatol* 120:520–524, 1984.

Masu S, Seiji M. Pigmentary incontinence in fixed drug eruptions. *J Am Acad Dermatol* 8:525–532, 1983.

Pigmented nevi

Rhodes AR, Silverman RA, Harrist TJ, et al. A histo-logic comparison of congenital and acquired nevome-lanocytic nevi. *Arch Dermatol* 121: 1266–1273, 1985.

Maize JC, Foster G. Age related changes in melanocytic naevi. *Clin Exp Dermatol* 4:49–58, 1979.

Nicholls EM. Development and elimination of pigmented moles, and the anatomical distribution of primary malignant melanoma. *Cancer* 32: 191–195, 1973.

Pratt CB, Palmer MK, Thatcher N, et al. Malignant melanoma in children and adolescents. *Cancer* 47: 392–397, 1981.

Ackerman AB, Mihara I. Dysplasia, dysplastic melano-cytes, dysplastic nevi, the dysplastic nevus syndrome, and the relationship between dysplastic nevi and malignant melanomas. *Hum Pathol* 16:87–91, 1985.

National Institutes of Health Consensus Development Conference. Precursors to malignant melanoma. *J Am Acad Dermatol* 10:683–688, 1984.

Weedon D, Little JH. Spindle and epithelioid cell nevi in children and adults. A review of 211 cases of the Spitz nevus. *Cancer* 40:217–225, 1977.

Hypopigmented macules

Fitzpatrick TB, Szabo G, Hori Y, et al. White leaf-shaped macules. *Arch Dermatol* 98:1–6, 1968.

Fryer AE, Osborne JP. Tuberous sclerosis—a clinical appraisal. *Pediatr Rev Commun* 1:239–255, 1987.

Nevus anemicus

Fleisher TL, Zeligman I. Nevus anemicus. *Arch Dermatol* 100:750–755, 1969.

Incontinentia pigmenti achromians

Happle R. Tentative assignment of hypomelanosis of Ito to 9q33-qter. *Hum Genet* 75:98–99, 1987.

Ishikawa T, Kanayama M, Sugiyama, et al. Hypomelanosis of Ito associated with benign tumors and chromosomal abnormalities: a neurocutaneous syndrome. *Brain Dev* 7:45–49, 1985.

Piebaldism

Wardenburg MF. A new syndrome combining develop-mental anomalies of the eyelids, eyebrows and nose root with congenital deafness. *Am J Hum Genet* 3:195–253, 1951.

The term *reactive erythemas* refers to a group of disorders characterized by erythematous patches, plaques, and nodules that vary in size, shape, and distribution. Unlike other specific dermatoses, these lesions represent cutaneous reaction patterns triggered by a variety of endogenous and environmental agents. In children the most common reactive erythemas include drug eruptions, urticaria, viral exanthems, erythema multiforme, erythema nodosum, vasculitis, photosensitive eruptions, and collagen vascular disorders.

DRUG ERUPTIONS

Two to 3 percent of all patients admitted to the hospital experience an adverse drug reaction, and about half of them develop a rash. Drug-induced rashes are also a frequent diagnostic problem in the outpatient setting. Although the skin rash often occurs alone, it may be accompanied by fever, arthritis, and other systemic findings. Almost half of the rashes are morbilliform, followed by urticaria in 25 percent, fixed drug reactions in 10 percent, erythema multiforme in 5 percent, and exfoliative, lichenoid, and acneiform eruptions in less than 5 percent each. Early recognition of drug-related rashes and discontinuation of the inciting agent may prevent progressive, life-threatening complications.

Morbilliform Drug Eruptions

Morbilliform rashes (measles-like, maculopapular, exanthematous) account for the majority of drug-induced rashes. Typically, after five to 10 days of drug therapy, red macules and papules erupt on the extremities and spread centrally to involve the trunk. Not infrequently, however, the trunk is the first area to be involved and the rash spreads centripetally (Fig. 7.1). Lesions may become confluent, but the perioral and perinasal areas are often spared. Conjunctival and oral mucosal erythema may be prominent. Although the rash is often asymptomatic, sometimes pruritus is severe. The skin may be the only organ system initially involved, but fever, arthralgias, and general malaise may follow. Occasionally the rash resolves despite continuation of the medication. However, in rare instances the lesions progress to erythema multiforme or toxic epidermal necrolysis, with widespread necrosis of the epidermis.

Almost any drug can trigger a morbilliform rash. Among the common categories implicated are antibiotics, anticonvulsants, and antihypertensives. Prompt diagnosis and discontinuation of the drug usually results in improvement in one to two days and resolution within a week. Occasionally the rash does not appear until several days after the drug course has been completed.

Unfortunately, morbilliform rashes often appear in febrile children who have been placed on antibiotics for treatment of presumed bacterial infections such as sinusitis and otitis media. The differentiation of a viral infection with associated exanthem from a drug rash is usually impossible, and many of these children are presumed to be allergic to antibiotics. In some patients,

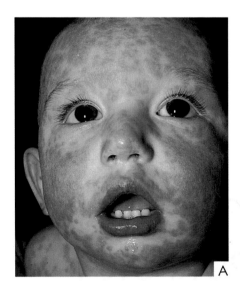
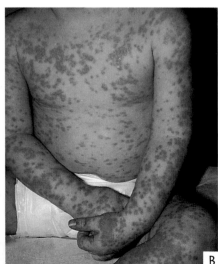

FIGURE 7.1 (A,B) A morbilliform reaction to phenobarbital developed in a toddler after two weeks of treatment with phenobarbital for febrile seizures. Lesions were most prominent on the face, upper trunk, and extremities. Note the perioral and perinasal sparing.

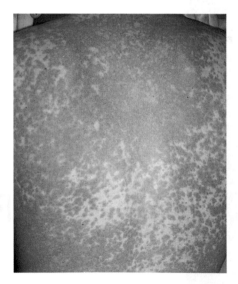

FIGURE 7.2 A teenager who was initially diagnosed with streptococcal pharyngitis was started on amoxicillin. Four days later a morbilliform rash erupted on the trunk and spread to the face and extremities. A monospot test was positive in the office, and the antibiotic was discontinued.

recognition of specific viral exanthems and serologic confirmation will support an infectious etiology. Moreover, some drugs may interact with certain viruses to produce an exanthem, such as the rash seen in up to 90 percent of children with mononucleosis who are accidentally treated with ampicillin (Fig. 7.2). The differential diagnosis also includes graft versus host disease (see Chapter 9) and Kawasaki disease, but the medical history and associated findings will help to exclude these disorders.

Erythema Multiforme

Erythema multiforme (EM) is a distinctive, acute hypersensitivity syndrome that can be caused by a number of drugs as well as by viruses, bacterial infections, foods, and immunizations. It may also arise in association with connective tissue disorders and malignancy. Medications and infectious diseases are the most common triggering factors in children.

The classic eruption is symmetrical, and may occur on any part of the body, although it typically appears on the dorsum of the hands and feet and on the extensor surfaces of the arms and legs (Fig. 7.3A). Involvement of the palms and soles is common. The initial lesions are dusky red macules or wheals that evolve into iris- or target-shaped plaques, the hallmark of EM. The annular configuration occurs as the central inflammatory process spreads peripherally and leaves behind a depressed, damaged epidermis. When epidermal injury is severe, full-thickness necrosis leads to formation of central bullae. In some cases, multiple concentric erythematous rings develop around dusky areas, forming bull's-eye lesions. The eruption continues in crops that last from one to three weeks. In most patients, mucous membrane involvement is minimal, the disease is self-limited, and systemic manifestations are confined to low-grade fever, malaise, and myalgia (EM minor).

Rarely, erythema multiforme progresses to become *Stevens–Johnson syndrome (EM major)*, with large areas of epidermal and mucous membrane necrosis and shedding (Fig. 7.3B and C) Hence, Stevens–Johnson syndrome is believed to represent the most severe end of the spectrum of EM. In this disorder the constitutional symptoms are severe, including high fever, cough,

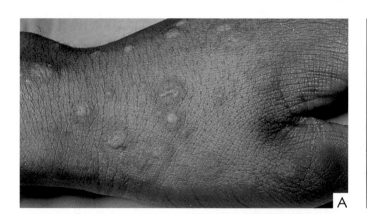

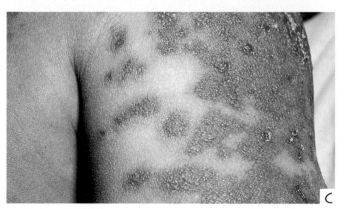

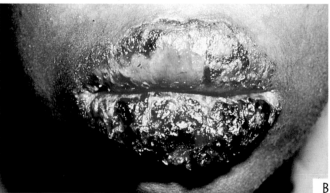

FIGURE 7.3 Erythema multiforme. (**A**) Typical target lesions erupted on the arms and legs of this nine-year-old boy with recurrent EM minor, probably resulting from a barbiturate in a cold remedy. He had only minimal mucous membrane involvement. (**B,C**) Severe mucous membrane lesions occurred in this adolescent with Stevens–Johnson syndrome. Note the thick hemorrhagic crusts on the lips and necrotic, hemorrhagic bullae on his arm.

sore throat, vomiting, diarrhea, chest pain, and arthralgias. Blister formation occurs early and is often hemorrhagic and extensive. Mucous membrane involvement, particularly of the oral, conjunctival, and urethral mucous membranes, is typical and often severe. It consists of formation of fragile, thin-walled bullae that rupture with minimal trauma, leaving ulcerations that are rapidly covered by exudate. Keratitis may result in ocular infection and formation of synechiae. Loss of the epidermal barrier results in fluid and electrolyte imbalances and a high risk of secondary bacterial infection. The mortality rate ranges between 5 percent and 25 percent.

Although the skin biopsy findings vary according to the clinical presentation, several characteristic findings allow histologic confirmation. A perivascular mononuclear cell infiltrate with some eosinophils is present in the papillary dermis. Variable hydropic degeneration of the basal cell layer is associated with the formation of colloid bodies and, in severe cases, with subepidermal blister formation. Dyskeratosis may be mild or widespread, ranging from discrete satellite cell necrosis to almost total necrosis of the epidermis.

In cases of drug-induced EM, it is imperative that the clinician identify the inciting agent. Failure to do so may result in the development of severe, recurrent disease on re-exposure to the medication. Herpes simplex infections are also associated with repeated episodes of EM, usually the minor variant.

During acute episodes, careful cleaning and protection of bullous lesions is imperative to reduce the risk of infection. Patients with Stevens–Johnson syndrome may require intensive supportive care in a burn unit.

Toxic Epidermal Necrolysis

Although originally described in adults, toxic epidermal necrolysis (TEN) has been reported in children, especially in association with drug hypersensitivity reactions. The condition usually begins with fever, sore throat, malaise, and a generalized sunburn-like erythema, followed by sloughing of large areas of skin (see

Chapter 4). The entire skin surface as well as the conjunctivae, urethra, rectum, oral and nasal mucosa, larynx, and tracheobronchial mucosa may become involved. Although a Nikolsky sign is present and the erythema is reminiscent of staphylococcal scalded-skin syndrome (SSSS), the site of cleavage in TEN is at the dermal–epidermal junction and results in full epidermal necrosis. Many investigators equate TEN with the most fulminant presentation of Stevens–Johnson syndrome because the inciting agents and the clinical courses are similar.

Frozen sections of sloughed epidermis can be used for rapid differentiation of TEN from SSSS while the practitioner awaits the definitive results of a skin biopsy. Intensive supportive measures are required to avoid fluid and electrolyte losses and secondary bacterial infection. Respiratory distress syndrome has been reported in severe cases.

Morbidity and mortality are comparable to those in patients with Stevens–Johnson syndrome. In uncomplicated cases, re-epithelialization of the skin occurs within several weeks and full recovery in four to six weeks. Scarring may develop in areas of secondary infection. Careful ongoing ophthalmologic evaluation is necessary to reduce the complications of severe conjunctival and corneal involvement.

Fixed Drug Eruption

Fixed drug eruption is a distinctive reaction pattern characterized by the sudden development of erythema multiforme-like annular, erythematous, edematous plaques, from 1 to over 5 cm in diameter, after exposure to any of a number of medications (Fig. 7.4). Intense edema may result in frank bulla formation. When the drug is withdrawn, the lesions flatten, the erythema fades, and prominent postinflammatory hyperpigmentation persists for weeks to months. On re-exposure to the allergen, old lesions reappear and new plaques may slowly progress.

Although the rash may develop at any site, the lips and genitals are most commonly involved. The most

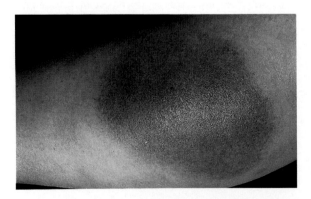

FIGURE 7.4 Fixed drug reaction. A red, edematous plaque recurred on the arm of a 16-year-old girl each month when she took a nonsteroidal anti-inflammatory agent for menstrual cramps. Some residual hyperpigmentation is present in the center of the plaque from prior flares.

frequent triggering agents include trimethoprim-sulfamethoxazole, aspirin, tetracycline, phenolphthalein (present in laxatives), barbiturates, and phenylbutazone.

Although the cause is not known, T lymphocytes that reside in the dermis are thought to be responsible for both the acute reaction and the cutaneous memory function of the fixed drug eruption. Histologic findings are similar to those of erythema multiforme, but pigment incontinence tends to be intense. This explains the impressive discrete hyperpigmentation, which may be the only clinical finding between episodes. Once the diagnosis is considered, the allergen can be identified and avoided.

Urticaria

Urticaria, commonly known as hives, is characterized by the sudden appearance of transient, well-demarcated wheals that are usually intensely pruritic, especially when they arise as part of an acute IgE-mediated hypersensitivity reaction (Fig. 7.5A–C). Individual lesions usually last for several minutes to several hours, but occasionally they may persist for up to 24 hours. Wheals may have a red center with an edematous white halo or the reverse, an edematous white center with a red halo. The size can vary from a few millimeters to giant lesions more than 20 cm in diameter. Central clearing with peripheral extension may lead to the formation of annular, polycyclic, and arcuate plaques that simulate erythema multiforme and erythema marginatum. The reaction may involve the mucous membranes and can spread to the subcutaneous tissue, producing "woody" edema known as angioedema (Fig. 7.6). Histopathology usually demonstrates a mild lymphocytic perivascular infiltrate with marked dermal edema.

Urticaria can be triggered by a variety of immunologic mechanisms, including IgE-antibody response, complement activation, and abnormal response to vasoactive amines. Most cases of acute urticaria, which lasts for less than six weeks, are caused by a hypersensitivity reaction to drugs, food, insect bites, contact antigens, inhaled substances, or acute infections. Physical agents including cold, heat, water, exercise and mechanical pressure can also trigger hives. In less than 5 percent of patients the process evolves into chronic urticaria, which lasts from six weeks to many years.

Specific drugs and foods known to cause hives should be avoided because of the risk of inducing anaphylaxis on subsequent exposure. Exhaustive laboratory

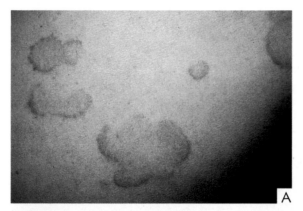

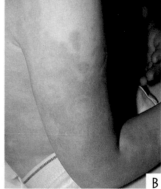

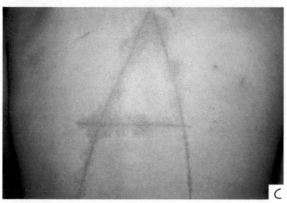

FIGURE 7.5 **(A)** Widespread urticaria developed during a course of amoxacillin for otitis media. Note the discrete annular plaques on the trunk of this three-year-old. **(B)** Wheals have become confluent on the trunk and extremities of this boy. **(C)** Dermatographism, which is common in patients with urticaria, was produced by the examiner on the back of an adolescent with chronic hives.

studies in an otherwise healthy child are unlikely to be rewarding. Laboratory evaluation should be guided by the findings on history and physical examination. Patients with chronic disease require intermittent re-examination, particularly if other problems such as arthritis, diarrhea, or fever develop.

Extensive urticaria associated with pruritus may respond readily to H_1 antihistamines such as diphenhydramine, hydroxyzine, or chlorpheniramine. Dosages should be pushed to twice the recommended level or until unacceptable adverse reactions are noted. Most children accommodate quickly to the sedation associated with these medications. In resistant cases, the addition of an H_2 antihistamine such as cimetidine or ranitidine and/or beta-adrenergic agonists such as ephedrine and terbutaline may be helpful. Several new nonsedating antihistamines, including astemizole and terfenadine, are particularly useful in chronic urticaria. Epinephrine may be lifesaving in urticaria and angioedema that involve the airway. Systemic corticosteroids should be reserved for patients with life-threatening disease.

Urticarial lesions may appear early in the course of serum sickness reactions triggered by infectious agents or drugs. Asymptomatic or painful red papules, expanding annular plaques, and target lesions suggestive of erythema multiforme are associated with fever, arthralgias, periarticular swelling, and occasionally frank arthritis. The skin lesions differ from classic urticaria by the lack of pruritus and persistence beyond 24 hours. This reaction has been reported recently with cefaclor but may also occur with a number of other antibiotics (Fig. 7.7). Skin biopsies usually demonstrate a lympho-histiocytic dermal inflammatory infiltrate, but occasionally vasculitis is present.

Erythema marginatum, one of the major criteria for rheumatic fever, which occurs in 20 percent of patients, may be confused with hives (Fig. 7.8). This eruption is characterized by transient, asymptomatic red papules which enlarge over several hours to form annular, scalloped, and serpiginous expanding plaques with narrow borders and central clearing. Successive crops appear on the trunk and extremities as old plaques fade. New lesions typically flare with evening fever spikes, and involvement is restricted predominantly to the trunk and proximal extremities. The absence of pruritus helps to distinguish erythema marginatum from hives, and skin biopsies show predominantly a perivascular neutrophilic infiltrate. The diagnosis of rheumatic fever is dependent on the recognition of other well-defined criteria.

Urticaria must also be distinguished from the figurate erythemas and other reactive erythemas discussed later in this chapter.

Exfoliative, Lichenoid, and Acneiform Drug Reactions

Drugs may also trigger reactions that mimic other cutaneous conditions. In an *exfoliative erythroderma*, widespread inflammation in the skin is associated with generalized erythema and scale. The entire surface is involved, including the scalp, palms and soles. Although this reaction pattern usually evolves from a primary cutaneous disorder such as atopic dermatitis, seborrheic dermatitis, psoriasis, or T-cell lymphoma, a number of medications including allopurinol, barbiturates, capto-

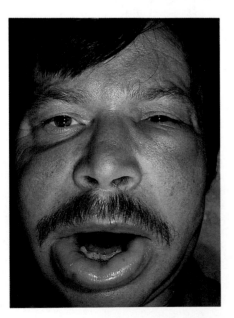

FIGURE 7.6 This young adult developed recurrent episodes of idiopathic angioedema. Fortunately, although his face and lips were frequently involved, he never experienced layrngeal edema or dyspnea.

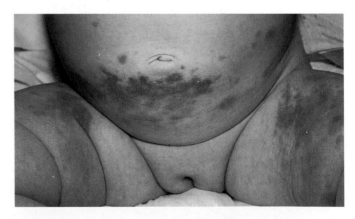

FIGURE 7.7 A 10-month-old girl developed urticaria on the lower trunk and thighs while being treated with cefclor for an ear infection. Although the drug was stopped, the annular plaques progressed and became purpuric centrally. The rash was accompanied by arthralgias, joint swelling, and fever consistent with a serum-sickness picture.

pril, carbamazepine, chloroquine, cimetidine, diltiazem, griseofulvin, gold, thiazide diuretics, isoniazid, hydantoins, D-penicillamine, quinidine, and sulfonamides have been implicated in some patients. A history of drug exposure, preceding rashes, and associated findings will provide clues to the cause of the erythroderma. Histopathology usually reveals a chronic dermatitis. However, the presence of eosinophils suggests a hypersensitivity reaction, while other distinct findings will point to an underlying skin disorder.

In *lichenoid drug reactions*, the clinical findings are usually indistinguishable from lichen planus (see Chapter 3). However, the dermal infiltrate may contain eosinophils, which is unusual for classic lichen planus. Withdrawal of medications may lead to improvement of the eruption over weeks to months. Drugs that have been reported to cause lichenoid reactions include thiazide diuretics, streptomycin, isoniazid, methyl-dopa, beta-blockers, naproxen, and captopril.

Acneiform drug reactions can be distinguished from typical acne vulgaris by the presence of uniform inflammatory papules and pustules (rather than the mixed comedones and inflammatory lesions seen in acne vulgaris), involvement of the usual acne areas (face, shoulders, upper trunk) as well as the lower trunk, arms, and legs, acute onset with introduction of the inciting drug, and resistance to standard therapy (see Chapter 8). Medications may also exacerbate pre-existing acne. Commonly implicated drugs include corticosteroids, ACTH, isoniazid, lithium, iodides, bromides, oral contraceptives, quinidine, and anticonvulsants. Although the eruption may improve with the use of systemic and topical acne preparations, severe or recalcitrant cases

may require that the medication be decreased or discontinued when possible.

VIRAL EXANTHEMAS

A number of viral infections have cutaneous manifestations that provide a clue to the diagnosis. In some of these infections the skin rash is the major finding. Early recognition of distinct exanthems also helps to differentiate viral infections from drug reactions, bacterial and rickettsial rashes, and other reactive erythemas.

In the early twentieth century, clinicians commonly referred to childhood exanthems by number. Scarlet fever and measles were known as first and second disease, but the two rashes were frequently confused. Rubella was established as an entity distinct from measles and was known as third disease. In 1900, Duke described fourth disease, which probably does not represent a distinct condition but a combination of rubella and scarlet fever. Fifth disease is recognized today as erythema infectiosum, and roseola finishes off the numbered exanthems as sixth disease. Many other viruses produce distinct reaction reaction patterns in the skin. Herpes and pox viruses are readily diagnosed by their characteristic vesiculobullous eruptions, while picornaviruses, which include the enteroviruses, are well known for their maculopapular exanthems.

Viruses trigger exanthems by a number of mechanisms. Direct infection of the skin occurs in varicella, enteroviruses, and herpetic infections. Other rashes, such as measles and rubella, are probably caused by a combination of viral spread to the skin and host immuno-

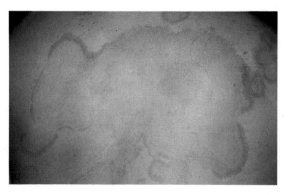

FIGURE 7.8 Erythema marginatum in a child with acute rheumatic fever. Note the scalloped margins and distribution on the trunk.

logic response. Some host-virus interactions are activated by exposure to certain drugs, exemplified by the generalized maculopapular eruption that occurs in more than 90 percent of patients with Epstein–Barr virus infection who are given ampicillin.

Measles and Rubella

In the pre-vaccine era, measles and rubella were common, and their exanthems became a paradigm for other "morbilliform" rashes. Although the usual late winter to early spring epidemics have been interrupted by widespread vaccination in industrialized nations, failure to immunize significant numbers of children during the last decade has resulted in a resurgence of cases in the United States.

Measles (rubeola, red measles, 10-day measles) is a highly contagious, potentially severe illness with a prodrome characterized by fever, malaise, dry cough, coryza, conjunctivitis, and severe photophobia (Fig. 7.9). Several days into the course, diagnostic Koplik's spots appear on the buccal and labial mucosae. Lesions consist of 1-mm to 3-mm bluish-white papules surrounded by red halos, which increase in number and fade over two to three days. Unfortunately, this characteristic enanthem is often transient and goes unnoticed.

On the third or fourth day of illness the exanthem first appears on the face as a blanching, red, maculopapular eruption which spreads cephalocaudad over three days, ultimately involving the palms and soles (Fig. 7.10A and B). Once generalized, the lesions become confluent on the face, trunk, and extremities in succession. Older lesions commonly develop a rusty hue caused by capillary leakage and hemosiderin deposition. The rash begins to fade after three days and clearing is complete three days later, giving a total of nine or 10 days' duration for the illness. One to two weeks after resolution of the rash widespread desquamation may appear.

Patients are contagious four days before the exanthem until four days after it appears. During the illness fever may be persistent and severe. Generalized adenopathy is common. Morbidity and mortality are highest in patients who are compromised by hereditary or acquired immunodeficiency and in those in Third World countries where malnutrition is rampant. Potential complications resulting from primary viral infection or secondary bacterial infection include otitis media, pneumonitis, meningitis, acute encephalitis, and obstructive laryngotracheitis. Atypical measles is an unusual syndrome that occurs in individuals who received killed measles vaccine, when it was available between 1963 and 1967, and are subsequently exposed to the measles virus. Unlike typical measles, the exanthem begins and remains primarily on the extremities and often develops a petechial component. Koplik's spots are absent, fevers are high, and pneumonitis is usually severe. This disorder probably represents a hypersensitivity reaction to the virus and is most frequently confused with Rocky Mountain spotted fever and collagen vascular disease.

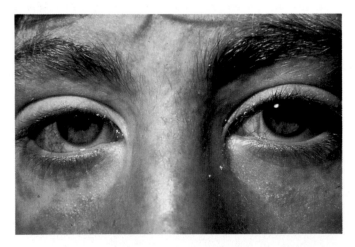

FIGURE 7.9 Rubeola/measles. During and after the prodroma period, the conjunctivae are injected and produce a clear discharge. This is associated with marked photophobia.

Rubella (German measles) is known as three-day measles because the pink maculopapular exanthem, which mimics a mild case of measles, usually evolves over one to three days (Fig. 7.11). In fact, nearly 25 percent of patients exhibit only mild upper respiratory symptoms with little or no rash.

Rubella is typically associated with several days of low-grade fever, adenopathy, headache, sore throat, and coryza. In young children fever may last for less than 24 hours. Forscheimer spots consist of transient, small, red papules on the soft palate which are seen in some patients at the beginning of the rash. This enanthem helps to distinguish this otherwise nonspecific eruption from other maculopapular viral exanthems.

As with measles, the peak incidence of rubella is in the late winter and early spring. Serological testing may be necessary to make a specific diagnosis, particularly if the patient is pregnant. Although complications are rare in children, the fetus is particularly susceptible to intrauterine infection during the first trimester, with complications including spontaneous abortion, diffuse cataracts, microphthalmia, glaucoma, deafness, and congenital heart disease. Up to 25 percent of infected newborns will develop severe disseminated disease with jaundice, pneumonitis, meningoencephalitis, bony abnormalities, thrombocytopenia, blueberry muffin lesions, and a maculopapular exanthem. Babies with congenital infection may shed virus in urine, stools, and

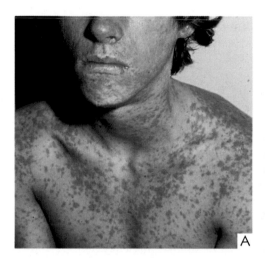
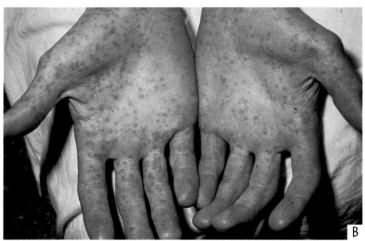

FIGURE 7.10 (A) The measles exanthem is a blotchy, erythematous, blanching maculopapular eruption that appears at the hairline and then spreads cephalocaudally over three days (B), ultimately involving the palms and soles. With evolution les-ions become confluent at proximal sites.

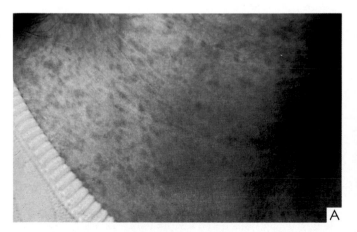
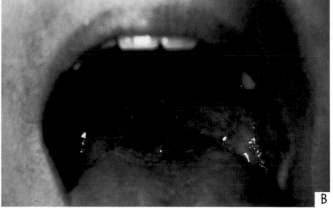

FIGURE 7.11 Rubella/German measles. (A) The exanthem of rubela usually consists of a fine pinkish-red maculopapular eruption that appears first at the hairline and rapidly spreads cephalocaudally. Lesions tend to remain discrete. (B) The presence of red palatal lesions (Forscheimer spots), seen in some patients on the first day of the rash, and occipital and posterior cervical adenopathy are suggestive findings of rubella.

respiratory secretions for up to a year and should be isolated from other infants and pregnant women.

Fifth Disease

In 1983, *erythema infectiosum (fifth disease)* was linked to human parvovirus B19. Since then investigators have defined the clinical features and epidemiology of infection in normal and compromised patients.

In its most commonly recognized clinical presentation, viral infection presents in school-aged children with asymptomatic "slapped-cheek" erythema on the face and a lacy or reticulated blanching erythema on the trunk and extremities (Fig. 7.12A and B). Although the exanthem usually fades over two to three weeks, lesions may recur for up to three months, especially when cutaneous blood flow is increased after fever or vigorous physical activity.

The prevalence of B19 antibody is about 5 to 10 percent in children under five years and rises to over 50 percent in adults. Human volunteer studies suggest that the virus is spread in respiratory secretions. After a five- to seven-day incubation period, infectivity peaks during the viremia, which lasts five to seven days. The end of viremia is marked by a rise in IgM and then in IgG antibody and is followed two to five days later by the appearance of the rash. Consequently, the risk of infection is low when the exanthem is diagnosed, and children can remain in school.

Associated symptoms, including fever and arthralgias, are usually mild or absent in young children. However, arthralgias or frank arthritis can be severe in adolescents and adults. At least 25 percent of patients with serological evidence of disease never develop the exanthem, and the arthropathy can develop before, after, or without the rash.

Early in the infection most patients experience a transient reticulocytopenia for seven to 10 days and a clinically insignificant drop in hemoglobin. This phenomenon, however, may trigger an aplastic crisis in patients with severe hemoglobinopathies. The virus has also been implicated as a cause of hydrops fetalis in pregnant women without other evidence of clinical disease. In hereditary or acquired immunodeficiency syndromes, B19 may produce persistent infection and chronic life-threatening anemia.

The reticulated exanthem of erythema infectiosum may be confused with *livedo reticularis*, a persistent, lacy, blanching violaceous erythema that occurs in a primary and secondary form (Fig. 7.13). In the idiopathic variant, lesions are symmetric and widespread, with poorly defined borders. Unlike cutis marmorata in neonates, the pattern does not resolve with warming. This exanthem occurs most commonly in young women who are otherwise healthy. The secondary variant is more common in men and has been reported in association with periarteritis nodosa, hepatitis, syphilis, and a number of other infections, connective tissue diseases, and malignancy.

Sixth Disease

Roseola or *exanthem subitum* (the "surprise" rash) has been recognized by pediatricians for over a century. The

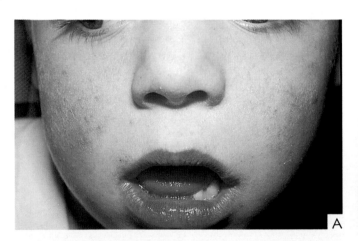

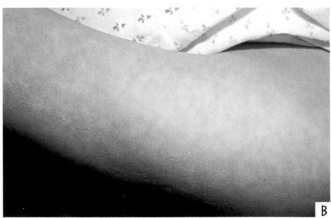

FIGURE 7.12 Fifth disease. (**A**) The typical "slapped-cheek" rash and (**B**) reticulated erythema on the trunk and extremities were present in this otherwise healthy five-year-old boy. The lesions flared intermittently for six weeks.

classic clinical course occurs in children between six months and three years old. After a three- to five-day illness marked by high spiking fevers, which occasionally trigger febrile seizures, a sudden end to the fever is followed by the appearance of a widely disseminated pink papular rash (Fig. 7.14). As in fifth disease, the end of viremia is marked by the development of the rash and a rise in antibody to the causative agent, human herpesvirus 6 (HH6). Consequently, the risk of infection is greatest during the febrile period and is minimal after appearance of the rash.

Serologic studies show an almost universal exposure of the population to HH6. Although only a third of infants develop clinical disease, the prevalence of antibody increases from less then 10 percent in children under six months of age to 75 percent to 90 percent in adults. Consequently, a large number of children develop asymptomatic infection. Conversely, seroprevalence studies of febrile infants demonstrate that viral infection may commonly produce a febrile illness without a rash.

HH6 has also been linked to a mononucleosis-like illness in young adults, and its role as an immunomodulator is being investigated in the immunodeficient host.

Papular Acrodermatitis

In 1956, Gianotti and Crosti described a distinctive exanthem associated with anicteric hepatitis, lymphadenopathy, and hepatitis B surface antigenemia, subtype ayw. The skin rash consists of flat-topped, 3-mm to 10-mm, skin-colored to red edematous papules involving the arms, legs, buttocks, and face (Fig. 7.15). Lesions on the calves and the extensor surfaces of the arms may become so edematous as to appear vesicular, and occasionally frank vesicles are present.

During the last decade it has become apparent that most cases in the United States are caused by other viruses, including enteroviruses, respiratory viruses,

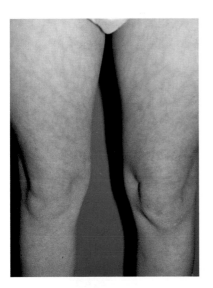

FIGURE 7.13
Widespread livedo reticularis was particularly prominent on the proximal extremities of this young adult with secondary syphilis.

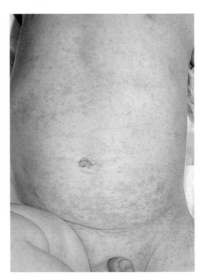

FIGURE 7.14
Roseola/exanthem subitum. A generalized, pink, maculopapular rash suddenly appeared on this infant after three days of high fever.

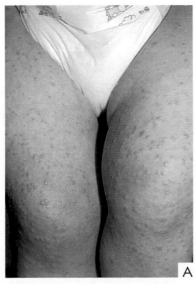
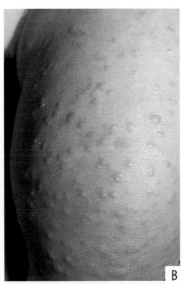

FIGURE 7.15 Papular acrodermatitis. **(A)** A symmetric, acrally distributed, red papular rash developed in this toddler with low-grade fever and loose stools. **(B)** Note the distinct, edematous papules on the close-up of the knee.

and Epstein–Barr virus. Serologic screening is still important because of the public health implications of hepatitis B infection. Since most children are asymptomatic, no treatment is necessary. However, parents should be counseled that the eruption may persist for up to several months.

Papular acrodermatitis can be differentiated from lichen planus, which is usually extremely pruritic. A negative history of recent drug exposure should exclude a lichenoid drug eruption. Other viral eruptions may be also be confused with papular acrodermatitis. Unfortunately, the histopathology is not specific and shows focal spongiosis and exocytosis in the epidermis overlying a perivascular, lymphocytic dermal infiltrate.

Other Viral Exanthems

Exanthems associated with the enteroviruses are quite variable and usually follow a shorter incubation period than the classic viral exanthems. Although they occur year 'round, the incidence peaks in the late summer and early fall. Maculopapular, vesicular, petechial, and urticarial eruptions are variably present, usually in association with fever (Fig. 7.16). Other symptoms may include meningitis, conjunctivitis, cough, coryza, pharyngitis, and pneumonia. Hand, foot, and mouth syndrome is a distinctive entity associated with papulovesicular lesions on the palms, soles, palate, and not infrequently the trunk, particularly the buttocks. Coxsackie viruses A5, A10, and A16, and echovirus 71 have been identified in patients with this syndrome. Papulovesicular rashes can be differentiated from varicella/zoster and herpes simplex infections by obtaining a Tzanck smear. The clinical course and, if necessary, cultures and serologic studies will help in making a specific diagnosis. Although meningococcal infections tend to peak during the winter and spring, occasional

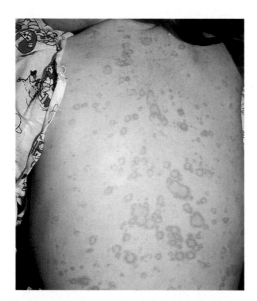

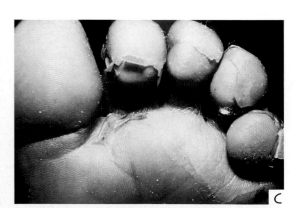

FIGURE 7.16 An urticarial viral exanthem spread from the trunk to the face and extremities in this infant. Lesions faded over several days.

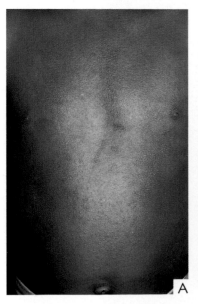

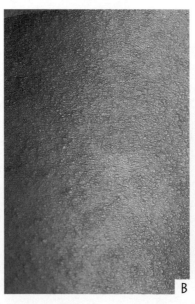

FIGURE 7.17 Scarlet fever. (A) A generalized, bright-red, fine papular rash developed in a seven-year-old boy with a streptococcal pharyngitis. (B) Note the sandpaper-like papules on his abdomen. (C) Ten days later he began to desquamate in large sheets around the tips of his toes and fingers.

cases occur during the summer and fall enteroviral season. Consequently, the child with a petechial exanthem and presumed enteroviral meningitis should be evaluated carefully to exclude a bacterial infection.

Infection with cytomegalovirus, Epstein–Barr virus, and respiratory viruses can be associated with macular, morbilliform, or urticarial exanthems which are difficult to differentiate from drug rashes. Children who require medications and develop intercurrent viral infections may remain on their medications under close observation. These minor viral exanthems usually fade in several days, whereas drug reactions tend to persist or intensify. However, drugs should be discontinued in any patients who develop urticaria, angioedema, erythema multiforme, or other signs of progressive allergic reactions.

SCARLANTINIFORM RASHES

The rash of scarlet fever provides a model for a number of important disorders which must be distinguished by other signs and symptoms. Bacterial toxins, viral infections, drugs, and Kawasaki syndrome have all been associated with scarlatiniform eruptions.

Scarlet Fever

Scarlet fever is characterized by a fine, red, papular, sandpaper-like rash that begins on the face and neck and generalizes to the trunk and extremities within one to two days (Fig. 7.17A–C). The skin is warm and flushed, and some patients complain of mild pruritus. Circumoral pallor is typical but not diagnostic. The rash ranges from a subtle pink to a fiery red color and usually follows the onset of streptococcal pharyngitis by 24

to 48 hours. The palms, soles, and conjunctivae are usually spared. "Pastia's lines" refers to the accentuation of the rash from linear petechiae which occur in the flexural creases of the arms, legs, and trunk. Other associated symptoms include nausea, vomiting, fever, headache, general malaise, and abdominal pain. In classic cases the pharynx is beefy red with palatal petechiae, purulent tonsillitis, and tender cervical adenopathy. Early in the course the lingual papillae poke through a white membrane (white strawberry tongue). Shedding of the membrane by the fourth to fifth day results in a bright-red strawberry tongue (Fig. 7.18). In many patients the throat infection is mild or completely asymptomatic. Scarlet fever may also be associated with streptococcal impetigo.

The rash is triggered by one of three antigenically distinct erythrotoxins which are produced by most strains of group A β-hemolytic *Streptococcus*. Development of antibodies against the streptococcal organism and erythrotoxin is protective and results in resolution of the symptoms and rash within four to five days. This is followed one to two weeks later by generalized desquamation, particularly marked on the fingertips and toes. Although both oral and cutaneous infections with nephritogenic streptococci can trigger glomerulonephritis, only pharyngeal infections have been associated with subsequent development of rheumatic fever. Treatment of patients with amoxicillin or penicillin (erythromycin in penicillin-allergic patients) may shorten the course of fever and other symptoms. If antibiotics are initiated within 10 days of the onset of pharyngitis, the risk of rheumatic fever can be reduced from 3 percent to less than 1 percent. Unfortunately, early treatment of nephritogenic strains has not been shown to decrease the incidence of poststreptococcal

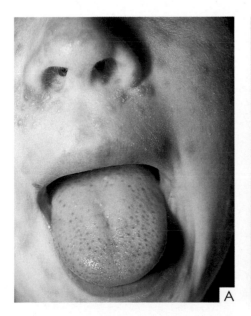 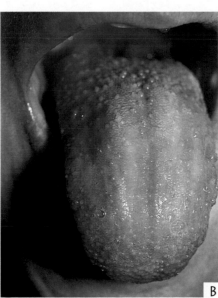

FIGURE 7.18 Scarlet fever. **(A)** A white strawberry tongue is usually followed by **(B)** a red strawberry tongue as the erythrotoxin-mediated enanthem evolves.

renal disease. Moreover, asymptomatic pharyngeal infection may escape detection until after the development of late complications.

Several other toxin-mediated syndromes may be confused with scarlet fever. Children with staphylococcal scarlet fever develop a rash that can be indistinguishable from streptococcal disease. A Nikolsky sign may be present but pharyngeal signs are usually absent. Cultures from the typical purulent conjunctivitis or the oral or nasal pharynx invariably demonstrate. *Staphylococcus aureus*. Unlike streptococcal scarlet fever, desquamation begins early in the course by the second day and is complete within a week. The clinical signs and course probably vary with the source of the infection, the amount of staphylococcal exotoxin present, and the host response. A similar eruption may accompany toxic shock syndrome. However, in the latter the eruption is usually accompanied by hyperemia of the conjunctivae and the oral and vaginal mucosa, a strawberry tongue, and severe multisystem disease. The early findings in both SSSS and toxic epidermal necrolysis may mimic scarlet fever. However, the presence of a Nikolsky sign and progression to widespread sloughing of skin quickly distinguish these disorders. Scarlatiniform viral exanthems can be caused by a number of different organisms. The course may be similar to scarlet fever and can be distinguished only by serologic studies and the absence of streptococci in throat or skin cultures.

Kawasaki Disease

Although the exact etiology of Kawasaki disease is unknown, the epidemiology, clinical findings, and course suggest an as yet unidentified infectious agent. Over 75 percent of patients are under four years old and 50 percent less than two years of age. Cases occur all year 'round, with slight peaks in the late spring and late fall. Epidemics have also been reported. Although all races can be affected, the increased incidence among Japanese and the intermediate risk among Japanese-Americans supports a genetic predisposition.

Kawasaki disease is defined clinically by the presence of five out of six major criteria, including fever, usually unresponsive to antipyretics for at least five days, conjunctivitis, pharyngitis, erythema and edema of the hands and feet, rash, and adenopathy (Fig. 7.19A–C). The acute phase, which lasts 10 to 14 days, begins with acute onset of fevers to between 39° and 40°C. The child is uncomfortable and irritable. The rash usually appears shortly after the fever and may take the form of a scarlatiniform, morbilliform, or urticarial exanthem. It is commonly accentuated in intertriginous

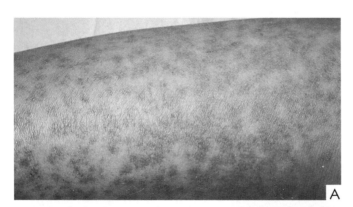

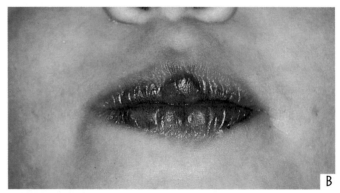

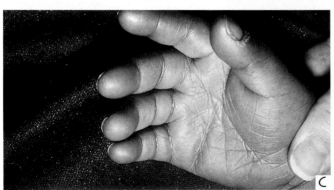

FIGURE 7.19 Kawasaki disease. Characteristic clinical findings demonstrated include (**A**) a generalized erythema multiforme-like rash, (**B**) erythema and fissuring of the lips, (**C**) palmar and plantar erythema with edema of the hands.

areas where maceration and scaling may be prominent, particularly on the perineum and inguinal creases. Facial swelling and pallor are commonly present. Other findings during the acute phase include nonpurulent conjunctival injection, erythema, edema, and cracking of the lips, palatal erythema and a strawberry tongue, painful erythema and edema of the hands and feet, and painful unilateral cervical adenopathy. Arthritis, diarrhea, abdominal pain, aseptic meningitis, hepatitis, urethritis, otitis, and hydrops of the gallbladder may also be present.

The subacute phase begins 10 to 14 days after the onset of symptoms as the fever and rash improve. It is during this period that carditis associated with coronary angiitis becomes apparent. Although up to 20 percent of children may have positive findings on echocardiography, only about 1 percent develop serious heart disease. By three weeks most patients experience a thrombocytosis of over 1 million platelets/ml, which may further increase coronary morbidity. One to two weeks after resolution of the rash, widespread desquamation occurs, particularly over the fingers and toes where the skin is shed in large sheets. Although there are no specific laboratory tests for Kawasaki disease, leukocytosis is common and acute-phase reactants, including C-reactive protein and erythrocyte sedimentation rate, are markedly elevated. The convalescent phase begins in the fourth or fifth week and ends when the sedimentation rate returns to normal. Children require cardiac re-evaluation at least through this stage and for a year or more if aneurysms are detected.

The differential diagnosis includes viral exanthems, toxin-mediated bacterial disorders, connective tissue disease, and a number of other reactive erythemas.

Acral erythema and edema are also typical of papular acrodermatitis and other viral exanthems, Rocky Mountain spotted fever, erythromelalgia, pernio, and acrodynia (pink disease). Papular acrodermatitis is eas-

ily differentiated from Kawasaki disease by the lack of fever and other systemic symptoms. The specific criteria and course of Kawasaki disease usually help to distinguish it from other viral infections that produce urticarial lesions and edema of the extrenities. The findings in rickettsial diseases are also distinctive.

ACRAL ERYTHEMA

Erythromelalgia

Erythromelalgia is an unusual entity characterized by paroxysms of painful erythema of the hands and feet which last minutes to hours (Fig. 7.20). Patients often complain of warmth of the distal extremities, followed by marked erythema and pain that are initially improved by elevation and then only by increasing periods of immersion in cold water. Although the primary variant is probably familial, secondary erythromelalgia can be triggered by polycythemia vera, lymphoproliferative disorders, hypertension, and disorders associated with hyperviscosity. When the underlying condition is treated, symptoms improve. Unfortunately, cases of primary disease are often recalcitrant, and cold-water exposure results in an "immersion foot" syndrome with progressive vascular injury, recurrent ulcerations, and secondary bacterial infection.

Pernio

Pernio is caused by cold exposure, usually above freezing, and recurrent trauma. It is commonly reported in temperate climates, where women and children are most commonly affected. Typical lesions consist of painful nodules and plaques overlying bony prominences on the hands and feet (Fig. 7.21). Histopathology demonstrates intense edema of the papillary dermis and endothelial swelling associated with a mononuclear perivascular infiltrate. Inflammation may extend to ves-

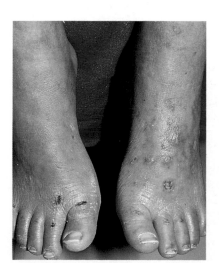

FIGURE 7.20
Erythromelalgia. Necrotic blisters and ulcerations recurred chronically in this 11-year-old girl who received relief from throbbing, debilitating foot pain by dunking her feet in near-freezing water for up to 12 hours a day. Her brother also had erythromelalgia, but his symptoms were mild and usually resolved with leg elevation alone.

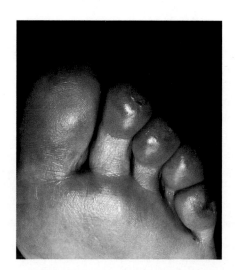

FIGURE 7.21
Pernio. Painful purple nodules developed on the sides of the feet and toes in this 18-year-old college student after scuba diving.

sels in the deep dermis and fat. Equestrians, scuba divers, and individuals who participate in fall and winter sports are particularly prone to develop lesions.

Acrodynia

Acrodynia, or pink disease, occurs in infants and toddlers as a result of chronic exposure to mercury. Painful persistent erythema and swelling of the hands and feet are accompanied by other signs of sympathetic stimulation, including tachycardia, hyperhidrosis, restlessness, and irritability. Treatment is directed toward removing the source of mercury exposure and institution of chelation therapy.

PURPURA

Bleeding into the skin can be an innocent finding in minor trauma or the first sign of a life-threatening disease. Early diagnosis and treatment, when necessary, require that the practitioner recognize and carefully evaluate any patient with purpura.

Cutaneous hemorrhage can be distinguished from hyperemia resulting from increased blood flow through dilated vesels by failure of the hemorrhagic area to blanch when pressure is applied across the surface

(diascopy). Diascopy can be demonstrated by pressing the skin apart between the thumb and index finger or by applying a glass or plastic slide. Pinpoint areas of hemorrhage are called petechiae; large confluent patches are referred to as ecchymoses. Purpura can be caused by extravascular, intravascular, and vascular phenomena.

Extravascular Purpura

Trauma is the most common cause of extravascular purpura in children. Nonblanching purple patches caused by accidental trauma vary in size from a few millimeters to many centimeters and are usually located over bony prominences such as the knees, elbows, the extensor surfaces of the lower legs, and the forehead, nose, and chin. Petechiae are only occasionally seen in otherwise healthy children, although they may occur on the face and chest after vigorous coughing or vomiting.

The presence of purpura on protected or nonexposed sites such as the buttocks, spine, genitals, upper thighs, and upper arms should suggest the possibility of deliberately induced trauma. In some cases the shape of the bruise provides a clue to the weapon used to inflict the injury.

Scars, sun damage, nutritional deficiency, inherited disorders of collagen and elastic tissue, and other factors that decrease the tensile strength of the skin may

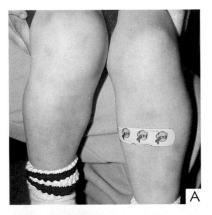
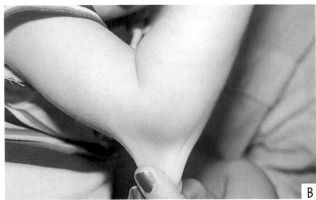
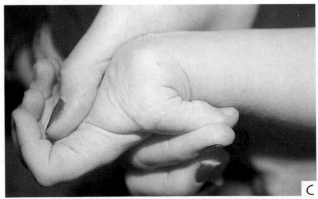
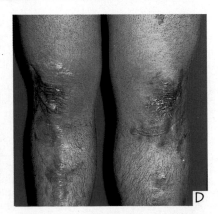

FIGURE 7.22 Ehler–Danlos syndrome. This child demonstrates a number of classic features of the disorder including **(A)** increased bruisability, **(B)** hyperelastic skin, and **(C)** hyperextensible joints. His father **(D)** had multiple widespaced purple scars over the shins which accumulated over the years from trauma.

increase the risk of bruising caused by extravascular phenomena even after minor trauma (Fig. 7.22).

Intravascular Purpura

Intravascular purpura can be caused by any disorder that interferes with normal coagulation. Petechiae and ecchymoses are present on the skin, mucosal bleeding may be seen, and in severe cases bleeding may occur in the kidneys, gastrointestinal tract, and central nervous system. Among the causes are idiopathic thrombocytopenic purpura, acute leukemia, aplastic anemia, sepsis, and clotting factor deficiencies.

Idiopathic Thrombocytopenic Purpura In children, idiopathic thrombocytopenic purpura (ITP) is the most common cause of intravascular purpura. Patients typically present in the late winter and early spring, a few weeks to several weeks after a viral illness, with purpura of all sizes and no history of trauma. When injuries occur, ecchymoses may be impressive. Bleeding of the gums occurs regularly with brushing, and occult blood may be detected in the urine and stool. Fortunately, severe bleeding is unusual and most cases are self-limited, with improvement in platelet counts from less than $10,000/mm^3$ to over $100,000/mm^3$ within one to two months. ITP is associated with the development of an IgG that binds to platelets and results in increased destruction by the reticuloendothelial system. Antiplatelet antibodies have also been reported in patients with lupus erythematosus, leukemia, lymphoma, and drug reactions (Fig. 7.23A and B). Moderate to severe cases usually respond to treatment with parenteral gammaglobulin. Resistant patients may require systemic corticosteroids and/or splenectomy.

Patients with ITP may be clinically indistinguishable from those with leukemia or thrombocytopenia. Associated symptoms, including fatigue, general malaise, fever, weight loss, and bone pain, should suggest the diagnosis of leukemia. In leukemia, blast cells may be discovered in the peripheral smear as well as the bone marrow. In ITP, the bone marrow demonstrates increased numbers of megakarocytes, whereas these cells are usually decreased in leukemia. In aplastic anemia, purpura may be the first sign of marrow failure. All blood elements are decreased in both the peripheral blood and the bone marrow. Severe bacterial infection is a common complication. Children with inherited clotting factor disorders bruise easily and may develop hemarthroses and bleeding into viscera. Petechiae are not usually seen in these patients.

Disseminated Intravascular Coagulation Bacterial sepsis, disseminated viral infection, malignancy, and medications occasionally trigger disseminated intravascular coagulation (DIC), with widespread bleeding into the skin and viscera. Ecchymoses may progress rapidly to cover large areas of the body surface over minutes to hours (Fig. 7.24). Unfortunately, necrosis may develop in the center of some areas of purpura. In survivors, healing occurs with scarring and occasionally loss of digits or limbs.

Patients are usually critically ill, and death may ensue quickly unless supportive measures, including urgent volume expansion, vasopressors, and parenteral antibiotic therapy, are begun immediately. Some intensivists recommend treatment with heparin and fresh frozen plasma. Laboratory studies demonstrate thrombocytopenia, decreased fibrinogen, prolonged bleeding time, and elevations in fibrin split products. In children meningo-

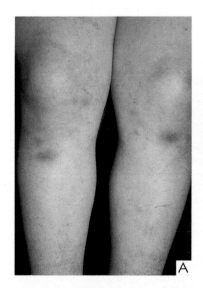

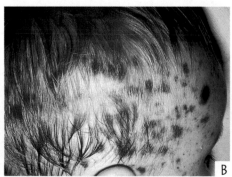

FIGURE 7.23 Intravascular purpura. (**A**) A child with idiopathic thrombocytopenic purpura and (**B**) acute lymphocytic leukemia shows bruises of varying sizes, typically found in individuals with low platelet counts.

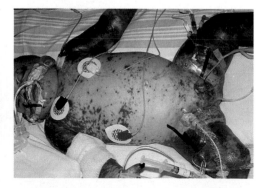

FIGURE 7.24 Purpura fulminans developed in this infant with meningococcemia. Widespread bleeding into the skin was noted, particularly on the extremities.

coccemia, *Haemophilus influenzae* type B, and streptococcal infections are the most common cause of DIC.

Vascular Purpura

Vascular purpura develops when an inflammatory process involves the vessel wall (vasculitis). In leukocytoclastic vasculitis the inflammation is predominantly neutrophilic. In later stages of leukocytoclastic vasculitis and lymphocytic vasculitis, vascular damage is caused by infiltrating mononuclear cells. Pyoderma gangrenosum shares features of leukocytoclastic and lymphocytic vasculitis, whereas Sweet's syndrome is characterized primarily by leukocytoclastic changes.

Leukocytoclastic Vasculitis Leukocytic vasculitis results from immune complex deposition on the basement membrane and subsequent complement activation. Infections, medications, autoimmune disorders, and malignancy may trigger vasculitis.

Henoch-Schönlein purpura (HSP), also known as anaphylactoid purpura or allergic vasculitis, is the most common form of leukocytoclastic vasculitis in children. The peak incidence occurs in children between four and eight years old. However, HSP has also been reported in infants and adults.

Although the rash is characterized by palpable purpura, the typical 2-mm to 10-mm purpuric papules may be preceded by several days of urticaria. Lesions most commonly pepper the buttocks and the extensor surfaces of the arms and legs (Fig. 7.25A–E). However, any site can be involved including the face, ears, and trunk. Crops erupt episodically for two to four weeks. Individual lesions usually fade over three to five days. Confluent ecchymoses occasionally evolve from small lesions, and occasionally necrosis and hemorrhagic bullae develop. Scalp edema and periarticular swelling (Schönlein's purpura) and paroxysmal abdominal colic with melena or frankly bloody stools (Henoch's purpura) may occur before, during, or after the rash. Vasculitis may also involve the kidneys, lungs, and central nervous system.

Recurrences affect about half of patients for up to several months. However, these episodes are usually mild. In most cases visceral disease is self-limited. However, acute renal failure develops rarely and intussusception may complicate vasculitis in the bowel. More subtle renal disease may persist for years.

Leukocytoclastic vasculitis involves small dermal blood vessels, usually postcapillary venules. The classic histologic findings include endothelial swelling, fibrin deposition within and around vessels, neutrophilic infiltrate within the vessel walls, and nuclear dust (scattered nuclear fragments from neutrophils). Vascular destruction with hemorrhage may be prominent. Fresh biopsies

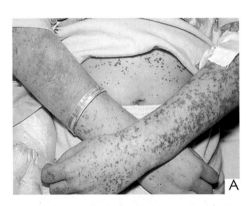
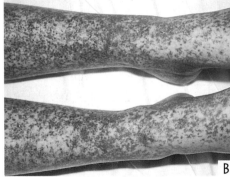
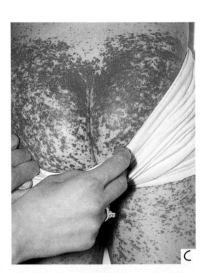
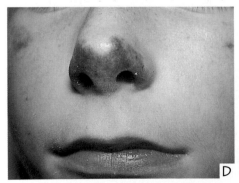
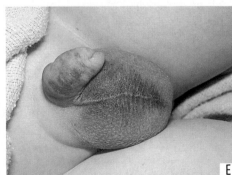

FIGURE 7.25 Henoch–Schönlein purpura. Vasculitic lesions typically erupt on the extensor surfaces of the (**A**) arms, (**B**) legs, and (**C**) buttocks. Any area, including the (**D**) face and (**E**) genitals, can be involved.

demonstrate IgA and C3 deposition around dermal blood vessels.

Although most children with HSP can be observed at home, patients with progressive renal disease or severe abdominal pain require hospitalization.

A normal blood count, platelet count, and coagulation studies will help to differentiate HSP from intravascular forms of purpura. Identification of typical clinical findings and course, histopathology, and other screening studies (e.g., antinuclear antibodies, rheumatoid factor, precipitin antibodies) will exclude lupus erythematosus and other connective tissue disorders.

Periarteritis nodosa (PAN) is a vasculitis that involves small- and medium-sized arteries. A systemic form that is extremely rare in children presents acutely with fever, weakness, abdominal pain, and cardiac failure. Despite treatment with high-dose corticosteroids and immunosuppressive agents, death may ensue quickly from renal failure, gastrointestinal bleeding, and bowel perforation. Cutaneous lesions including livedo reticularis, erythema, and purpura on the lower extremities are not diagnostic.

Cutaneous polyarteritis nodosa is more likely to come to the attention of the dermatologist. In this distinct variant, cutaneous findings predominate and the viscera are usually spared. Crops of painful nodules and annular plaques blossom on the arms and legs, particularly the hands and feet, and less commonly on the trunk, head, and neck (Fig. 7.26A–C). Urticaria, livedo, and cutaneous ulcerations may also develop. Episodes can last for several weeks and tend to recur for years. Although severe systemic disease is not a feature, fever and arthralgias frequently accompany flares in disease activity. The diagnosis of cutaneous PAN is made by establishing the clinical pattern and the histopathology, which demonstrates a leukocytoclastic vasculitis of medium-sized arteries. Patients usually respond quickly to prednisone, but resistant cases may require methotrexate or azathioprine. Nodules localized to the palms and soles melt away with intralesional corticosteroids.

The painful nodules of cutaneous PAN may be difficult to differentiate from erythema nodosum, cold panniculitis, and lupus panniculitis, particularly early in the course. Associated clinical findings and histopathology, however, are distinctive in these disorders.

Lymphocytic Vasculitis Rather than being a distinct entity, lymphocytic vasculitis represents a reaction pattern in the skin associated with a number of disorders in which lymphocytic inflammation predominates.

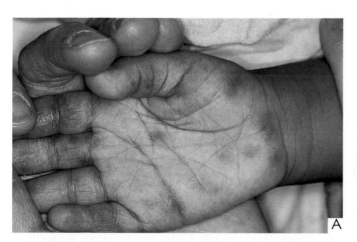

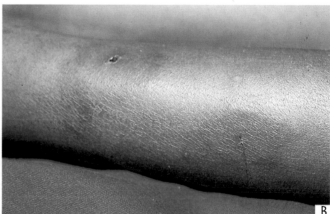

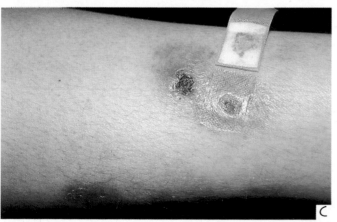

FIGURE 7.26 Periarteritis nodosa. Over several days a three-year-old girl developed painful nodules on the trunk, face, and extremities. Lesions on the hands (**A**) were associated with arthritis. (**B**) Some of the nodules on the legs developed central necrotic vesicles. (**C**) An eight-year-old boy with chronic cutaneous PAN complained of recurrent painful ulcerated nodules on his shins.

Lymphocytic vasculitis has been described in cutaneous drug reactions, vasculitic lesions of Sjögren's syndrome, and as a late phase of leukocytoclastic vasculitis. *Progressive pigmented purpuric dermatosis* (PPPD) is the only disorder in which lymphocytis vasculitis occurs consistently.

PPPD is characterized by the development of localized patches of petechiae and larger patches of purpura, particularly on the lower extremities. Hemosiderin deposition and postinflammatory hyperpigmentation lead to shades of brown, gold, and bronze color as lesions evolve (Fig. 7.27A and B). Confluent patches may form a reticulated pattern. Although lesions are usually flat and asymptomatic, fine scale and lichenoid papules may be associated with mild pruritus.

Skin biopsies from active areas demonstrate lymphocytes around and within the walls of superficial dermal capillaries. Mild hemorrhage and hemosiderin deposition are also present.

Clinically and histologically it may be impossible to distinguish PPPD from a drug reaction. Occasionally, practitioners have reported children with large patches over the lower back or buttocks for suspected abuse. Unfortunately no treatment has proven satisfactory, and lesions may persist for years. Systemic and topical steroids may arrest progression temporarily.

Infectious Vasculitis Although overwhelming infection by a number of bacterial organisms can trigger rapidly fatal DIC with widespread bleeding into the skin, mucous membranes, and viscera, many patients develop discrete vasculitic lesions. In fact, the presence of 0.5-cm to 2-cm angulated, pink to red hemorrhagic macules, papules, pustules, and plaques is associated with a relatively good prognosis (Fig. 7.28). Over several hours lesions become hemorrhagic and central necrosis with bulla formation or ulceration may develop. Prompt recognition of this condition and the initiation of antibiotics and supportive care may be lifesaving.

Although the rash may be caused by hematogenous dissemination of the organism to the skin, some lesions result from immune complex deposition in dermal vessels. For example, Osler's nodes, tender nodules on the finger or toe pads, and Janeway spots, small, painless nodules on the palms, probably represent an immune-mediated phenomenon. *Neisseria meningitidis, Haemophilus influenzae* type B, *Streptococcus (Pneumococcus) pneumoniae, Streptococcus* sp., and

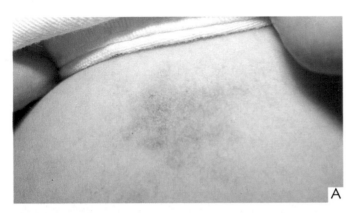

FIGURE 7.27 Progressive pigmented purpuric dermatosis. **(A)** An early lesion on the thigh of a 10-year-old boy shows mild purpura and reticulated, bronze hyperpigmentation.

(B) Reticulated hyperpigmented patches have slowly advanced across the leg of a 15-year-old girl for years.

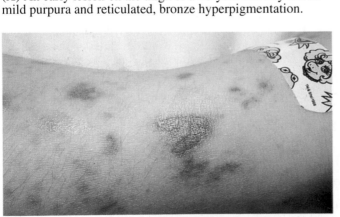

FIGURE 7.28 Sharply angulated purpuric and necrotic papules developed on the extremities of a seven-year-old with meningococcemia. He presented with meningitis and responded quickly to parenteral antibiotics.

Staphylococcus aureus have been cultured from blood and skin in normal hosts with infectious vasculitis. Rocky Mountain spotted fever may produce a similar clinical picture. In immunosuppressed individuals these organisms, as well as opportunistic bacteria and fungi, should also be considered.

Ecthyma gangrenosum, characterized by a punched-out ulceration with a central opalescent eschar and a hemorrhagic border, is caused by *Pseudomonas* septicemia (Fig. 7.29). Lesions typically appear on the lower abdominal wall, thighs, and groin in leukemics, burn patients, and other debilitated individuals who have been on antibiotics. Although most patients are severely ill with multiple lesions, in some cases only one or several indolent ulcers are present. Other Gram-negative organisms, as well as fungi such as *Candida* and *Aspergillus*, may produce the same type of skin lesions.

The diagnosis can be made by searching for organisms in Gram stains obtained from pustules and necrotic ulcers. Identification of specific organisms from blood and tissue cultures is required for selection of appropriate antibiotics. Skin biopsies show a necrotizing vasculitis with a variable number of bacteria within vessels and neutrophils. Aplastic patients may show minimal inflammation with large numbers of organisms.

Sweet's Syndrome *Sweet's syndrome*, also referred to as *acute febrile neutrophilic dermatosis*, is characterized by violaceous 0.5-cm to 3-cm nodules and plaques that erupt abruptly on the face and extremities. Recurrent crops of nodules over one to eight months are heralded by high fever, arthralgias, and occasionally periarticular swelling and arthritis (Fig. 7.30). Necrotic vesicles and bullae may also form. Although Sweet's syndrome is self-limited, symptoms may be debilitating. Skin lesions, arthralgias, and fever usually melt away with systemic corticosteroids; however, recurrences are common when the medication is tapered.

Although initially described in middle-aged women, a number of cases have been reported in infants and children. About 10 percent of adult cases are associated with myeloproliferative disorders, especially acute myelocytic or myelomonocytic leukemia. Children with this syndrome require a thorough physical examination

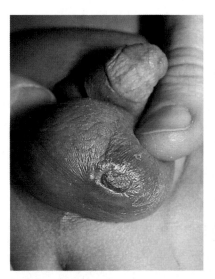

FIGURE 7.29 An infant with an inherited immunodeficiency experienced recurrent episodes of Gram-negative septicemia. *Pseudomonas* grew from cultures obtained from blood and the necrotic, crusted ulcer on the scrotum.

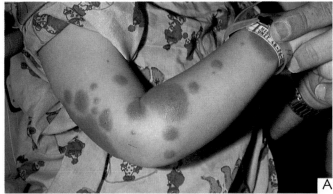

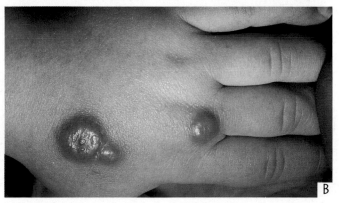

FIGURE 7.30 (A,B) Sweet's syndrome. A two-year-old girl developed fever, arthritis, leukocytosis, and widely disseminated red to violaceous plaques and nodules, which demonstrated intense neutrophilic inflammation on skin biopsy. An extensive evaluation failed to reveal any underlying disease. Although she responded quickly to systemic corticosteroids, it took nearly a year to wean her because of frequent recurrences.

and laboratory evaluation, including a blood count, peripheral smear, and bone marrow, to exclude an underlying disorder.

Sweet's syndrome may be confused with erythema multiforme, erythema nodosum, viral exanthems, Henoch–Schönlein purpura, infectious vasculitis, and polyarteritis nodosa. Although Sweet's syndrome may be suspected because of the cutaneous lesions and the clinical course, a skin biopsy of a fresh lesion will demonstrate diagnostic findings including a dense perivascular neutrophilic infiltrate and intense edema in the upper dermis, some leukocytoclasia without true vasculitis, and in some cases subepidermal bulla formation.

Pyoderma Gangrenosum In pyoderma gangrenosum (PG), painful pustules or nodules develop central necrosis and an enlarging ulcer with a hemorrhagic, purple, undermined advancing border (Fig. 7.31A and B). Ulcers range in size from about 1 cm when they first appear to over 10 cm as they evolve. One or several lesions may appear, and any area including the face, trunk, and extremities can be involved. Pathergy, or the development of new lesions at sites of trauma such as venipunctures, is a reliable diagnostic clue. An underlying systemic disease such as inflammatory bowel disease, myelogenous leukemia, or rheumatoid arthritis is associated with cutaneous lesions in 50 percent of the cases.

Skin biopsies show typical but nondiagnostic findings, including a lymphocytic vasculitis at the advancing border and necrosis with abscess formation and reactive polymorphous inflammation extending into the subcutaneous tissue.

PG usually responds to treatment of the underlying condition. Idiopathic cases can be treated with antibiotics, systemic corticosteroids, or dapsone. Resistant cases may require immunosuppressive agents such as azathioprine, methotrexate, or cyclosporine.

FIGURATE ERYTHEMA

A number of disorders are characterized by the development of annular plaques with a well-defined advancing red border and central clearing. Typical but nondiagnostic histologic findings include a tight perivascular mononuclear cell infiltrate in the superficial dermis with occasional extension to the mid and deep dermis. The overlying epidermis is normal or shows mild spongiosis. *Erythema annulare centrifugum* (EAC) and *erythema chronicum migrans* (ECM) are the most commonly recognized figurate erythemas in children.

Erythema Annulare Centrifugum

In EAC, one notes one or multiple asymptomatic, expanding, annular or serpiginous red plaques with a well-defined raised border and trailing scale on the inner aspect of the border (Fig. 7.32A and B). As lesions progress from less than 1 cm to over 20 cm over several weeks, new plaques may arise within the borders, producing concentric rings. The eruption typically spreads from the central trunk to the proximal extremities (centrifugal), and lesions continue to evolve for months to years.

Although EAC probably respresents a hypersensitivity reaction to the same sort of phenomena that trigger urticaria and erythema multiforme, a number of reports suggest a common association with chronic dermatophyte infection (e.g., tinea pedis, tinea cruris). EAC occurs most commonly in adults, but cases may erupt

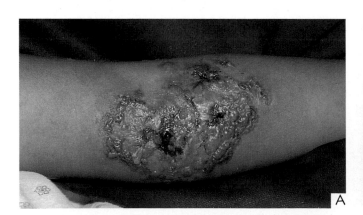

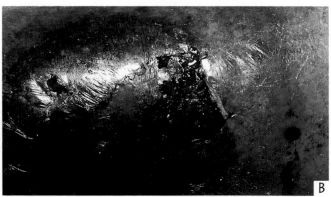

FIGURE 7.31 Pyoderma gangrenosum. **(A)** A nine-year-old boy developed a painful, expanding, crusted necrotic plaque on his arm. An exhaustive medical evaluation was unrevealing until a bone-marrow biopsy demonstrated chronic myelogenous leukemia. **(B)** A similar plaque in a teenager with Crohn's disease shows marked central hemorrhagic necrosis and an undermined purple border. Lesions in both children healed after aggressive treatment of the underlying disorders.

throughout childhood. Annular erythema of infancy is undoubtedly a clinical variant of this disorder.

EAC can be distinguished from urticaria by the persistence of individual lesions and the lack of pruritus. The chronic course and the absence of viral symptoms should help to exclude an urticarial viral exanthem. Granuloma annulare can be excluded by the finding of epidermal changes (erythema and scale) in EAC. Although there are no specific laboratory tests for EAC, a skin biopsy typically shows a tight lymphocytic perivascular infiltrate (coat-sleeve pattern) in the mid and deep dermis. Dermatitic changes may also be present in the epidermis.

When a fungal infection is identified, oral griseofulvin or ketoconazole may lead to clearing of the rash. Otherwise, no specific treatment is indicated.

Erythema Chronicum Migrans

In erythema chronicum migrans (ECM), which marks the onset of Lyme disease, a single papule begins three to 30 days after a deer tick bite and expands quickly to form an enlarging red plaque with central clearing (Fig. 7.33). New lesions may continue to evolve successively or in crops over several months. Plaques over 4 cm in diameter are typical, and some may exceed 30 cm. Mild influenza-like symptoms including headache, sore throat, arthralgias, and malaise are commonly associated with the skin rash. If untreated, resolution of skin lesions is followed several months later by a periarticular arthritis involving the knees, elbows, and/or wrists in 50 percent of patients. In 15 percent of cases neurologic abnormalities, including meningoencephalitis, neuropathy, or Bell's palsy, occur two weeks to eight months after the tick bite. Cardiac symptoms, which appear in 5 percent of patients, may mimic rheumatic fever.

Lyme disease is caused by the spirochete *Borrelia burgdorferi*, which can be carried by *Ixodes dammini* and related ticks. These ticks are widely distributed throughout the United States and Europe, and in some places, such as coastal New England and the Great Lakes states, the infection has become endemic. The ticks are the size of a pinhead, and up to 50 percent of patients do not recall the bite.

The incidence of Lyme disease is highest in children, but all ages can be affected. Although the diagnosis is usually made clinically, new, more reliable serologic tests may aid in differentiation of the annular plaques of ECM from urticaria, viral exanthems, erythema marginatum, and erythema annulare centrifigum.

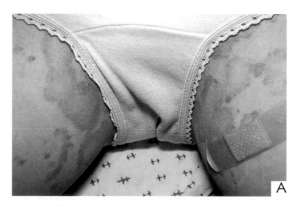

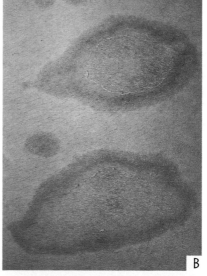

FIGURE 7.32 Erythema annulare centrifigum. **(A)** Symmetric, annular red plaques slowly expanded on the anterior thighs of a 10-year-old girl. **(B)** Another child with large lesions on the trunk demonstrates the bright-red border with a fine trailing scale and central clearing.

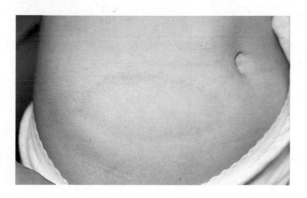

FIGURE 7.33 Erythema chronicum migrans. A solitary indurated pink plaque with central clearing grew over several weeks from a small red papule at the site of a tick bite. The lesion, as well as associated arthralgias and intermittent low-grade fever, resolved within 48 hours of starting oral amoxacillin.

Skin biopsy specimens obtained from the expanding border or the center of lesions may demonstrate spirochetes with special silver stains. Otherwise, the histopathologic findings are not diagnostic and show changes typical of insect bite reactions.

Any individual in an endemic area who develops an annular eruption, especially if it is associated with viral symptoms and a tick bite, should be treated to reduce the risk of arthritis and other late complications. Although treatment recommendations vary, a three-week course of tetracycline 250 mg q.i.d. or doxycycline 100 mg b.i.d. is the choice for older children and adults, and penicillin V or amoxicillin at a dose of 25 to 50 mg/kg/day with a maximum of 1 to 2 g daily, is used in children less than eight years old. Children allergic to penicillin can be treated with 30 mg/kg/day of erythromycin up to 250 mg t.i.d.

Avoiding tick-infested areas or wearing protective clothing will reduce the risk of exposure. Tick repellents containing diethyl toluamide (DEET) are also effective. However, excessive use of DEET, particularly in infants and young children, has been associated with neurotoxic reactions. New low-concentration lotions (Skedaddle, 7.25 percent, and OFF, 10 percent) are probably as effective as traditional repellents with concentrations over 50 percent and have a much better safety profile. Tick inspections after hikes and camping trips and removal of ticks within 24 to 48 hours of attachment will also reduce transmission of the spirochete.

PANNICULITIS

Panniculitis refers to a group of disorders in which an inflammatory process involves the fat lobules, intervening fat septae, or both. Clinically, patients present with deep-seated, poorly defined, tender violaceous nodules. The overlying epidermis is usually intact, although it may be taut and shiny. If necrosis develops ulcerations may occur.

Erythema Nodosum

Erythema nodosum (EN) is the most common panniculitis affecting children, usually appearing in adolescents. Typically, painful red subcutaneous nodules and plaques from 1 cm to 5 cm in diameter erupt on the shins, but lesions may also involve the arms and thighs, and rarely the trunk and face (Fig. 7.34). Nodules usually fade over several weeks, but recurrences are frequent. In some cases, crops recur for months.

Over 100 years ago the development of EN with tuberculosis was recognized. More recently, EN has been associated with a number of infections including viral pharyngitis, streptococcal pharyngitis, histoplasmosis, coccidiomycosis, and other deep fungi and atypical mycobacteria. Noninfectious inflammatory conditions such as sarcoidosis, inflammatory bowel disease, and lupus erythematosus may trigger the reaction.

The finding of a septal panniculitis without fat necrosis is characteristic of erythema nodosum. Early in the course neutrophilic inflammation is common. Later, lymphocytes, histiocytes, and giant cells predominate. Vessels show endothelial cell swelling, inflammation in the vascular walls, and hemorrhage.

In most children EN is self-limited and treatment, when necessary, is tailored to the underlying disorder. Leg elevation and nonsteroidal anti-inflammatory agents may help to reduce the pain.

Cold Panniculitis

In infants and young children, cold injury results in crystallization and rupture of fat cells and subsequent inflammation. Persistent, indurated red nodules and

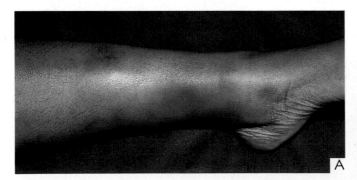
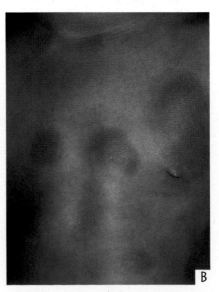

FIGURE 7.34 Erythema nodosum. **(A)** Tender, deep-seated nodules appeared on the shins of a 16-year-old girl two weeks after starting birth control pills. The lesions resolved when the medication was discontinued. **(B)** An 18-month-old boy developed (biopsy proven) erythema nodosum on the chest and abdomen after a cold. The nodules resolved over several weeks without therapy.

plaques apppear most commonly on the cheeks (popsicle panniculitis), but the trunk and extremities may also be involved (Fig. 7.35). Ulceration and atrophy do not usually develop, and nodules resolve without treatment in several weeks to several months.

Although the cause is not known, the increased saturation of fatty acids in the subcutaneous fat of infants compared with adults makes their fat more prone to solidification at low temperatures.

Fat necrosis of the newborn is a variant of cold panniculitis that occurs within the first month of life. Several circumscribed lesions appear on the trunk and proximal extremities in an otherwise healthy infant. Nodules heal without scarring, but transient depression of the skin surface is common and ulceration occasionally occurs.

Cold injury may also produce *sclerema* of the newborn. In this process, widespread woody induration of the skin develops in a severely ill infant. This process is probably a complication of multisystem failure and associated cooling of the skin and fat resulting from decreased cutaneous perfusion. In skin biopsies from these infants, edema of the fibrous septae is seen without necrosis of fat cells. Fat necrosis of the newborn and cold panniculitis in older infants and children are associated with necrosis of fat cells and granulomatous inflammation.

Morphologically, cold panniculitis may be confused with bacterial cellulitis (Fig. 7.36). However, in cellulitis the indurated plaques are warm, tender, and progressive, and the patients are febrile and toxic appearing. Other nodular erythema, such as periarteritis nodosa and erythema nodosum, can usually be distinguished by the clinical course and skin biopsy findings when necessary.

Lupus Panniculitis

In lupus panniculitis, persistent purple, painless nodules from 1 cm to 5 cm in diameter develop on the face, extremities, and buttocks (Fig. 7.37). Although these lesions usually occur in a child with other signs of systemic lupus erythematosus, they may be the first or only manifestation of the disease. Individual lesions may persist for months to years, and ulceration and scarring are common. Unfortunately, lupus panniculitis is often resistant to treatment with antimalarials, and the use of systemic steroids and immunosuppressive agents should probably be guided by systemic symptoms.

Histopathologic findings are nonspecific and show lymphohistiocytic inflammation within the fat lobules and hyalinization of fat cells. Inflammation and vasculitis may also occur in the fat septae.

PHOTOSENSITIVITY

Photosensitivity is a term used to describe a group of conditions marked by abnormal reactions to light. Sunburn is a phototoxic reaction that is caused by exposure to naturally occurring short-wavelength ultraviolet (UVB) light. Longer-wavelength UVA light is only weakly phototoxic; however, all individuals deliberately or accidentally exposed to high enough doses of topical or oral UVA photosensitizing agents may also develop burns. In photoallergic reactions, susceptible individuals who are exposed to certain photosensitizing chemicals or drugs develop an immunologically mediated rash which is activated by light. A number of genetic and metabolic disorders are associated with photosensitivity, and the recognition of cutaneous findings may be

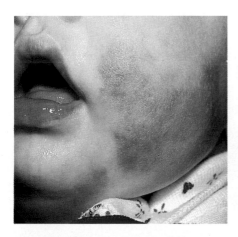

FIGURE 7.35 Cold panniculitis appeared on the cheeks and chin of this six-month-old one day after he was given an ice-filled teething ring.

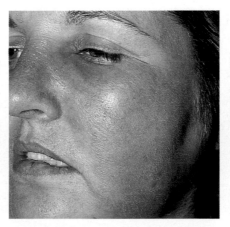

FIGURE 7.36 Facial cellulitis/erysipelas. A painful, indurated red plaque spread within several hours across the cheek of a 17-year-old girl. She also had a fever and tender cervical adenopathy, which resolved on parenteral penicillin.

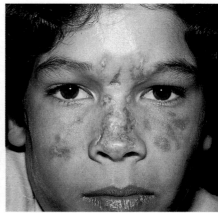

FIGURE 7.37 Lupus panniculitis. A 13-year-old boy presented with chronic, recurring deep-seated nodules and plaques, which healed with punched-out scars.

a clue to diagnosis. Photodermatoses include several specific conditions with unusual reactions to light. In some of these dermatoses the action spectra or the wavelengths that trigger skin findings have been described. Finally, other diseases may be exacerbated by light. Recognition of this phenomenon may be important in management of these conditions.

Phototoxic and Photoallergic Reactions

Exposure of the skin to sunlight causes a number of biologic reactions. Small amounts of UVB activate the conversion of 7-dehydrocholesterol into vitamin D_3. Large amounts of ultraviolet light produce the erythema and swelling known as sunburn (Fig. 7.38A and B). Intense reactions may result in the development of second-degree burns on sun-exposed surfaces. Healing is marked by desquamation, thickening, and hyperpigmentation of the skin.

Although UVB is 100 times more erythemogenic than UVA, the large quantity of UVA (1000 times more than UVB) that reaches the ground contributes substantially to sunburn (10 percent to 15 percent). On overcast days, when 15 percent to 20 percent of UVB is absorbed and scattered by the cloud cover, the role of UVA is even greater. The minimal dose of light required to produce a discrete area of sunburn is referred to as the minimal erythema dose (MED). The MED tends to increase with increasing skin types. Individuals with skin type 1 always burn and never tan. These people have blonde or red hair, blue eyes, and often demonstrate freckling in sun-exposed sites. Skin type 2 denotes individuals who always burn at first, but sometimes tan after repeated sun exposure. Type 3 people occasionally burn, but tan readily. Olive-complexioned individuals who always tan fall into type 4. Types 5 and 6 include members of darkly pigmented races.

Factors that potentiate the development of sunburn include increasing elevation above sea level, wind, low humidity, and factors that result in thinning of the epidermis, such as the application of peeling agents (Retin A, salicylic acid, lactic acid). Damage to DNA is the initiating event in the development of the erythema response. The subsequent production of inflammatory mediators (e.g., prostaglandins, histamine) triggers the clinical response. Factors that interfere with normal DNA repair mechanisms (hereditary defects in DNA repair enzymes, or antimetabolites such as methotrexate) result in an exaggerated or prolonged erythema response.

Wrinkling, elastosis, lentigines, and other "age"-related changes in the skin result from long-term exposure to sunlight, and the majority of an individual's lifetime exposure occurs during childhood. It has been estimated that the incidence of basal cell carcinoma and squamous cell carcinoma could be reduced by 75 percent to 80 percent if people used sun-protective clothing, sunscreens (chemicals that absorb UV light), and sun blocks (agents that reflect sunlight) beginning in early childhood. Although most sunscreens (e.g., paraaminobenzoic acid, PABA esters, cinnamates) provide good coverage against UVB, only Photoplex with parsol absorbs adequately in the UVA range. The sun-protective factor (SPF) of a product is determined by calculating the MED of sunscreen-protected skin divided by the MED of unprotected skin. In infants, who should never be left in the sun, sunscreens are only rarely necessary. Parents of ambulatory children, particularly those with light pigmentation, should receive

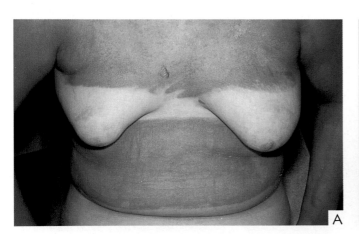

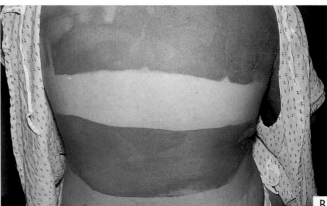

FIGURE 7.38 (A,B) Phototoxic reaction. A severe sunburn developed in sunexposed areas after this teenager applied a topical photosensitizing cream to her skin and spent the day outdoors. Note the areas of sparing under her bathing suit.

aggressive counseling about sun protection. People with skin types 1 and 2 should use screens with an SPF of 15 to 30, whereas darker pigmented individuals are safe with lower SPFs, particularly after gradually increasing sun exposure produces protective darkening of the skin.

Unlike phototoxicity, photoallergic reactions involve an immunologic response in a small number of individuals who are sensitized to certain chemicals or drugs in the presence of sunlight. In many cases a type IV delayed hypersensitivity reaction results in the development of an eczematous dermatitis rather than a sunburn in a sun-exposed distribution. A number of medications have been implicated in the production of both phototoxic and photoallergic reactions. Some of the most common photosensitizers include furocoumarins, nalidixic acid, dyes, salicylanilides, fragrances, para-aminobenzoic acid, phenothiazines, sulfonamides, tetracyclines, thiazides and related sulfonamide diuretics, and nonsteroidal anti-inflammatory agents. Patients taking these drugs should be warned to protect themselves against the risk of photosensitivity.

Rarely, photo-activated eczematous reactions persist for months or years. A *persistent light reaction* usually evolves from a previous photo-contact allergic dermatitis, but oral medications have been implicated as well. In *actinic reticuloid*, the chronic dermatitis often spreads to involve covered sites, the lesions become lichenified and nodular, and skin biopsies may show lymphoma-like infiltrates in addition to a chronic dermatitis. In these patients the dermatitis can be reproduced on normal patches of skin by exposure to UVA, UVB, and sometimes visible light, and MEDs at various wavelengths of UV light are markedly decreased. Some patients with atopic dermatitis note a flare of disease activity in sun-exposed sites. These individuals can be differentiated from patients with photo-activated

eczematous reactions by the absence of exposure to photosensitizing drugs and topical agents, negative photo-patch tests, and an abnormal MED to UVB only.

Photodermatoses

Polymorphous Light Eruption Several photo-induced dermatoses can be identified by distinctive clinical and histological findings. Polymorphous light eruption (PMLE) is the most common dermatosis, appearing in up to 10 percent of individuals. In PMLE, crops of red macules, papules, vesicles, or plaques typically erupt on exposed areas several hours to several days after intensive sun exposure in the early spring (Fig. 7.39). The morphology of the lesions varies from patient to patient. However, the rash tends to be monomorphous in a given individual. PMLE appears most commonly in adolescents and young adults and may recur each spring for years. Although the rash usually progresses for several weeks, complete regression occurs within three to four weeks despite continued light exposure. In fact, phototherapy (PUVA) has been used to deliberately trigger the reaction and treat or "harden" the skin in a controlled setting to avoid inconvenient expression of the rash. PMLE is most common in temperate or northern climates, where the "hardening" of the skin tends to wane during the winter months. In the sunbelt states and tropics, where sun exposure occurs year 'round, the rash is less common and often spares the face and "V" of the neck, which are most prominently exposed.

The histopathology of PMLE typically shows an intense lymphocytic perivascular infiltrate in the upper and mid dermis. Dermal edema may also be prominent. Differential diagnosis from lupus erythematosus can be difficult clinically and histologically. The histology of lupus usually demonstrates inflammation at the dermal–epidermal junction, and the dermal infiltrate often

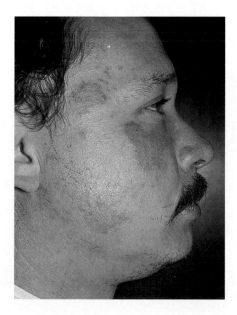

FIGURE 7.39 Polymorphous light eruption. Red papules and plaques erupted on the face of this young adult the day after a trip to the beach in the spring.

surrounds adnexal structures as well as vessels. However, early in the course of lupus the histology may be nonspecific, clinical findings may be confined to the skin, and serological studies may be negative.

Solar Urticaria Although urticaria after sun exposure can be caused by medications or associated with systemic illness such as lupus or prophyria, a rare group of otherwise healthy individuals develops hives within minutes of sun exposure. Although lesions can become quite itchy and extensive, symptoms usually abate with continued light exposure. Various wavelengths of light, including ultraviolet and visible radiation, have been associated with hives.

In many cases solar urticaria is caused by a type I IgE-mediated reaction, and lesions result from the release of histamine and other vasoactive substances. In time inflammatory mediators become depleted and the lesions subside. Unfortunately, antihistamines only partially suppress solar urticaria. However, persistent light exposure can be maintained with phototherapy to keep the reaction under control.

Genetic Disorders

A number of inherited and metabolic disorders are associated with photosensitivity. In xeroderma pigmentosum, Bloom's syndrome, Cockayne's syndrome, and Rothmund–Thompson syndrome, light alone triggers an abnormal reaction in the skin. Disorders that result in pigment dilution, such as albinism, phenylketonuria, and other aminoacidopathies, markedly increase the sensitivity to phototoxic reactions. In congenital porphyrias, porphyria cutanea tarda, and Hartnup syndrome endogenous metabolites function as potent photosensitizers (Fig. 7.40A and B). In many of these disorders the clinical findings may provide the key to diagnosis.

Photo-exacerbated Disorders

Many disorders are triggered or aggravated by sunlight. For example, although careful exposure to sun may result in improvement of psoriasis and repigmentation in vitiligo, sunburn often produces a Koebner phenomenon that causes exacerbation of both disorders (Fig. 7.41A–C). Sun exposure, particularly sunburn, is also

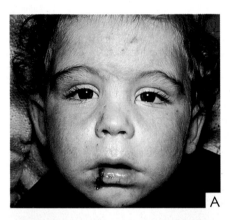

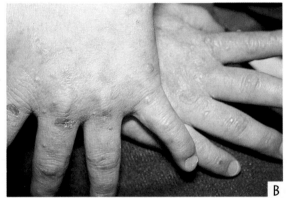

FIGURE 7.40 Congenital erythropoietic porphyria. Severe photosensitivity from accumulation of cutaneous porphyrins results in recurrent blistering and scarring in sun-exposed areas. (**A**) Note scarring, erosions, and hirsutism on his face and (**B**) scarring with milia formation on his hands.

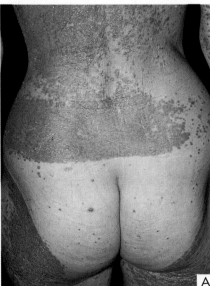

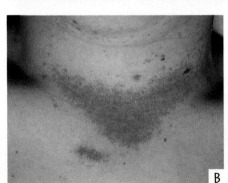

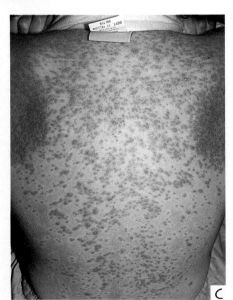

FIGURE 7.41 Photoexacerbated conditions. (**A**) This young woman with psoriasis developed recurrent skin lesions in sun-exposed areas after a sunburn (Koebner phenomenon). (**B**) Vasculitic plaques of Henoch-Schönlein purpura erupted in sun-exposed sites. (**C**) Photoexacerbation was evident in this child with varicella. The bathing trunk area was relatively spared.

known to exacerbate acne vulgaris, acne rosacea, erythema multiforme, viral exanthems, pemphigus and other bullous disorders, lichen planus, lupus erythematosus, pityriasis alba, and herpes labialis.

COLLAGEN VASCULAR DISEASE

Collagen vascular disorders present with a myriad of confusing and overlapping cutaneous findings. Although the clinical picture and laboratory markers may help to define a specific entity, often the practitioner is unable to make a definitive diagnosis. A number of autoantibody systems have been identified in these diseases. Antibodies target vascular endothelium and epithelial basement membrane zone structures, resulting in cutaneous and visceral inflammation. In the skin, inflammation produces distinctive reaction patterns.

Lupus Erythematosus

Lupus is a chronic multisystem disorder which can affect any organ system. Although as recently as 20 years ago *systemic lupus erythematosus* (SLE) was considered to be progressive, often with a fatal outcome, the aggressive use of systemic steroids and immunosuppressive agents has greatly improved the prognosis. Early intervention requires immediate recognition of variable and sometimes subtle signs and symptoms. Cutaneous findings may suggest the diagnosis.

SLE is the most common variant of lupus in childhood. Although the incidence is only 1 in 200,000 in childhood, nearly 25 percent of all cases begin before age 20. In young children boys are affected almost as often as girls. However, in adolescence, when the incidence begins to rise, girls account for 80 to 90 percent of cases. Other forms of lupus that are uncommon in childhood include benign cutaneous (discoid) lupus, lupus panniculitis, and neonatal lupus.

Discoid lupus lesions are the most common skin rash found in childhood SLE (Fig. 7.42A and B). This eruption is characterized by red, coin-shaped plaques from 0.5 cm to 5 cm in diameter, with central atrophy and hypopigmentation and peripheral hyperpigmentation. Adherent scale, follicular plugging, and telangiectasias, especially in areas of atrophy, may be prominent. Although these plaques can develop on any area, sun-exposed sites, including the face in a malar distribution, scalp, ears, neck, upper trunk, and extensor surfaces of the arms, are most commonly involved. Discoid lesions may be the sole cutaneous finding in SLE. However, when discoid lesions occur without systemic disease the disorder is referred to as *discoid lupus erythematosus* (DLE). About 15 percent to 20 percent of patients with DLE eventually go on to develop SLE. These patients must be counseled and followed accordingly. Discoid plaques may progress and heal with extensive scarring. Topical steroids, systemic steroids, and antimalarials are the mainstay of therapy, depending on the severity of the systemic disease.

Other cutaneous findings in SLE include urticarial or psoriasis-like malar rashes, scarring and nonscarring scalp hair loss, nail-fold telangiectasias, livedo reticu-

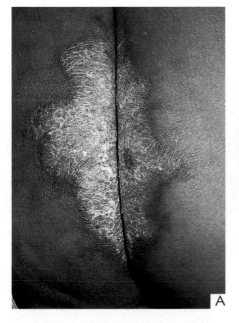
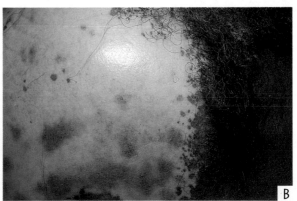

FIGURE 7.42 Discoid lupus erythematosus. **(A)** An atrophic, scaly red plaque with a hyperpigmented border in the gluteal cleft showed histologic changes typical of lupus. **(B)** Atrophy, scarring alopecia, and telangiectasias persisted in an old lesion.

laris, and palpable purpura resulting from small-vessel vasculitis (Fig. 7.43A–E). Severe Raynaud's phenomenon with digital infarcts may also develop. Mucous membranes may also be affected, with the development of nasal and oral ulcerations and painful erosions on the lip.

In addition to cutaneous features, the most comom presenting complaints in SLE are fevers and arthralgias. Other common findings include pulmonary disease (pleuritis or pneumonitis, 66 percent), cardiac manifestations (pericarditis, myocarditis, or endocarditis, 50 percent), lupus nephritis (60 percent), and central nervous system disease (50 percent).

Serologic findings can be very useful in establishing the diagnosis of lupus and other collagen vascular diseases (Fig.7.44). Almost 100 percent of patients with

SLE have a positive antinuclear antibody. The rate of positivity varies, however, with the substrate used for the test. In the past a subset of SLE patients was identified as ANA negative. Many of these patients have subsequently tested positive with Hep 2 cells, which are derived from a human tumor line, as a substrate. Although there is no direct correlation between ANA titers and disease activity, patients with high-titer ANAs tend to have active SLE. A number of other antibodies are also present in lupus patients and may correlate with certain aspects of disease activity. One of these antibody systems, Ro (SSA) and La (SSB), which is directed against a small cytoplasmic ribonuclear protein, is associated with photosensitivity, neonatal lupus, and an annular psoriasiform eruption on sun-exposed areas (see Fig. 7.43B and C). Ro and La are also found

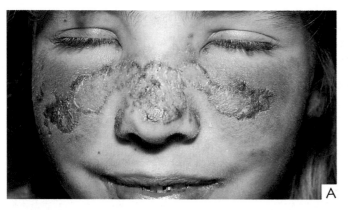

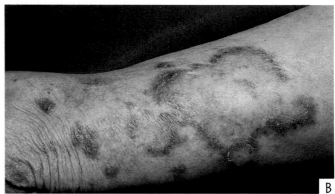

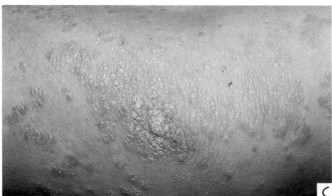

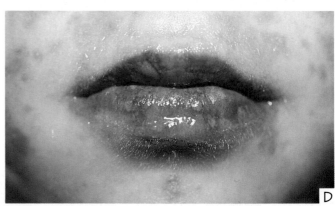

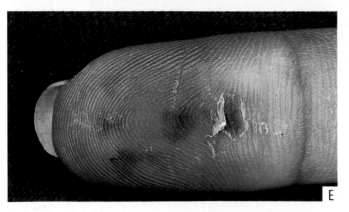

FIGURE 7.43 Lupus erythematosus. (**A**) A 13-year-old girl with SLE developed malar erythema, edema, and erosions associated with a flare of nephritis after spending a day in the sun at the beach. Other lesions typical of lupus include (**B**) annular scaly patches and plaques, (**C**) psoriasis-like plaques, (**D**) erosions on the oral mucosa and vermillion border, and (**E**) Raynaud's phenomenon with digital infarcts.

Figure 7.44 Antinuclear and Anticytoplasmic Antibodies in Collagen Vascular Disorders

Designation	Antigen	Frequently Associated Disease States
Antinuclear Antibodies		
dsDNA	Double-stranded DNA	Lupus erythematosus, nephritis
ssDNA	Single-stranded DNA	Lupus erythematosus, other nonrheumatic diseases
ENA	Estractable nuclear antigen	Subtypes as below
Sm	RNAase-resistant glycoprotein U1, U2, U4, U5, U6 small ribonucleoprotein	Lupus erythematosus, nephritis
RNP	RNAase-sensitive ribonucleoprotein (U1 small ribonucleoprotein)	Lupus erythematosus, discoid LE Mixed connective tissue disease, Raynaud's phenomenon
Leukocyte specific		Rheumatoid arthritis, Felty's syndrome
SSC (RAP)	Trypsin-sensitive protein	Rheumatoid arthritis
RANA		Rheumatoid arthritis
NANA	Nucleolar ANA	Systemic sclerosis
PM-1 (Mi)	Trypsin-sensitive protein	Polydermatomyositis
DNP	DNA-histone	Drug-induced lupus erythematosus Rheumatoid arthritis Lupus erythematosus
Centromere	Kinetochore	CREST syndrome
Centriole	Centriole	Sclerosis–Raynaud's phenomenon
Scl-70	Nonhistone nuclear protein	Systemic sclerosis, CREST syndrome
Anticytoplasmic Antibodies		
ssRNA	Single-stranded RNA	Systemic sclerosis
Ro (SSA)	Acidic glycoprotein	Lupus erythematosus, photosensitivity, Sjögren's syndrome
Ribosomal	Ribosome	Lupus erythematosus
La (SSB)	RNA-protein	Lupus erythematosus, Sjögren's syndrome

Adapted from Dahl MV, *Clinical immunopathology*. Chicago: Yearbook Medical Publishers, 1988:243.

in Sjögren's syndrome in the absence of SLE. Patients with photosensitivity should be counseled about sunscreens, protective clothing, and judicious sun exposure. Occasionally systemic disease can be triggered by excessive sun exposure.

The symptoms of *juvenile rheumatoid arthritis* (JRA) may suggest the diagnosis of lupus. However, the rash of JRA is urticarial and evanescent, peaking with fever spikes (Fig. 7.45). Unlike the destructive arthritis of JRA, the arthritis in lupus is often transient and does not impair function. Many of the other reactive erythemas may share features with lupus. However, the diagnosis of lupus is dependent on clearly defined criteria.

Dermatomyositis

Dermatomyositis (DM) accounts for only 5 percent of pediatric collagen vascular disease. However, cutaneous lesions are distinctive and mark the onset of nonsuppurative inflammation in the muscle. Unlike the adult variant, DM in childhood is self-limited and is not associated with underlying malignancy. Unfortunately, the calcinosis cutis that follows the disease can be debilitating.

Most cases of childhood DM occur between four and 12 years of age. As in lupus there is a female predominance (2:1). There is no known inheritance pattern or racial predisposition.

Cutaneous findings may precede myositis by up to a year, and the onset of signs and symptoms is usually insidious. Conversely, progressive symmetric proximal muscle weakness may precede the rash by months. Patients often complain of easy fatigability with routine tasks such as brushing teeth, combing hair, and climbing stairs. Muscle tenderness may be accompanied by anorexia, malaise, and fever. Dysphagia, dysphonia, and dyspnea occur in 10 percent of patients and signal palatal, esophageal, and thoracic involvement.

Nearly 75 percent of children with DM develop a diagnostic rash (Fig. 7.46A and B). Periorbital findings include a periorbital dermatitis, with or without edema, giving a violaceous hue and known as heliotrope. A psoriasis-like rash involves the extensor surfaces of the elbows, knees, and knuckles. Over the distal interphalangeal joints these changes are referred to as Gottron's papules (Fig. 7.47A and B). A malar rash reminiscent of lupus is variably present. Periungual and facial telangiectasias may become prominent (Fig. 7.48A). Atrophy, fibrosis, hypopigmentation, and hyperpigmentation progress gradually, resulting in poikiloderma.

Up to 50 percent of children develop dystrophic calcification in skin and muscle probably secondary to necrosis and scarring of the involved tissues (Fig. 7.48B). In some patients, painful, chronic uleration of calcified nodules, recurrent cellulitis, and progressive contractures continue to limit recovery even after active inflammation resolves. Complications may also occasionally result from gastrointestinal, cardiac, and pul-

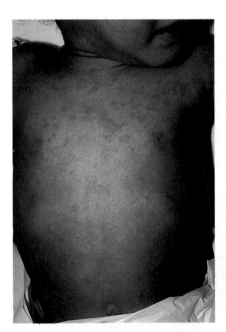

FIGURE 7.45 An evanescent, pink urticarial rash on the trunk accompanied high spiking fevers in a two-year-old boy with juvenile rheumatoid arthritis.

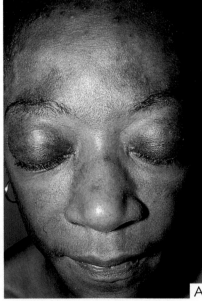

FIGURE 7.46 Dermatomyositis. **(A)** Heliotrope. A young woman with dermatomyositis presented with violaceous erythema and edema of the upper eyelids. **(B)** A 10-year-old boy with a psoriasis-like dermatitis on the elbows and knees for six months developed rapidly progressive proximal muscle weakness.

monary involvement. Treatment consists of aggressive use of systemic corticosteroids and physical therapy to preserve muscle function. In severe cases methotrexate or other immunosuppressives may be required. Persistent, widespread telangiectasias and calcinosis cutis are resistant to therapy.

Clinical diagnosis is usually confirmed by detection of elevated muscle enzymes, typical electromyographic findings, and muscle biopsy. In DM, as in lupus, the inflammatory process targets blood vessels in the involved tissues. Skin biopsies from the heliotrope rash, Gottron's papules, and the psoriasiform dermatitis demonstrate perivascular and dermal–epidermal junction changes indistinguishable from lupus.

Scleroderma

Although scleroderma is uncommon, accounting for only 5 percent of collagen vascular disease in childhood, the most common variant, localized scleroderma or morphea, can be very subtle and is probably underdiagnosed.

Localized morphea can present in a round plaque, linear, guttate, or generalized pattern (Fig. 7.49A–C). Sclerotic plaques with an ivory-white center and an advancing lilac-colored border characterize scleroderma. During the course hyperpigmentation may also become marked. In the most common form, one or several lesions from 1 cm to 10 cm in diameter appear on the trunk. In generalized morphea similar widespread

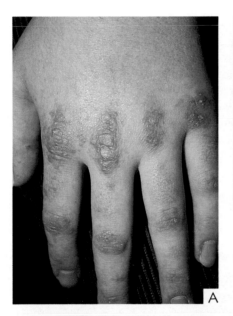

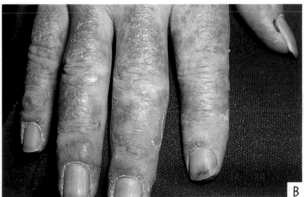

FIGURE 7.47 Gottron's papules (**A**) in a child with dermatomyositis are contrasted with a psoriasis-like dermatitis (**B**) on the hands of a patient with systemic lupus. Note the sparing of the knuckles in lupus.

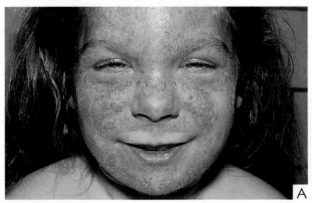

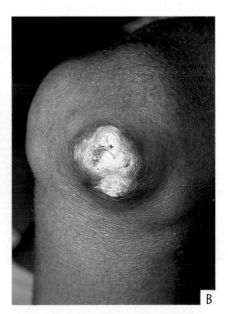

FIGURE 7.48 (**A**) Dermatomyositis. Despite resolution of cutaneous inflammation and myositis with systemic corticosteroids, telangiectasias progressed on the face of this six-year-old girl. (**B**) Extensive cutis calcinosis, particularly over bony prominences, resulted in chronic, painful draining ulcers and cellulitis in this 12-year-old boy with burned-out dermatomyositis. Note the white, chalk-like calcium deposits at the base of an ulcer on his knee.

lesions develop on the trunk and extremities. Occasionally multiple small, oval lesions reminiscent of lichen sclerosis et atrophicus erupt on the upper trunk in the guttate variant. Morphea can also progress in a linear pattern, particularly on the scalp, face, and extremities. Coup-de-sabre describes a subset of linear morphea cases in which a furrow extends vertically from the scalp across the forehead and down the face (Fig. 7.50). Involvement of the underlying soft tissue and bone may lead to severe disfigurement. Over months to years lesions heal, with softening of the involved areas and atrophy. In children, cutaneous disease without systemic symptoms is not associated with progression to systemic sclerosis.

Laboratory findings in localized scleroderma are not specific. Occasionally eosinophilia is present on a blood count, and rheumatoid factor may be elevated. Antinuclear antibodies may be present in 10 to 15 percent of cases, but are of no prognostic importance. Skin biopsies from new lesions or from the advancing borders of etablished lesions show lymphocytic inflammation between collagen bundles and around blood vessels in the deep dermis, extending into the subcutis. Some areas of fat may be replaced by newly formed collagen. In late sclerotic plaques, thick, homogeneous collagen extends from the dermal–epidermal junction into the subcutaneous tissue. Adnexal structures appear to be enveloped in collagen, and little if any inflammatory infiltrate remains.

Unfortunately, therapy has been disappointing. The use of penicillamine, even in severe localized disease, is controversial. Short courses of high-dose corticosteroids (1–2 mg/kg/day) may help to shut off rapidly progressive linear morphea when it endangers important structures. Physical therapy may be necessary when lesions extend across joints.

Progressive systemic sclerosis (PSS) is rare in childhood, and the clinical course is similar to that of adult cases. Raynaud's phenomenon is present in 90 percent of patients and may precede the onset of systemic disease by years. Classic findings in the skin include tightening of the skin associated with woody induration, edema, telangiectasias, and pigmentary changes. Other organ system involvement includes musculoskeletal, gastrointestinal, pulmonary, cardiac, and renal effects. Most patients with PSS develop antinuclear antibodies, and nearly 50 percent have antinucleolar antibodies. A number of other antibody systems are also present in some cases of PSS and may have special prognostic value.

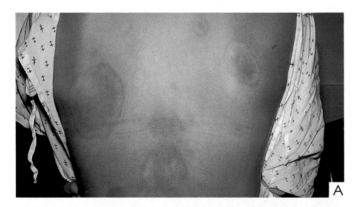

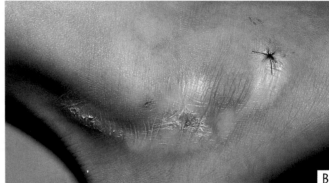

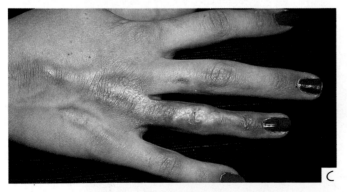

FIGURE 7.49 Scleroderma. **(A)** Multiple fibrotic plaques with central pigmentary changes and peripheral erythema slowly enlarged on the back of an adolescent girl. **(B)** An atrophic, fibrotic, hypopigmented plaque extended around the ankle of a 10-year-old girl for two years. Fortunately, she did not experience functional impairment. **(C)** Linear morphea produced fibrosis and atrophy of the soft tissue of this young woman's right fourth finger.

Lichen Sclerosis et Atrophicus

Lichen sclerosis et atrophicus (LSA) occurs most commonly in postmenopausal women. However, about 10 percent of cases appear in children under seven years of age. Although the cause is unknown, the association with morphea suggests an immunologic basis.

The anogenital area is the most common site of involvement. Typically, small, white, flat-topped papules arise on the cutaneous and mucous membrane surfaces of the labia, perineum, and perianal area. Confluent white atrophic patches may extend symmetrically in a figure-8 pattern around the vagina and rectum (Fig. 7.51A and B). Scaling, vesiculation, and hemorrhage may be prominent, particularly after accidental trauma or rubbing and scratching from pruritus. A mild watery discharge may be present. In some patients extragenital patches on the trunk and extremities pre-

dominate (Fig. 7.52A and B). In these lesions follicular dimpling caused by hyperkeratosis with follicular plugging is characteristic. Truncal patches also share clinical and histologic features with morphea, and lesions typical of both entities have been described simultaneously in the same patient.

Histopathologic findings are often diagnostic. In addition to scale and follicular plugging, there is thinning of the mid epidermis, hydropic degeneration of the basal layer, edema and homogenization of the upper dermis, and a band-like lymphohistiocytic infiltrate beneath the zone of homogenization.

Clinically, LSA should not be confused with child abuse, candidiasis, or streptococcal perianal or vaginal dermatitis. Cultures can be obtained to exclude bacterial and herpetic infections. The symmetric pattern and characteristic morphology of LSA should also help to

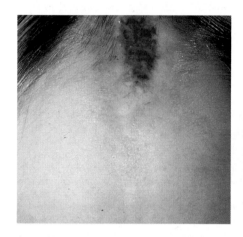

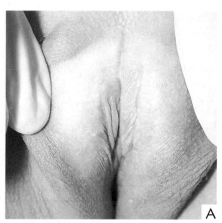

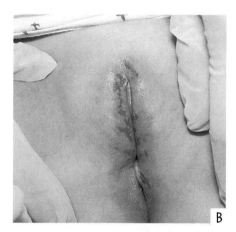

FIGURE 7.50 An unusual variant of morphea affecting the scalp, termed "coup-de-sabre" (stroke of the saber) extends from the mid-frontal scalp down the forehead to the nasal bridge.

FIGURE 7.51 Lichen sclerosis et atrophicus. (**A**) A pruritic, atrophic hypopigmented patch involved the genital skin and mucous membranes in this

five-year-old girl. (**B**) This girl presented with itchy recurrent erosions and a serosanguinous discharge. Note lesions extending around the vagina and anus.

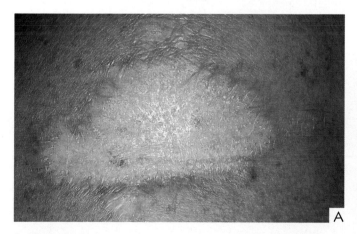

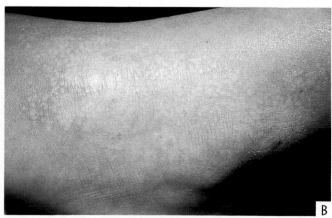

FIGURE 7.52 Lichen sclerosis et atrophicus. Atrophic, hypopigmented scaly papules coalesced into confluent

patches on the (**A**) trunk and (**B**) extremities of a 10-year-old girl.

eliminate child abuse as a serious consideration. In vitiligo, which may also present in a symmetric pattern in the anogenital area, the skin is completely normal except for depigmentation (Fig. 7.53). Inflammatory bowel disease may present with vaginal and perianal nodules, sinus tracts, and ulcers (Fig. 7.54). Other symptoms of gastrointestinal disease may be absent. Skin biopsies in these cases demonstrate granulomas typical of Crohn's disease. Primary bullous dermatoses may also present a diagnostic dilemma. If the clinical presentation is not distinctive, a skin biopsy with direct immunofluorescence may be necessary to make the diagnosis.

Necrobiosis Lipoidica

In necrobiosis lipoidica, reddish-yellow, indurated plaques typically appear on the shins in diabetics (Fig. 7.55A and B). As the lesions expand from less than 1 cm to 4 cm or larger over months, the center of the plaque becomes shiny and atrophic. Telangiectasias extend from the center. Although lesions may remain stable and will occasionally heal without treatment, most persist or slowly progress, and minor trauma may result in chronic, painful ulcerations. Some patients improve with topical or intralesional steroids injected into the expanding red border.

About 75 percent of patients with necrobiosis are female and over 50 percent have diabetes mellitus (necrobiosis lipoidica diabeticorum). In some cases necrobiosis precedes the onset of clinical diabetes by years. Although the cause is unknown, investigators have suggested that some sort of vascular insult triggered by diabetes initiates the necrobiotic changes in collagen. Histologically, granulomatous inflammation is present around altered and degenerating collagen, which extends in large bands into the deep reticular dermis. The overlying epidermis is atrophic and ulceration may be present. Thickening of vascular walls, endothelial cell proliferation, and occasionally vascular occlusion are seen throughout the dermis. The yellow color is imparted by deposition of lipid around necrobiotic collagen.

Necrobiosis lipoidica can usually be differentiated from granuloma annulare, which does not develop epidermal changes. In some patients fibrotic or atrophic plaques in scleroderma or lichen sclerosis et atrophicus mimic necrobiosis. The clinical course and skin biopsy findings, however, are distinctive.

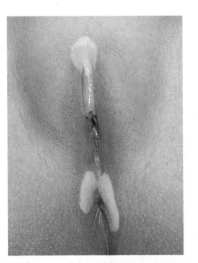

FIGURE 7.53
Vitiligo developed around the vagina and anus of a two-year-old girl, mimicking the pattern of lichen sclerosis et atrophicus.

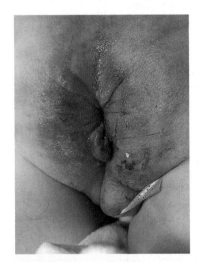

FIGURE 7.54
Inflammatory bowel disease. A two-year-old girl was treated for chronic diaper dermatitis and candidiasis for months before the diagnosis of Crohn's disease was considered. A biopsy of the perianal skin showed granulomas.

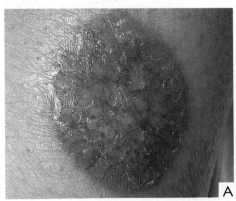

A

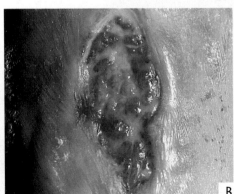

B

FIGURE 7.55
Necrobiosis lipoidica. (A) A plaque on the shin of a 17-year-old diabetic demonstrates the typical red border and yellow, shiny atrophic center with telangiectasias. (B) This patient developed a chronic painful ulcer after repeated trauma. The ulcer healed after several months of treatment with occlusive dressings.

ALGORITHM FOR EVALUATION OF REACTIVE ERYTHEMA

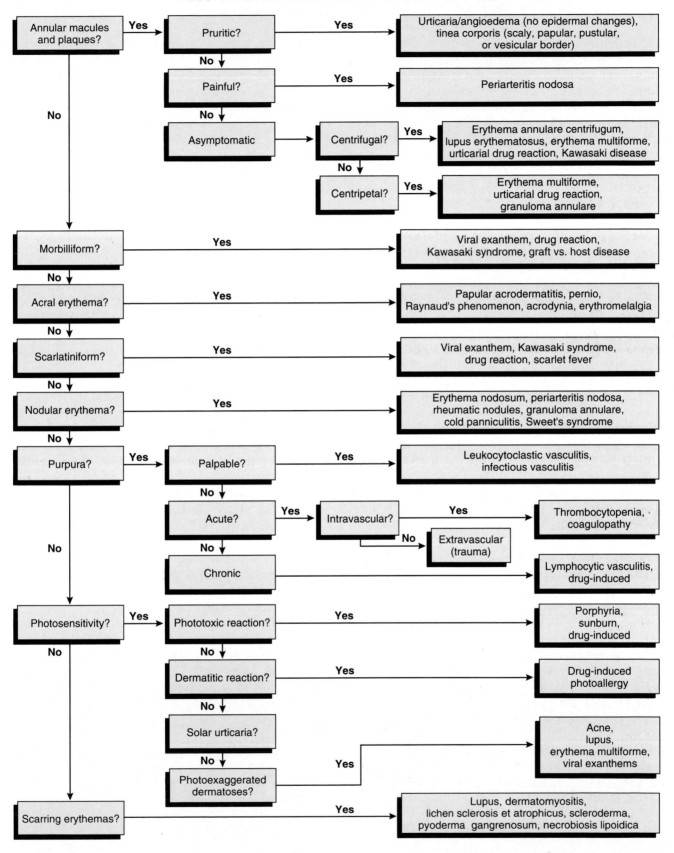

BIBLIOGRAPHY

Drug eruptions
Hood AF, Bronner A. Cutaneous complications of chemotherapeutic agents. *J Am Acad Dermatol* 9:645–663, 1983.

VanArsdel PP. Allergy and adverse drug reactions. *J Am Acad Dermatol* 6:833–845, 1982.

Wintroub BU, Stern R. Cutaneous drug reactions: pathogenesis and clinical classification. *J Am Acad Dermatol* 13:167–179, 1985.

Erythema multiforme
Nethercott JR, Choi CK. Erythema multiforme (Stevens–Johnson syndrome)—chart review of 123 hospitalized patients. *Dermatologica* 171:383–396, 1985.

Rasmussen JE. Erythema multiforme in children: response to treatment with sytemic corticosteroids. *Br J Dermatol* 95:181–186, 1976.

Special symposium: corticosteroids for erythema multiforme? *Pediatr Dermatol* 6:299–250, 1989.

Stevens AM, Johnson FC. A new eruptive fever associated with stomatitis and ophthlmia, report of two cases in children. *Am J Dis Child* 24:526–533, 1922.

Urticaria
Champion RH, Roberts SO, Carpenter RG, et al. Urticaria and angioedema. A review of 554 cases. *Br J Dermatol* 81:588–597, 1969.

Kauppinen K, Juntunen K, Lanki H. Urticaria in children. Retrospective evaluation and follow-up. *Allergy* 39:469–472, 1984.

Legrain V, Taieb A, Sage T, Maleville J. Urticaria in infants: a study of forty patients. *Pediatr Dermatol* 7:101–107, 1990.

Twatog FJ. Urticaria in childhood: pathogenesis and management. *Pediatr Clin North Am* 30:887–898, 1983.

Viral exanthems
Anand A, Gray ES, Brown TB, et al. Human parvovirus infection in pregnancy and hydrops fetalis. *N Engl J Med* 316:183–186, 1987.

Anderson LJ. Human parvovirus B19. *Pediatr Ann* 19:509–516, 1990.

Asano Y, Nakashima T, Yoshikawa T, et al. Severity of human Herpesvirus 6 viremia and clinical findings in infants with exanthem subitum. *J Pediatr* 118:891–895, 1991.

Cherry JD. Viral exanthems. *Curr Probl Pediatr* 13:5–44, 1983.

Hall CB. Herpes and the rash of roses: a new virus, HHV6, as the cause of an old childhood disease, roseola. *Pediatr Ann* 13:517–521.

Lepow ML. Measles vaccine and measles control. *Pediatr Ann* 13:543–550.

Kawasaki disease
Fujita Y, Nakamura U, Sakata K, et al. Kawasaki disease in families. *Pediatrics* 84:666–669.

Nakamura Y, Fuzita Y, Nagai M, et al. Cardiac sequelae of Kawasaki disease in Japan: statistical analysis. *Pediatrics* 88:1144–1147, 1991.

Neuburger JW, Takahashi M, Burns JC, et al. The treatment of Kawasaki syndrome with intravenous gamma globulin. *N Engl J Med* 315:341–347.

Taubert KA, Rowley AH, Shulman ST. Nationwide survey of Kawasaki disease and acute rheumatic fever. *J Pediatr* 119:279–282, 1991.

Acral erythema
Kurzrock R, Cohen PR. Erythromelalgia: review of clinical characteristics and pathophysiology. *Am J Med* 91:416–422, 1991.

Lokich JK, Moore C. Chemotherapy-associated palmar-plantar erythrodysesthesia syndrome. *Ann Intern Med* 101:798–800, 1984.

Michiels JJ, Abels J, Steketee J, et al. Erythromelalgia caused by platelet-mediated arteriolar inflammation and thrombosis in thrombocytopenia. *Ann Intern Med* 102:466–471, 1985.

Page EH, Shear NH. Temperature-dependent skin disorders. *J Am Acad Dermatol* 18:1003–1019, 1988.

Purpura fulminans
Auletta MJ, Headington JT. Purpura fulminans. A cutaneous manifestation of severe protein C deficiency. *Arch Dermatol* 124:1387–1391, 1988.

Robboy SJ, Mihm MC, Colman RC, et al. The skin in disseminated intravascular coagulation. *Br J Dermatol* 88:221–229, 1973.

Henoch–Schönlein purpura
Ekenstam E, Callen JP. Cutaneous leukocytoclastic vasculitis. *Arch Dermatol* 118:412–416, 1984.

Salibfury FT. Henoch–Schönlein purpura. *Pediatr Dermatol* 1:195, 1984.

Sams WM Jr. Necrotizing vasculitis (Review). *J Am Acad Dermatol* 3:1–13, 1980.

Sanchez NP, Van Hale HM, Su WPD. Clinical and histopathologic spectrum of necrotizing vasculitis. *Arch Dermatol* 121:220–224, 1985.

Periarteritis nodosa

Jones SK, Lane AT, Golitz LE, Weston WL. Cutaneous periarteritis nodosa in a child. *Am J Dis Child* 139:920–922, 1985.

Moreland LW, Ball GV. Cutaneous polyarteritis nodosa. *Am J Med* 88:426–430.

Ozen S, Besbas N, Saatci U, Bakkaloglu. Diagnostic criteria for polyarteritis nodosa in childhood. *J Pediatr* 120:205–209, 1992.

Progressive pigmented purpuric dermatosis

Newton RC, Raimer SS. Pigmented purpuric eruptions. *Dermatol Clin* 3:165, 1985.

Price ML, Jones EW, Calnan CD, Macdonald DM. Lichen aureus: a localized persistent form of pigmented purpuric dermatitis. *Br J Dermatol* 112:307–314, 1985.

Septicemia

Dalldorf FG, Jennette JC. Fatal meningococcal septicemia. *Arch Pathol* 101:6–9, 1977.

Dorff GI, Geimer NF, Rosenthal DR, et al. *Pseudomonas* septicemia. Illustrated evolution of its skin lesion. *Arch Intern Med* 128:591–595, 1971.

Sweet's syndrome

Hazen PG, Kark EC, Davis BR, et al. Acute febrile neutrophilic dermatosis in children: report of two cases in male infants. *Arch Dermatol* 119:998–1002, 1983.

Itami S, Nishioka K. Sweet's syndrome in infancy. *Br J Dermatol* 103:449–451, 1980.

Levin DL, Esterly NB, Herman JJ, Boxall LB. The Sweet syndrome in children. *J Pediatr* 99:73–78, 1981.

Pyoderma gangrenosum

Gilman AL, Cohen BA, Wrbach AH, Blatt J. Pyoderma gangrenosum: a manifestation of leukemia in children. *Pediatr* 81:846–848, 1988.

Hayani A, Steuber CP, Mahoney DH, Levy ML. Pyoderma gangrenosum in childhood leukemia. *Pediatr Dermatol* 7:296–298, 1990.

Erythema annulare centrifigum

Bressler GS, Jones RE. Erythema annulare centrifigum. *J Am Acad Dermatol* 4:597–602, 1981.

Erytherma marginatum

Sahn EE, Maize JC, Silver RM. Erythema marginatum: an unusual histopathologic manifestation. *J Am Acad Dermatol* 21:145–147, 1989.

Troyer C, Grossman ME, Silvers DN. Erythema marginatum in rheumatic fever: early diagnosis by skin biopsy. *J Am Acad Dermatol* 8:724–728, 1983.

Erythema chronicum migrans

Cristofaro RL, Appel MH, Gelb RI, et al. Musculoskeletal manifestations of Lyme disease in children. *J Pediatr Orthop* 7:527–530, 1987.

Eichenfield AH, Goldsmith DP, Benach JL, et al. Childhood Lyme arthritis: experience in an endemic area. *J Pediatr* 109:753–758, 1986.

Rose CD, Fawcett PT, Singsen BH, Dubbi SB, Doughty RA. Use of western blot and enzyme-linked immunosorbent assays to assist in diagnosis of Lyme disease. *Pediatrics* 88:465–470, 1991.

Steere AC. Lyme disease. *N Engl J Med* 321:586–596, 1989.

Panniculitis

Horsfield GI, Yardley HJ. Sclerema neonatorum. *J Invest Dermatol* 44:326–332, 1965.

KorAnsky JS, Esterly NB. Lupus panniculitis (profundus). *J Pediatr* 948:241, 1981.

Laurance B, Stone GH, Philpott MG, et al. Aetiology of erythema nodosum in children. *Lancet* 2:14–X, 1961.

Rotman H. Cold panniculitis in children. *Arch Dermatol* 94:720–724, 1966.

Photosensitivity

Harber LC, Bickers DR. *Photosensitivity diseases*, 2nd ed. Toronto: B.C. Decker, 1989.

National Institutes of Health consensus development conference statement: sunlight, ultraviolet radiation, and the skin. 7:1–10, 1989.

Stern RS, Weinstein MC, Baker SG. Risk reduction for nonmelanoma skin cancer with childhood sunscreen use. *Arch Dermatol* 122:537–545, 1986.

Lupus erythematosus

Glideen RS, Mantzouranis EC, Borel Y. Systemic lupus

erythematosus in childhood: clinical manifestations and improved survival in fifty-five patients. *Clin Immunol Immunopathol* 29:196–210, 1983.

Jones EM, Callen JP. Collagen vascular diseases of childhood. *Pediatr Clin N Am* 38:1019–1039, 1991.

Dermatomyositis

Pachman LM. Juvenile dermatomyositis: a clinical overview. *Pediatr Rev* 12:117–125, 1990.

Rockerbie NR, Woo TY, Callen JP, Giustina T. Cutaneous changes of dermatomyositis precede muscle weakness. *J Am Acad Dermatol* 20:629–632, 1989.

Silver RM, Maricq HR. Childhood dermatomyositis: serial microvascular studies. *Pediatrics* 83:278–283, 1989.

Woo TY, Callen JP, Voorhees JJ, et al. Cutaneous lesions of dermatomyositis are improved by hydroxychloroquine. *J Am Acad Dermatol* 10:592–600, 1984.

Scleroderma

Christianson HB, Dorsey CS, O'Leary PA, Kierland RR. Localized scleroderma: a clinical study of 235 cases. *Arch Dermatol* 74:629–639, 1956.

Moore EC, Cohen F, Farooki Z, Chang C. Focal scleroderma and severe cardiomyopathy: patient report and brief review. *Am J Dis Child* 145:229–231, 1991.

Lichen sclerosis et atrophicus

Clark JA, Mulb SA. Lichen sclerosis et atrophicus in children. A report of 24 cases. *Arch Dermatol* 95:476–482, 1967.

Loening-Baucke V. Lichen sclerosis et atrophicus in children. *Am J Dis Child* 145:1058–1061, 1991.

Necrobiosis lipoidica

Ullman S, Dahl MV. Necrobiosis lipoidica. *Arch Dermatol* 113:1671–1673, 1977.

Wood MG, Beerman H. Necrobiosis lipoidica, granuloma annulare, and rheumatoid nodule. *J Invest Dermatol* 34:139–147, 1960.

chapter eight

DISORDERS OF THE HAIR
AND NAILS

Diseases of the hair and nails are an important part of pediatric dermatology. Both hair and nails are composed of keratin, produced by the hair follicle and nail matrix. Some diseases are specific to these structures, whereas others affect the skin and other organ systems as well. In many cases, important diagnostic clues to skin and systemic disease can be found in related abnormalities of the hair and nails.

HAIR DISORDERS

Embryology and Anatomy

Hair follicles first appear on the face of the developing fetus at the end of the first trimester. They develop as a downbudding of the epidermis in association with proliferating mesenchyme, which eventually becomes the dermal papilla. The development of scalp and body hair follicles is delayed until about the fourth month. By 17 weeks, emergent hair shafts can be found over the face and at 18 weeks over the scalp. The growth of hair shafts occurs in a cephalocaudad direction. No new hair follicles develop, nor are follicles destroyed, after birth. However, the hair density decreases somewhat as the body surface area increases.

In the premature infant the scalp, forehead, and trunk are covered with variable amounts of fine, soft, long, lightly pigmented lanugo hair (Fig. 8.1). Lanugo is usually shed in utero at seven to eight months gestation. A second covering of subtle lanugo is shed shortly after birth and is replaced by short, fine, lightly pigmented vellus hair. Terminal hair is thicker and more darkly pigmented, and usually grows on the scalp, eyebrows, and eyelashes before puberty and the sites of sexual hair after puberty.

At term most infants have full scalp coverage with normal terminal hair. However, shortly before birth or up to four months postnatally, infants undergo a period

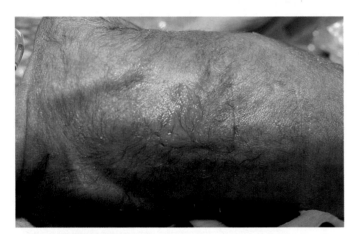

FIGURE 8.1 Lanugo hair. A 31-week preemie had extensive lanugo hair covering most of the back. At term, this hair is usually shed before delivery.

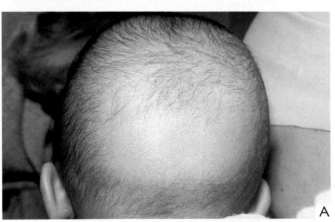

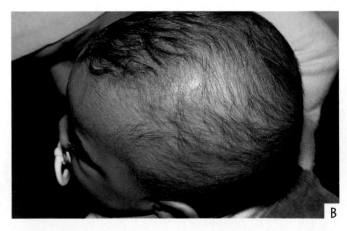

FIGURE 8.2 (**A,B**) These infants demonstrate the physiologic hair shedding that occurs in dark-haired babies at three to five months of age. In (**A**), note the band of exaggerated alopecia, probably brought on by trauma, girdling the occiput.

of brisk shedding when the infantile pattern shifts to a normal adult pattern of hair growth (Fig. 8.2A and B). In blonds and redheads the process is often complete before birth, and the hair is sparse at delivery. Shedding may be delayed in dark-haired individuals and may occur rapidly during early infancy. Parents should be reassured that this is a normal physiologic process.

The normal hair cycle consists of three components (Fig. 8.3). When the hair enters anagen (the active growth phase) the hair follicle enlarges into the deep dermis, where it surrounds the developing dermal papilla. Matrix cells proliferate and migrate into the upper part of the bulb to form the hair shaft. The length of anagen is genetically determined and varies according to anatomic location. Anagen in the scalp varies from two to three years. Catagen is a transitional phase, which lasts about three weeks, during which matrix cell growth ceases and the end of the hair bulb shrinks,

forms a club shape, and rises up the hair follicle. Finally, during telogen, the hair is attached to the upper portion of the hair follicle for three to four months before being shed. Telogen hairs are pushed out by the new anagen hair shafts arising from the base of the follicle.

In the newborn, scalp hair growth is synchronous, with all hairs in a given area in the same phase of the hair cycle. Between four months and about two years of age the normal dyssynchronous pattern becomes established. In this adult pattern approximately 85 percent to 90 percent of hairs in any given location are in anagen, 10 percent to 15 percent in telogen, and fewer than 1 percent in catagen.

Congenital and Hereditary Disorders

The normal pattern of hair growth and shaft morphology may be disturbed in a number of hereditary disorders and congenital syndromes (Fig. 8.4).

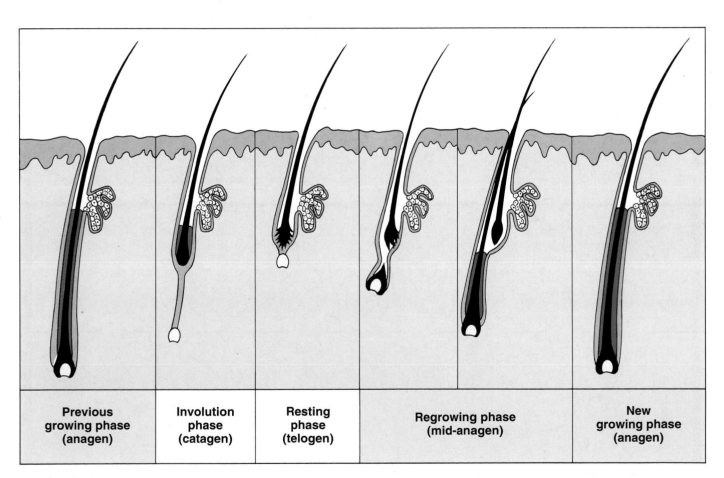

| Previous growing phase (anagen) | Involution phase (catagen) | Resting phase (telogen) | Regrowing phase (mid-anagen) | New growing phase (anagen) |

FIGURE 8.3 Normal hair cycle.

Figure 8.4 Selected Hair Anomalies

Alopecia (localized)

Harmartomatous nevi
Pigmented nevi
Halo scalp ring
Incontinentia pigmenti
Aplasia cutis congenita

Alopecia (generalized)

Hypohidrotic ectodermal dysplasia
CHILD syndrome
Clouston's syndrome
Cockayne's syndrome
Dyskeratosis congenita
Hallermann–Streiff syndrome
Hay–Wells syndrome
Homocystinuria
Menkes' syndrome
Oculodentodigital syndrome
Progeria
Trichorhinophalangeal syndrome
Trichothiodystrophy
Cartilage–HAIR hypoplasia
Papillon–Lefèvre syndrome
Acrodermatitis enteropathica

Hair shaft anomalies

Pili torti (twisted hair)
Björnstad's syndrome
Trichothiodystrophy
Menkes' syndrome
Monilethrix (beaded hair)
Arginosuccinicaciduria
Menkes' syndrome
Trichorrhexis nodosa
Arginosuccinicaciduria
Menkes' syndrome
Trichothiodystrophy
Trichorrhexis invaginata (bamboo hair)
Netherton's syndrome
Kinky hair
Tricho-dento-osseous syndrome
Menkes' syndrome
Uncombable hair syndrome
Wooly hair nevus

Hirsutism (localized)

Congenital pigmented nevus
Congenital smooth muscle and pilar hamartoma

Hirsutism (generalized)

Berardinelli lipodystrophy syndrome
Cerebro-oculo-facio skeletal syndrome
Coffin–Siris syndrome
Cornelia de Lange syndrome
Fetal hydantoin syndrome
Frontometaphyseal dysplasia
Mucopolysaccharidoses
Leprechaunism
Marshall–Smith syndrome
Trisomy 18
Schinzel–Giedion syndrome
Fetal alcohol syndrome

Localized patches of alopecia may be associated with perinatal trauma or hamartomatous malformations (Fig. 8.5A–D). In halo scalp ring, transient hair loss or permanent scarring results from local edema and vascular compromise produced by trauma to the scalp during labor. Scarring alopecia is a frequent complication of aplasia cutis congenita and incontinentia pigmenti, in which localized vasospasm, thrombosis, or vasculitis causes necrosis and ulceration of the skin. A number of nevi, such as hemangiomas, epidermal nevi, pigmented nevi, and connective tissue nevi, may also interrupt normal hair growth patterns.

Generalized sparse or abnormal hair growth should suggest an inherited hair shaft anomaly or genodermatosis (Fig. 8.6). Monilethrix is a relatively common developmental hair defect that results in brittle, beaded

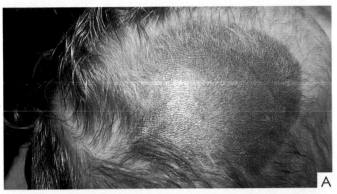
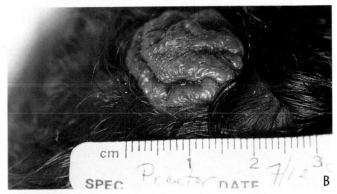
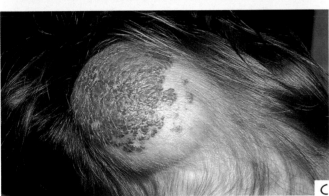
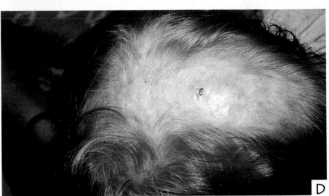

FIGURE 8.5 Congenital localized alopecia. (**A**) Marked hair thinning was present in a congenital pigmented nevus on the scalp. By 12 months of age the hair overlying the nevus was dark, long, and coarse. (**B**) An area of complete alopecia was noted at birth in a cerebriform nevus sebaceus.

(**C**) A one-year-old had sparse hair overlying an involuting hemangioma on the scalp. (**D**) A patch of permanent scarring alopecia extended across the mid-scalp of a child with amniotic band syndrome.

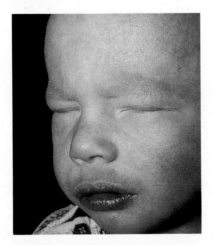

FIGURE 8.6 Ulerythema of the eyebrows and cheeks. In this variant of keratosis pilaris, inflammation of the pilosebaceous structures is associated with progressive alopecia and atrophy of involved hair follicles. This may occur as an isolated disorder of keratinization or in association with other anomalies.

hair (Fig. 8.7A and B). The condition is transmitted as an autosomal dominant trait, and clinical manifestations usually appear after two to three months of age, when vellus hairs are replaced by abnormal beaded hairs. Although the scalp is most severely affected, hair on any area of the body can be involved. The condition persists throughout life but may improve in adolescence or adulthood.

Care must be taken not to confuse monilethrix with pili torti, another structural defect in which the hair shaft is twisted on its own axis (Fig. 8.8A and B). Pili torti can be localized or generalized, and also appears with the first terminal hair growth of infancy. It may occur as an isolated hair defect or in association with a multisystem disorder such as Menke's syndrome, an inherited disease of copper metabolism which also affects the central nervous, cardiovascular, and skeletal systems.

In the ectodermal dysplasia syndromes, a heterogeneous group of genodermatoses, sparse hair is associated with dysmorphic facies and abnormalities of other structures including nails, sweat glands, and teeth (Fig. 8.9). In the hypohidrotic variants, early diagnosis may prevent fatal hyperthermia, which may develop during otherwise self-limited childhood infections.

Trichothiodystrophy is a distinctive hair shaft defect of autosomal recessive inheritance. It is characterized by increased fragility, splitting of the hair, low sulfur content, and alternating light and dark transverse bands on polarizing microscopy. Clinically, the hair is sparse, dull, and brittle. Multisystem features, including a progeria-like appearance, mental retardation, growth retardation, hypogonadism, photosensitivity, cataracts, and other neurologic abnormalities, have been reported with trichothiodystrophy.

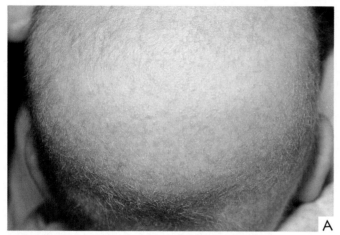
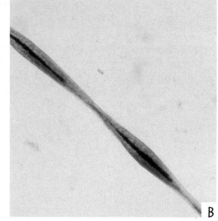

FIGURE 8.7 Monilethrix. (**A**) Short broken hairs give the appearance of diffuse alopecia. (**B**) Microscopically, one can see periodic narrowing of this hair shaft. Hairs are brittle and break off at constricted points near the scalp.

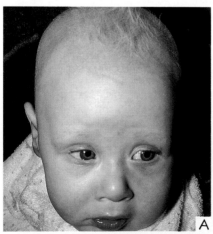
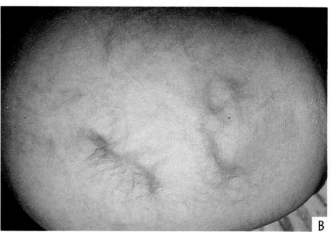

FIGURE 8.8 (A,B) Menke's syndrome. This child presented with light-pigmented skin, blue eyes, sparse hair demonstrating pili torti, seizures, and loss of developmental landmarks. Copper and ceruloplasmin levels in the serum were low.

Children with congenital hair disorders require a careful medical and neurodevelopmental evaluation. Family history will aid in establishing a pattern of inheritance. Hairs should be examined microscopically to detect specific anomalies.

Acquired Alopecia

Acquired alopecias can be distinguished by the presence or absence of clinical scarring. In nonscarring processes inflammation may be clinically evident, subtle, or absent. Nonscarring disorders can be further subdivided on the basis of localized or diffuse involvement.

Scarring Alopecia A number of inflammatory disorders can involve the hair follicle primarily or by spread from contiguous skin. In lichen planus and lupus of the scalp, hair structures are usually involved early in the course of the disease (see Chapter 7). Folliculitis decalvans, a noninfectious folliculitis, also produces slowly but relentlessly enlarging areas of cicatricial alopecia. Physical agents including allergens, irritants (acids and alkalis), thermal burns, and blunt trauma may cause necrosis of the skin and nonspecific scarring. Examples include alkali burns from hair grooming products, surgical scars, and radiation-induced injuries.

Patients with scarring alopecia deserve a careful examination of the skin, nails, and mucous membranes to identify clues to diagnosis. When the cause is not readily apparent, a skin biopsy should be considered. Delay in diagnosis and treatment may result in widespread patches of disfiguring, scarring alopecia.

Nonscarring Alopecia Most hair loss in children occurs without scarring. Clinically, the practitioner can distinguish between nonscarring alopecia associated with inflammation (e.g., erythema, scale, vesicles, pustules) and those disorders in which the scalp appears otherwise normal. The most common cause of inflammatory alopecia in children is tinea capitis. On the other hand, the scalp usually appears normal in telogen and anagen effluvium, alopecia areata, and traumatic hair loss.

Tinea Capitis Tinea capitis is the most common cause of hair loss in children between the ages of two and ten years (Fig. 8.10). For unknown reasons, this form of ringworm is endemic among black school children, although it is occasionally found in white children.

There are a variety of clinical presentations of tinea capitis. In some children, mild redness and scaling of the scalp reminiscent of seborrhea are seen in areas of partial alopecia. In other cases, widespread hair breakage caused by endothrix, or invasion of the hair shaft by the fungus, creates a "salt and pepper" appearance, with short residual hairs poking above the surface as black dots on the surface of the scalp. Occasionally, the scalp lesions are annular, like patches of tinea corporis. In

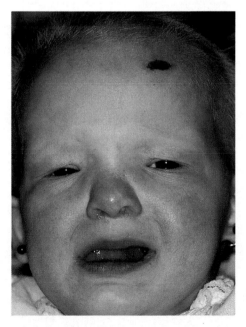

FIGURE 8.9 Hypohidrotic ectodermal dysplasia. This toddler demonstrates the typical findings of sparse hair, absent eyebrows and lashes, absent teeth, prominent forehead and supraorbital ridges, pointed chin, and midfacial hypoplasia.

some children, senstitization to the infecting organism leads to erythema, edema, and pustule formation. As the latter rupture and the area weeps, thick, matted, yellow crusts form, simulating impetigo. Less commonly, intense inflammation causes formation of raised, tender, boggy plaques studded with pustules, known as kerions. Large and occasionally painful occipital, postauricular, and preauricular adenopathy occurs with inflammatory

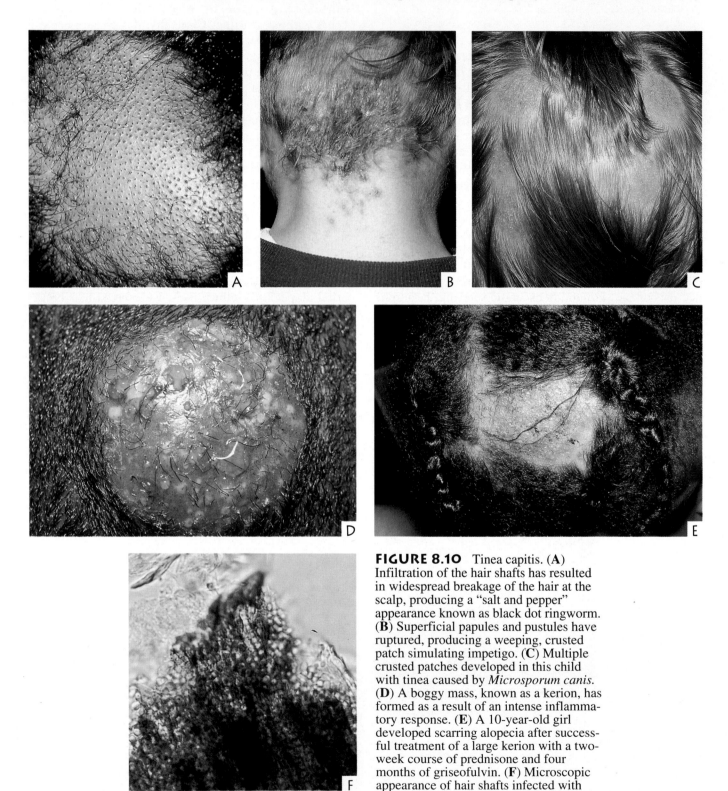

FIGURE 8.10 Tinea capitis. (**A**) Infiltration of the hair shafts has resulted in widespread breakage of the hair at the scalp, producing a "salt and pepper" appearance known as black dot ringworm. (**B**) Superficial papules and pustules have ruptured, producing a weeping, crusted patch simulating impetigo. (**C**) Multiple crusted patches developed in this child with tinea caused by *Microsporum canis*. (**D**) A boggy mass, known as a kerion, has formed as a result of an intense inflammatory response. (**E**) A 10-year-old girl developed scarring alopecia after successful treatment of a large kerion with a two-week course of prednisone and four months of griseofulvin. (**F**) Microscopic appearance of hair shafts infected with fungi. Note the tight packing of fungal arthrospores that cause hair shaft fragility and breakage (KOH mount for endothrix.)

tinea. Unless they are treated promptly and aggressively with oral antifungal agents and, in severe cases, oral corticosteroids, kerions may heal with scarring and permanent hair loss. Incision and drainage are not indicated, as loculations are small and septae thick.

Fungal infection of the scalp is readily confirmed by a KOH preparation of infected hairs. The best hairs for examination are those that are broken off at the surface. A good specimen can be obtained by scraping hairs and scale onto a glass slide with a #15 blade. A toothbrush can be used to brush hairs and scale from large areas of the scalp directly onto fungal medium for culture. Before 1970, most cases of tinea capitis in this country were caused by *Microsporum* species which fluoresce bright blue-green with a Wood's light. Unfortunately, this screening tool is of little value today because the endothrix infection produced by *Trichophyton tonsurans* does not fluoresce.

Topical antifungal agents do not penetrate deep enough to be effective in treatment of tinea capitis. However, oral griseofulvin and ketoconazole administered over two to four months are effective. Although this usually eradicates infection, the risk of reinfection is high. Recurrent infection should prompt a careful examination and possible culture of other family members to identify untreated cases. Concurrent use of selenium sulfide 2.5% shampoo or ketoconazole shampoo may help to minimize the risk of recurrence and spread to siblings and classmates.

Although most children who present with scalp pustules have tinea capitis, bacterial folliculitis should also be considered, particularly when the pustules are small, superficial, not associated with hair loss, and appear at the base of hairs under tension along parts in the hair. This disorder, termed impetigo of Bockhart, is easily treated by regular shampooing and loosening of the hair (Fig. 8.11). Occasionally an oral antibiotic is required. Seborrhea may be difficult to distinguish from tinea.

However, in seborrhea the scaly patches are usually symmetric and only mildly pruritic. A black school child with patches of scalp "seborrhea" deserves a KOH preparation and fungal culture to exclude tinea.

Telogen and Anagen Effluvium *Telogen effluvium* is the most common form of noninflammatory, nonscarring, diffuse hair loss in children (Fig. 8.12). In this form of alopecia some sort of systemic insult, such as severe illness, high fever, surgery, or certain drugs, triggers an abnormally high number of anagen hairs to switch over to telogen. This is followed three to five months later by diffuse, brisk shedding of telogen hairs. Although quite distressing, telogen effluvium is temporary and rarely produces more than 50 percent hair loss. In fact, the hair loss marks the end of the process as new anagen hairs replace those being shed. In some children telogen loss occurs repeatedly after recurrent ear infections and upper respiratory infections. Even in these cases the prognosis for full recovery is excellent. No treatment or laboratory studies are usually required. Early in the course, diagnosis can be confirmed by examination of hairs pulled from the scalp, which should demonstrate an increased percentage of telogen hairs. Parents should also be reminded that hair grows only about 1 cm each month, so that return to pretelogen effluvium hair length may take many months.

In *anagen effluvium,* sudden loss of growing hairs is caused by abnormal cessation of the anagen phase. Various toxins and antimetabolites trigger this diffuse process, which may involve up to 90 percent of scalp hairs over several days to several weeks. The extent of hair loss is determined by the toxicity of the agent and by the dose and length of exposure. In anagen effluvium, the hair shafts taper and lose adhesion to the follicle.

This type of alopecia is most common after systemic chemotherapy. Patients can be identified by the few long remaining telogen hairs scattered throughout the

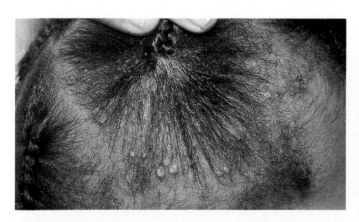

FIGURE 8.11 Impetigo of Bockhart. A toddler with tightly braided plaits developed follicular pustules in the area of greatest traction.

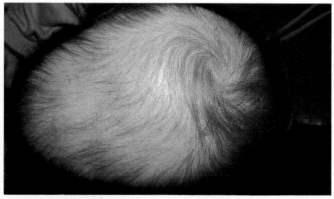

FIGURE 8.12 Telogen effluvium. An otherwise healthy six-year-old developed diffuse thinning of scalp hair three months after febrile illness. After a six-week period of brisk shedding, his hair regrew to normal thickness.

scalp. Other toxins including lead, arsenic, thallium, and x-irradiation can also cause anagen loss. Full hair regrowth usually occurs when the toxic agent is discontinued.

Alopecia Areata *Alopecia areata* is a form of asymptomatic localized alopecia that presents with round patches of complete hair loss anywhere on the body including the scalp, eyebrows, lashes, extremities, and trunk (Fig. 8.13). Occasionally hair loss progresses to involve the entire scalp (alopecia totalis) and body (alopecia universalis). The insult that triggers alopecia areata is unknown but probably is immunologic in origin. Although clinical signs of inflammation are absent, skin biopsies from sites of active disease show perifollicular lymphocyte infiltration as well as deposition of antibody and immune complexes.

Clues to diagnosis include the absence of inflammation and scaling in involved areas of the scalp and the presence of short (3 to 6 mm), easily epilated hairs at the margins of the patch. Under magnification these hair stubs resemble exclamation points, as the hair shaft narrows just before its point of entry into the follicle. Another finding in many patients with alopecia areata is Scotch plaid pitting of the nails, consisting of rows of pits crossing in a transverse and longitudinal pattern.

The course of alopecia areata is unpredictable; in adolescents and young adults hair loss usually resolves over months to years, without permanent alopecia. In infants and young children, particularly when alopecia is diffuse, the prognosis is more guarded. Treatment should include safe measures without risk of systemic toxicity. Topical steroids, local irritants (e.g., tar preparations, anthralin), topical minoxidil, topical sensitizers

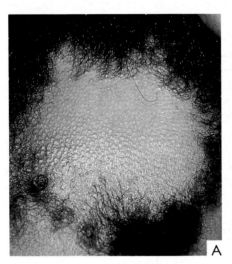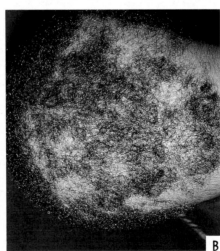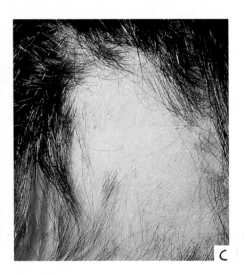

FIGURE 8.13 Alopecia areata. (**A**) A round patch of alopecia without scale or inflammation appeared on the scalp of a 10-year-old boy. The shiny complete alopecia is typical of alopecia areata. (**B**) Multiple patches of various sizes and in various stages of development cover the scalp of a healthy five-year-old. The lack of scale or inflammation helps to distinguish this presentation from tinea capitis. (**C**) In this closeup, small broken hairs which pull out easily are seen at the margins of a new, progressive patch.

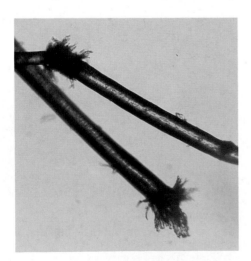

FIGURE 8.14 Trichorrhexis nodosa. A brittle hair shaft defect usually caused by overmanipulation of the hair or chemical use. The frayed broom appearance is typical.

(e.g., diphencyclopropenone), and ultraviolet light therapy have been used with some success. Although oral corticosteroids may induce hair regrowth, it has not been demonstrated that these medications change the prognosis of alopecia areata. Consequently, their use should be restricted to short courses in selected patients with widespread, rapidly progressive disease.

Traumatic Hair Loss Alopecia caused by breakage of the hair shaft is often due to an acquired structural defect of the hair, and is easily diagnosed by microscopic examination. The most comon defect is *trichorrhexis nodosa*. This can develop at any age and presents as brittle, short hairs that are perceived by the patient as not growing. By gentle pulling, one can demonstrate that many hairs are easily broken. Microscopically, the distal ends of the hairs are frayed, resembling a broom (Fig. 8.14) Other hairs may have nodules resembling two brooms stuck together. The fragility is caused by damage to the outer cortex of the hair shaft, resulting in the loss of structural support. Without this support the weaker fibrous medulla frays like an electrical cord with broken insulation. This disorder is most common in blacks, arising from the trauma of combing tightly curled hairs. It may also occur after repeated trauma to the cortex from hair straighteners, bleaches, and perma-

nents. Since the growth of the hair shaft is normal, the disorder is self-limited, and normal hairs regrow when the source of damage is eliminated.

Traction alopecia is a form of traumatic alopecia common in young girls and women whose hairstyles, such as ponytails, plaits, and braids, maintain a tight pull on the hair shafts (Fig. 8.15A and B). This traction causes shaft fractures and follicular damage. If prolonged, permanent scarring alopecia can result.

Hair pulling is a common disorder in toddlers, school-aged children, and adolescents, which mimics many other forms of alopecia (Fig. 8.16 A–E). It presents with bizarre patterns of hair loss, often in broad, linear bands on the vertex or sides of the scalp where the hair is easily twisted and pulled out. Rarely, the entire scalp, eyebrows, and eyelashes are involved. The most important clue is the finding of short, broken-off hairs along the scalp, with stubs of different lengths in adjacent areas. This is caused by repetitive pulling and/or twisting of the hair which fractures the longer shafts. Once broken, the hairs are too short to be rebroken until they grow longer.

Hair pulling is often confused with alopecia areata. However, in hair pulling patches of hair loss are never completely bald, and the hair shafts are usually difficult to remove from the scalp. In addition, there are no asso-

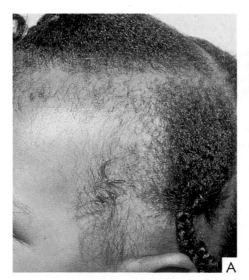

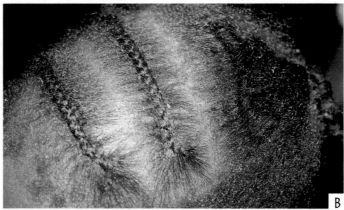

FIGURE 8.15 Traction alopecia. Alopecia is most prominent at the periphery of the scalp (**A**) and along the parts in the hair (**B**). These areas are under the most traction.

ciated nail abnormalities. Skin biopsy of the scalp from an area of recent hair pulling may demonstrate large numbers of catagen hairs, perifollicular hemorrhage, and trichomalacia or small, wavy, ghost-like hairs adjacent to normal hairs.

Although hair pulling may occur in children with severe obsessive–compulsive psychiatric disease, most cases are associated with habitual behavior or situational stress (Fig. 8.17). Parents and children may vigorously deny that the hair loss could be caused by the

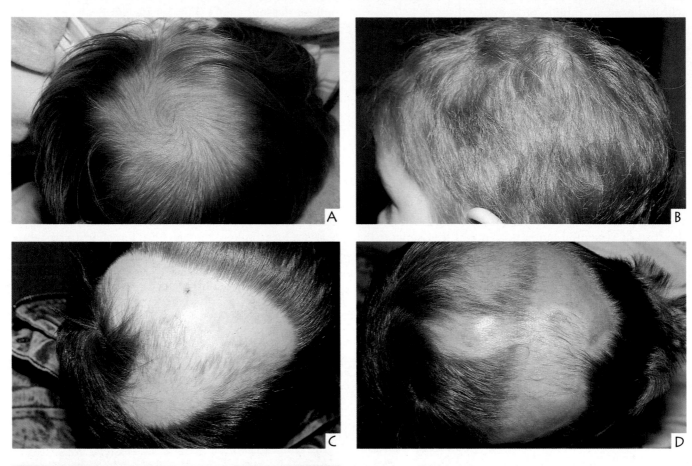

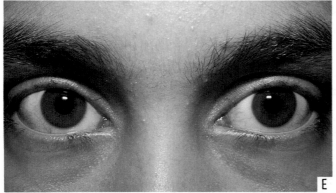

FIGURE 8.16 Hair pulling. (**A**) Alopecia from hair pulling is found most commonly on the occiput. (**B**) Hairs broken off and regrowing at various lengths may produce a moth-eaten appearance. (**C,D**) Bizarre patterns that defy anatomical landmarks are typical. In (**D**), note the rectangular area of regrowth in the mid scalp which followed one month of covering with an occlusive dressing. (**E**) Eyebrow and eyelash involvement may be difficult to distinguish from alopecia areata.

child, and therefore the diagnosis rests on a high index of suspicion and recognition of the clinical findings. In young habitual hair twirlers, positive reinforcement of socially acceptable alternative behaviors may succeed in extinguishing hair pulling.

Acne

Acne vulgaris, a disorder of the pilosebaceous apparatus, is the most common skin problem of adolescence (Fig. 8.18A–C). Lesions may appear on the face as early as age eight, but they usually begin to develop during the second decade of life with the onset of puberty. Other areas with prominent sebaceous hair follicles, including the upper chest and back, may become involved.

The exact pathogenesis of acne is unknown. However, abnormalities in follicular keratinization are believed to produce the earliest acne lesion, the microcomedo. Over time, microcomedones can grow into clinically apparent open comedones (blackheads) and closed comedones (whiteheads). The entire process is fueled by androgens, which stimulate sebaceous gland differentiation and growth and the production of sebum. The proliferation of *Propionibacterium acnes* in noninflammatory comedones and the rupture of comedo contents into the surrounding dermis may trigger the development of inflammatory papules, pustules, and cysts. Cystic acne is characterized by nodules and cysts scattered over the face, chest, and back. This variant frequently leads to disfiguring scarring.

Although therapy must be individualized, patients with mild to moderate comedonal and/or inflammatory acne respond well to a combination of topical retinoic acid (Retin-A), benzoyl peroxide, and antibiotics. Moderate to severe papulopustular acne warrants the use of oral antibiotics in combination with topical agents. Oral 13-*cis*-retinoic acid (Accutane) should be reserved for patients with severe, scarring cystic acne recalcitrant to conservative measures. Because of its association with a high incidence of severe birth defects, Accutane must be prescribed with great caution in adolescent girls who may be at risk for pregnancy.

Fortunately, acne is usually self-limited, winding down in late adolescence and early adult life. However, some middle-aged adults continue to require aggressive treatment for stubborn disease.

Evaluation of a patient with acne should include a careful medical and family history and physical examination. Although no special laboratory studies are usu-

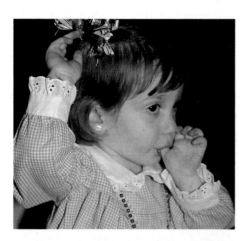

FIGURE 8.17 Hair pulling occurs frequently as a habitual behavior. At bedtime and naptime this happy, healthy toddler twirls her hair and sucks her thumb.

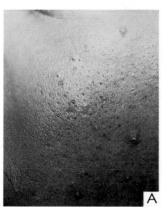
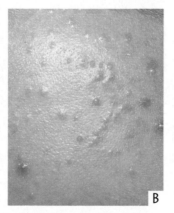
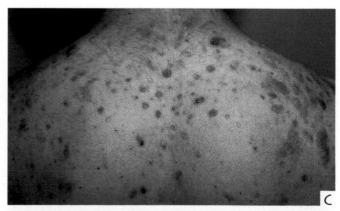

FIGURE 8.18 Acne. (**A**) Open comedones (blackheads) dot the cheek. (**B**) Closed comedones (whiteheads) covered the forehead of this 14-year-old girl. (**C**) Red papules, pustules, comedones, and cysts with scarring extended over the upper trunk of a 16-year-old boy. His nodulocystic acne went into remission after treatment with 13-*cis*-retinoid acid (Accutane).

ally necessary, signs and symptoms of precocious puberty or hyperandrogenism warrant further investigation. A history of severe acne in a first-degree relative should also serve as a warning for potentially serious disease.

Acneiform reactions differ from classic acne vulgaris by the presence of uniform lesions in a widespread distribution which may extend to involve the arms, legs, and lower trunk (Fig. 8.19). Endogenous hypersteroidism (e.g., Cushing's syndrome), prednisone, anabolic steroids, isoniazid, anticonvulsant agents, and lithium may trigger acneiform eruptions. When the medication cannot be decreased or discontinued, traditional management with topical and oral acne preparations may be helpful.

Acne vulgaris may be confused with bacterial or fungal folliculitis. In folliculitis, pustules predominate and the distribution is often restricted to areas of occlusion (Fig. 8.20). Gram stains, KOH preparations, and cultures should also help to distinguish folliculitis from acne. Occasionally an acne patient on longstanding antibiotics develops an acute worsening of acne in association with a Gram-negative folliculitis. This probably results from selection of a resistant Gram-negative organism. Pustules usually resolve with an alternative antibiotic or 13-*cis* retinoid acid.

Acne rosacea can be differentiated from acne vulgaris by the presence of red papules, pustules, cysts and extensive telangiectasias, and the absence of comedones (Fig. 8.21). Rosacea occurs most commonly in middle age, but some patients date the onset of lesions to adolescence or early adulthood.

Hidradenitis suppurativa may develop in association with cystic acne or as a separate entity (Fig. 8.22A and B). Hidradenitis is a severe, noninfectious inflammatory process that involves apocrine follicular structures in the axilla, groin, suprapubic, and perianal areas. As with acne, hyperkeratosis of the follicular epithelium is probably the initiating event. In the acute form, tender red pustules and deep-seated nodules become fluctuant and discharge pus. Over time, many patients develop chronic draining abscesses, sinus tracts, and severe scarring. Early in the course, hidradenitis improves with oral antibiotic therapy. Chronic disease responds only moderately to antibiotics, 13-*cis* retinoic acid, and systemic corticosteroids. Severe cases heal only after surgical excision of apocrine glands, scars, and sinus tracts in affected areas.

Hypertrichosis and Hirsutism

Hypertrichosis refers to localized patches of increased hair growth, whereas *hirsutism* is a term used to describe

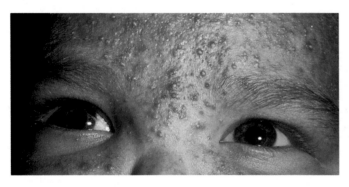

FIGURE 8.19 Acneiform eruption. Uniform pustules on an inflamed base covered the face, upper trunk, and proximal extremities of this eight-month-old who was on ACTH for infantile spasms. Lesions resolved when the ACTH was tapered several months later.

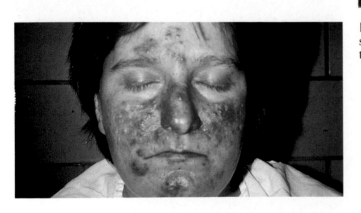

FIGURE 8.20 Hot-tub folliculitis. Painful red papules and pustules erupted in a bathing suit distribution in a teenage girl 24 hours after lounging in a neighbor's hot tub. *Pseudomonas* grew from pus obtained from one of the lesions. Fortunately, she remained well, and the folliculitis resolved over three days without treatment.

FIGURE 8.21 Acne rosacea. This young adult demonstrates the classic rash with red papules, pustules, cysts, and telangiectasias.

excessive hair growth, usually in children and women, in an adult male pattern (Fig. 8.23 A–C).

Congenital hypertrichosis has been noted in pigmented nevi and other cutaneous hamartomas. Generalized increase in hair at birth may occur as a normal physiologic variant. However, unusual patterns or persistence beyond early infancy should prompt a careful evaluation for potentially serious hereditary aberrations (e.g., hypertrichosis lanuginosa, Cornelia de Lange syndrome).

Acquired localized hypertrichosis occurs frequently in Becker's nevi (hairy epidermal nevus) and in patches of chronic physical trauma, chemical irritation, or thermal injury. The application of topical corticosteroids or androgens may also stimulate localized hair growth. Widespread hypertrichosis can appear in hypothyroidism, porphyria, and after the use of certain medications such as phenytoin, cyclosporine, and minoxidil.

Hirsutism may appear as a physiologic variant in an otherwise healthy child. However, an endogenous or exogenous source of androgens should be excluded. Cushing's, adrenogenital, and Stein–Leventhal syndromes may present with hirsutism. Endocrinologic evaluation should be guided by careful history and physical examination.

NAIL DISORDERS

As with hair disorders, abnormalities of the nails may provide a clue to the diagnosis of multisystem hereditary or acquired disease. Patients may also seek the advice of practitioners for nail problems because of pain or cosmetic concerns.

Embryology and Anatomy

Nails are first delineated as a fold in the skin of the developing fetus at ten to 11 weeks. By the fifteenth week the nail plate has already begun to keratinize, well before other epidermal structures. At birth the nail is fully formed.

The major part of the nail is composed of the hard nail plate which arises from the matrix beneath the proximal nail fold (Fig. 8.24). The pink color of the nail bed is derived from the extensive plexus of vessels that lies beneath the normally transparent nail plate. A white

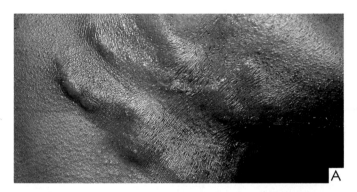
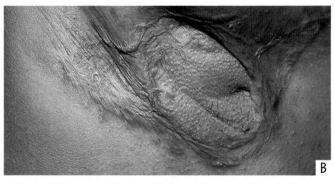

FIGURE 8.22 Hidradenitis suppurativa. An adolescent boy with severe involvement of the axillae (**A**) underwent extensive surgery with excellent results (**B**). Note the painful cysts and communicating sinus tracts in the preoperative photo.

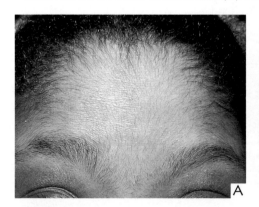
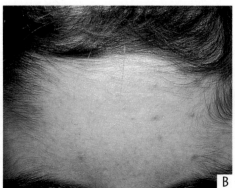
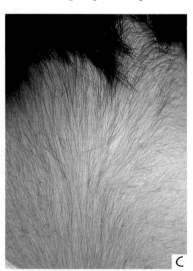

FIGURE 8.23 Hypertrichosis. (**A**) Excessive hair was noted at birth on the face of a two-year-old girl with microcephaly, hypertelorism, developmental delay, and other dysmorphic features.

A ten-year-old liver transplant recipient developed generalized hypertrichosis demonstrated here on the forehead (**B**) and back of the neck (**C**).

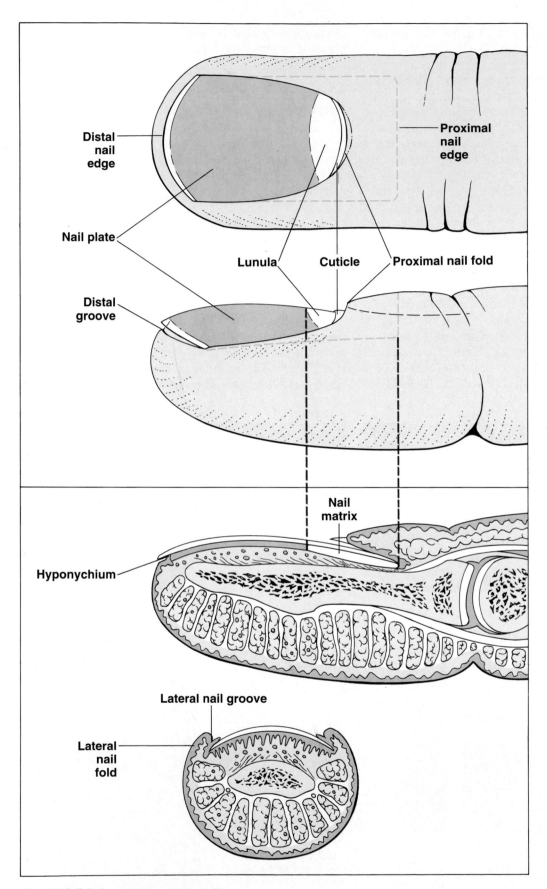

FIGURE 8.24 Anatomy of the nail.

crescent-shaped lunula, which extends from under the proximal nail fold, represents the distal portion of the nail matrix. As the nail plate emerges from the matrix, its lateral borders are enveloped by the lateral nail folds. The skin underlying the free end of the nail is referred to as the hyponychium, which connects the nail bed with the adjacent skin on the tips of the digits. Abnormalities in any part of the nail anatomy can result in characteristic clinical findings.

Congenital and Hereditary Disorders

Absence, hypoplasia, or dysplasia of the nails may occur as an isolated phenomenon or as part of an ectodermal dysplasia or other genodermatosis (Fig. 8.25).

Isolated Malformations *Clubbing* and *spooning (koilonychia)* of the nails may occur as autosomal dominant abnormalities without other anomalies. Although *congenital ingrown toenails* may be caused by congeni-

---

Figure 8.25 Selected Nail Anomalies

Anonychia

DOOR syndrome
Nail–patella syndrome
Hallermann–Streiff syndrome
Coffin–Siris syndrome
Klein's syndrome

Chromosomal anomalies

Monosomies 4p, 9p
Trisomies 3q partial, 7q,
  8, 8p, 9p, 13, 18, 21
Turner's syndrome
Noonan's syndrome
Group G-ring chromosome

Koilonychia (spoon nails)

Mal de Meleda keratoderma
Monilethrix
Nail–patella syndrome
Incontinentia pigmenti
Trichothiodystrophy

Miscellaneous disorders with nail dystrophy

Epidermolysis bullosa
Acanthosis nigricans
Acrodermatitis enteropathica
Diabetes
Gingival fibromatosis
Hyper-IgE syndrome
Hyperuricemia
Lesch–Nyhan syndrome
Tuberous sclerosis

Hereditary ectodermal dysplasias

(Variable findings in which alopecia, dental
  defects, nail defects, or anhidrosis occur in
  combination with one sign affecting other
  structures of epidermal origin)

Hyperplastic nails

Palmar–plantar keratodermas
Icthyosis
Pachonychia congenita
Group G-ring chromosome

Drug-induced malformations

Phenytoin, trimethadione, paramethadione
  Hyperpigmentation
  Hypoplasia
Warfarins
  Hypoplasia
Fetal alcohol syndrome
  Hypoplasia

tal malalignment of the great toenails (and resolve only with surgical realignment), a self-limited variant has also been described (Fig. 8.26). In the spontaneously regressing type, the ingrown nail may result from trauma or paronychia.

Ectodermal Dysplasias In *pachonychia congenita,* an autosomal dominant disorder with variable penetrance, hyperkeratosis of the nail bed, which develops in the first few months of life, is followed by vertical thickening and elevation of the nail plate with yellow-brown

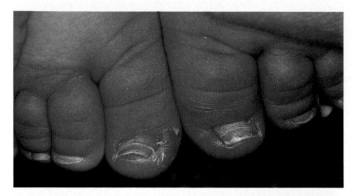

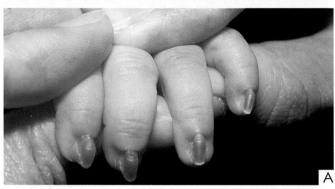

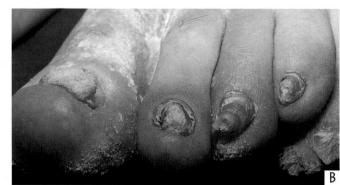

FIGURE 8.26 Congenital ingrown nails. This infant had involvement of both toe nails which improved without treatment by six months of age.

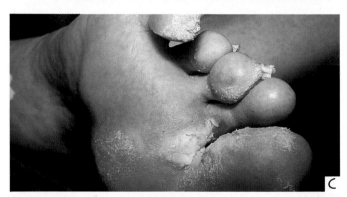

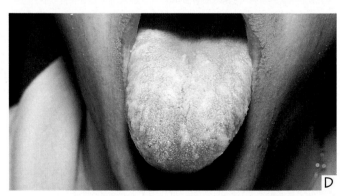

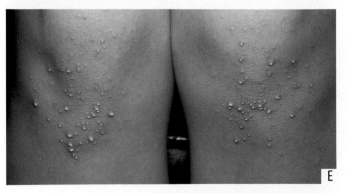

FIGURE 8.27 Pachonychia congenita. (**A**) At three months of age all 20 of this child's nails showed early changes of pachonychia, with yellowing and pinched up hyperplasia. (**B,C**) His father had marked involvement of all nails, as well as painful callosities on the dorsal and plantar aspects of the feet. (**D**) Leukokeratosis without a risk of malignant degeneration usually appears in infancy or early childhood and may involve the tongue, gingivae, and oral mucosae. (**E**) Hyperkeratotic papules on the extensor surfaces of the extremities are also common, particularly over the knees and elbows.

discoloration (Fig. 8.27A–E). Minor trauma may induce painful separation of the nail plate from the nail bed and bleeding. Hyperhidrosis of the palms and soles, as well as callosities and blistering, are common. Other findings include leukokeratosis of the oral mucosae (not associated with malignant degeneration), thickening of the tympanic membranes leading to deafness, leukokeratosis of the cornea, and cataracts. Hyperkeratotic papules on the extensor surfaces of the extremities, dermoid cysts, and steatocystoma multiplex have also been reported.

Dyskeratosis congenita may be confused with pachonychia congenita (Fig. 8.28). However, in dyskeratosis congenita, which can be either X-linked, autosomal dominant, or autosomal recessive, the nail plate is thinned, with longitudinal ridging and pterygium formation. Poikiloderma with reticulated pigmentation, telangiectasias, and atrophy is most prominent on the neck and trunk. Leukoplakia of the oral mucosae may be associated with the development of squamous-cell carcinoma and other malignancies of the gastrointestinal tract. Pancytopenia occurs in 50 percent of affected individuals during the second and third decades, and resembles Fanconi's anemia. Hypoplasia of the nails may also be a feature of *hidrotic ectodermal dysplasia* and *Coffin–Siris syndrome.*

Genodermatoses and Systemic Disease *Nail–patella syndrome* is an autosomal dominant disorder that presents with congenital absence or hypoplasia of the nails and patellae (Fig. 8.29). Glomerulonephritis occurs in a small percentage of cases and is rarely fatal. Heterochromia of the iris, keratoconus, and cataracts have also been reported.

Periungual fibromas, which arise from the proximal nail groove, are a common finding in patients with *tuberous sclerosis.* Although they do not appear until later childhood or adult life, they may provide the first clue to diagnosis in individuals who are otherwise mildly affected.

Congenital hypoplasia of the nails in infants with intrauterine exposure to anticonvulsant agents, alcohol, warfarin, or other teratogens should prompt a thorough evaluation for other drug-induced stigmata.

Acquired Nail Disorders

Paronychia *Paronychia* is a common childhood disorder. It presents as a red, tender swelling of the proximal or lateral nail fold. In the acute form, exquisite pain, sudden swelling, and abscess formation around one nail is caused by bacterial invasion after trauma to the cuticle (Fig. 8.30). Chronic paronychia may involve one or several nails. There is usually a history of frequent exposure to water (dishwasher's or thumbsucker's paronychia). Tenderness is mild, and a small amount of pus can sometimes be expressed. In chronic cases the nail may be discolored and dystrophic (Fig. 8.31A and B). The causative organisms are *Candida*, usually *C. albicans.*

Acute paronychia responds quickly to drainage of the abscess and warm tapwater soaks. Occasionally oral antistaphylococcal antibiotics are required. Chronic lesions resolve with topical antifungal agents and avoidance of water. Parents of toddlers must be reassured that recurrent *Candida* paronychia will eventually heal without scarring when thumbsucking ends. Intermittent, chronic use of antifungal creams in young children is effective and safe.

Nail Dystrophy *Nail dystrophy,* distortion and discoloration of normal nail plate structure, may result from any traumatic or inflammatory process that involves the

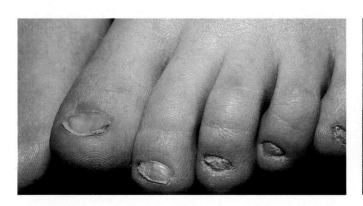

FIGURE 8.28 Dyskeratosis congenita. Unlike pachonychia congenita, the nails are usually thin, fragile, and hypoplastic.

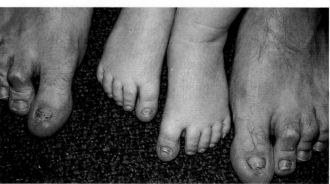

FIGURE 8.29 Nail–patella syndrome. Both father and son had hypoplastic patellae and dystrophic, hypoplastic nails.

nail matrix, nail bed, or surrounding tissues. Although *onychomycosis*, caused by dermatophyte fungal infection, is the most common cause of nail dystrophy in adults, it is unusual in children before puberty (Fig. 8.32). Dystrophic nails occur frequently as a complication of trauma or underlying dermatosis, such as psoriasis or atopic dermatitis (Fig. 8.33).

Trauma to the nail may cause a *subungual hematoma*, resulting in a brown-black discoloration (Fig. 8.34). This is particularly likely after crush injuries. Usually the diagnosis is simple, unless trauma is subtle. When a large, painful hematoma is produced,

it should be evacuated using electrocautery or carbon dioxide laser to relieve pain and reduce the risk of infection. Pigmentation at the base of the great toenail, caused by jamming the toe into the end of the shoe at a sudden stop, is called "turf toe" and results in mild subungual hemorrhage. This must be distinguished from melanoma and *melanonychia* (Fig. 8.35A and B). Hemorrhage can be identified by the presence of purple-brown pigment in the distal nail and normal proximal outgrowth of the nail. In melanonychia, gray-brown streaks of pigment extend longitudinally in a uniform fashion from the proximal nail fold of one or several

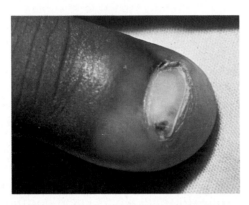

FIGURE 8.30 Paronychia. An acute staphylococcal paronychia developed after this child picked at a hangnail.

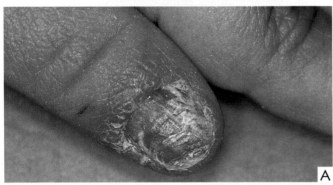

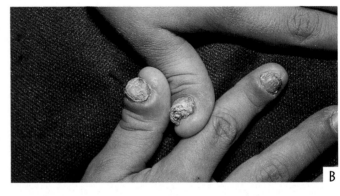

FIGURE 8.31 Chronic paronychia. (**A**) A chronic *Candida* paronychia recurred for over a year on the finger of an otherwise healthy toddler. Note the erythema at the base of the nail and loss of the cuticle. (**B**) All 20 nails were discolored and

hyperplastic in this eight-year-old boy with chronic mucocutaneous candidiasis. The chronic paronychiae and nail dystrophy resolved on long-term treatment with oral ketoconazole.

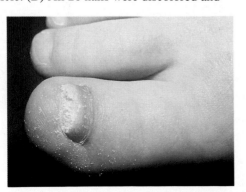

FIGURE 8.32 Onychomycosis. This four-year-old boy developed a single dystrophic toenail which grew *Trichophyton rubrum* on fungal culture. His father had chronic athlete's foot.

areas on one or several nails of dark-pigmented individuals. Irregular or changing pigment streaks may require a nail biopsy to confirm their innocent nature.

Nail biting, grooming, and chronic manipulation of any sort may also result in nail dystrophy. Repeated trauma to the cuticle can result in *leukonychia* (transverse white lines) and *median nail dystrophy* (central longitudinal ridging) (Fig. 8.36A and B).

Twenty nail dystrophy is a disorder of otherwise healthy school-aged children characterized by yellow-

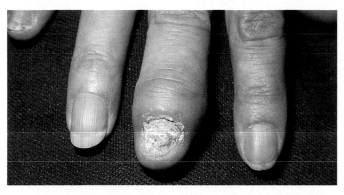

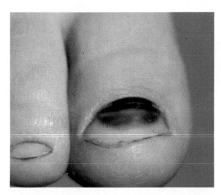

FIGURE 8.34 Traumatic subungual hematoma. Discoloration due to traumatic hemorrhage under the toenail is common in children and athletic adults. It is a result of jamming the toe into the end of the shoe while running or stopping (turf toe).

FIGURE 8.33 Psoriatic nails. Psoriasis produced typical pitting and onycholysis in a patient with psoriatic arthritis.

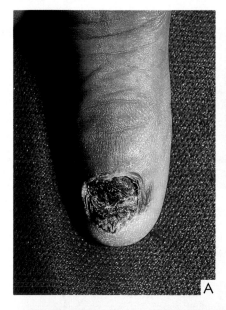

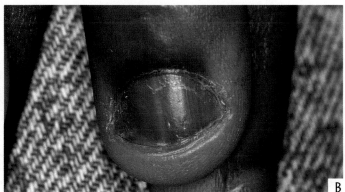

FIGURE 8.35 (**A**) In this patient with an acral melanoma, which arose in the nail matrix or nail bed, the nail has become dystrophic and the nail bed is infiltrated with pigmented malignant cells. (**B**) In melanonychia, neat, hyperpigmented streaks are seen extending vertically across the nail from the proximal nail fold.

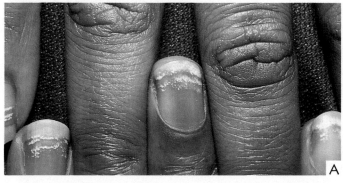

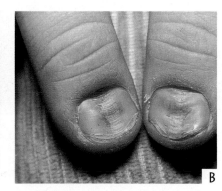

FIGURE 8.36 (**A**) Leukonychia consists of transverse white lines which grow out along the nail plate and frequently result from trauma to the nail at the cuticle. (**B**) Median nail dystrophy developed in this teenaged boy who admitted to picking chronically at his nails.

ing, pitting, increased friability, and other dystrophic changes, which progresses over six to 18 months to involve most or all of the nails. Although the course is variable, in many cases the dystrophy resolves wthout scarring over a period of several years. This disorder probably includes a number of conditions that cannot be distinguished unless other cutaneous findings appear.

Nail dystrophy may accompany other skin disorders and can help with their diagnosis. For example, alopecia areata is associated with characteristic Scotch-plaid pitting of the nails (Fig. 8.37). Psoriasis in the nail matrix results in scattered pits that are larger, deeper, and less numerous than those found in alopecia areata (see Fig. 8.33). Psoriasis of the nail bed, especially

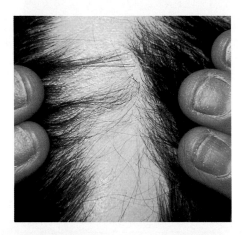

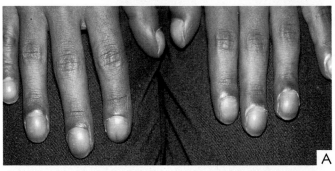
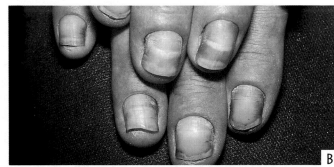

FIGURE 8.37 Broad, shallow Scotch-plaid pitting of the nails was associated with alopecia areata in this teenager.

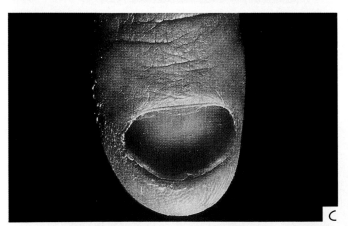
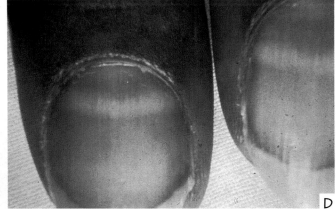

FIGURE 8.38 Nail changes and systemic disease. (**A**) Clubbing may occur as an isolated inherited defect or a complication of chronic lung or heart disease. (**B**) Yellow nail syndrome with chronic yellowing and slow growth was noted in this patient with Hodgkin's disease. (**C**) Koilonychia developed in a young woman with chronic iron deficiency anemia. (**D**) Broad, white transverse bands (Mee's lines) in the nail plate are seen with acute arsenic poisoning.

under the distal nail, causes separation of the nail plate fron the underlying skin (*onycholysis*) and oil-drop discoloration with heaped-up scaling. Onycholysis alone, without pits or discoloration, may be causesd by trauma, infection, nailpolish hardeners, or phototoxic reactions to drugs such as tetracycline.

Nail Changes and Systemic Disease Finally, nail findings may provide a clue to the diagnosis of underlying medical disorders (Fig. 8.38 A–D). For example, clubbing may be associated with chronic pulmonary disease or congenital heart disease with a right-to-left shunt. *Splinter hemorrhages* in the nail bed should be recognized as a physical sign of subacute bacterial endocarditis. Cyanosis of the nail beds in Raynaud's phenomenon and periungual telangiectasias may support a diagnosis of collagen vascular disease. Thickened, yellow, slow-growing nails occur in chronic pulmonary disease and lymphedema. Koilonychia has been reported in hemochromatosis and iron deficiency.

ALGORITHM FOR EVALUATION OF DISORDERS OF THE HAIR

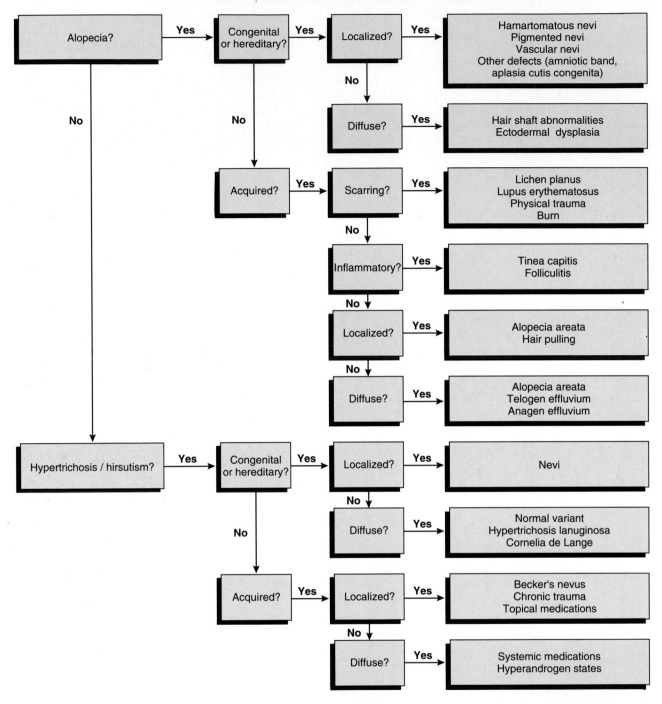

ALGORITHM FOR EVALUATION OF DISORDERS OF THE NAILS

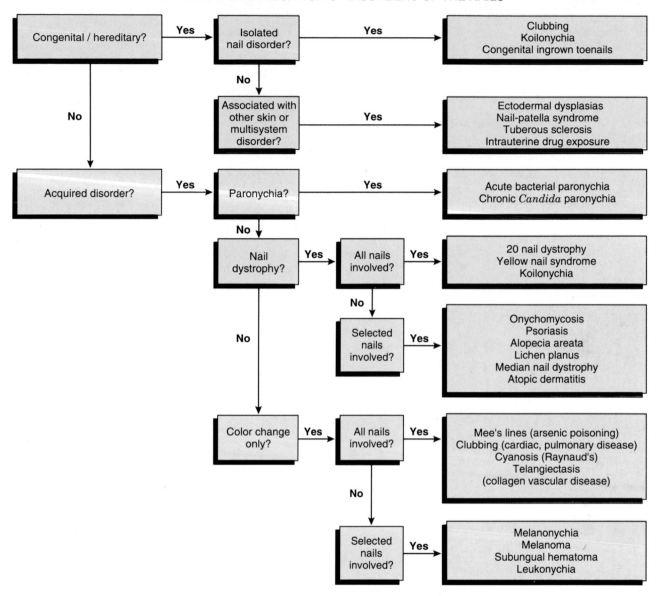

Congenital / hereditary? — **Yes** → Isolated nail disorder? — **Yes** →
Clubbing
Koilonychia
Congenital ingrown toenails

Isolated nail disorder? — **No** → Associated with other skin or multisystem disorder? — **Yes** →
Ectodermal dysplasias
Nail-patella syndrome
Tuberous sclerosis
Intrauterine drug exposure

Congenital / hereditary? — **No** → Acquired disorder? — **Yes** → Paronychia? — **Yes** →
Acute bacterial paronychia
Chronic *Candida* paronychia

Paronychia? — **No** → Nail dystrophy? — **Yes** → All nails involved? — **Yes** →
20 nail dystrophy
Yellow nail syndrome
Koilonychia

All nails involved? — **No** → Selected nails involved? — **Yes** →
Onychomycosis
Psoriasis
Alopecia areata
Lichen planus
Median nail dystrophy
Atopic dermatitis

Nail dystrophy? — **No** → Color change only? — **Yes** → All nails involved? — **Yes** →
Mee's lines (arsenic poisoning)
Clubbing (cardiac, pulmonary disease)
Cyanosis (Raynaud's)
Telangiectasis
(collagen vascular disease)

All nails involved? — **No** → Selected nails involved? — **Yes** →
Melanonychia
Melanoma
Subungual hematoma
Leukonychia

BIBLIOGRAPHY

Hair disorders

Baden HP. *Diseases of the hair and nails.* Chicago: Yearbook Medical Publishers, 1987.

Barth JH. Normal hair growth in children. *Pediatr Dermatol* 4:173–184, 1987.

Caserio R, Hordinsky MK. Disorders of hair. *J Am Acad Dermatol* 19:895–903, 1988.

Frieden IJ. Genetic hair disorders. In: Alper JC, ed. *Genetic Disorders of the Skin.* St. Louis: Mosby Year Book, 1990:209–221.

Hurwitz S. Hair disorders. In: Schachner LA, Hansen RC, eds. *Pediatric Dermatology.* New York: Churchill Livingstone, 1988:575–612.

Rook A, Dawber R. *Diseases of the hair and scalp.* Oxford: Blackwell Scientific, 1982.

Uno H. The histopathology of hair loss. *Curr Concepts* (Upjohn):3–47, 1988.

Whiting DA. The diagnosis of alopecia. *Curr Concepts* (Upjohn):3–41, 1990.

Whiting DA. Structural abnormalities of the hair shaft. *J Am Acad Dermatol* 16:1–25, 1987.

Nail disorders

Baden HP, Zaias N. *Nails.* In: Fitzpatrick TB, Eisen AZ, Wolff K, Freedberg IM, Austen KF, eds. *Dermatology in General Medicine*, 3rd ed. New York: McGraw–Hill, 1987:651–666.

Baran R, Dawber RPR. *Diseases of the nails and their management.* Oxford: Blackwell Scientific, 1984.

Daniel CR, Scher RK. Nail changes secondary to systemic drugs and ingestants. *J Am Acad Dermatol* 17:1012–1016, 1987.

Norton LA. Genetic nail disorders. In: Alper JC, ed. *Genetic Disorders of the Skin.* St. Louis: Mosby Year Book, 1990:195–208.

Scher RK, Norton LA, Daniel CR. Disorders of the nails. *J Am Acad Dermatol* 15:523–528, 1986.

Silverman R. Nail and appendageal abnormalities. In: Schachner LA, Hansen RC, eds. *Pediatric Dermatology.* New York: Churchill Livingstone, 1988:613–642.

chapter nine

FACTITIAL DERMATOSES

The term *factitial* is defined as "artificial" or "not natural." In dermatology, factitial disorders usually include a number of specific psychodermatoses. However, in this chapter the definition is expanded to include a number of entities that do not fit neatly into other chapters. After the discussion of disorders with psychiatric implications, the cutaneous findings of child abuse will be reviewed, and the chapter will conclude with sections on graft versus host reaction and acquired immunodeficiency syndrome, diseases that have been, at least in part, created by human agency.

PSYCHODERMATOLOGY

Secondary psychiatric disorders as well as psychophysiologic disorders are common in pediatric practice. Fortunately, primary psychiatric disorders and neurologic disorders that mimic psychiatric disease are relatively infrequent.

Secondary Psychiatric Disorders

Localized skin conditions that involve strategically important areas such as the head and neck, or chronic, widespread rashes, may cause secondary psychiatric disorders. In this group of diseases, disfigurement results in low self-esteem, social phobia, and paranoia. In severe cases major depression may occur. Common skin problems associated with secondary psychiatric disorders include psoriasis, cystic acne, alopecia areata, vitiligo, port-wine stains, and large pigmented nevi.

Disfiguring lesions in infants and young children are a source of parental stress. However, if they are treated before a critical period in psychological development, long-term sequelae may be avoided in affected children. Although these critical periods have not been well defined, many pediatricians agree that, when possible, treatment should be completed before patients begin school. For instance, facial pigmented nevi can be excised before kindergarten, and pulsed dye laser treatment of port-wine stains can begin shortly after birth. Treatment of chronic, recurrent disorders such as psoriasis and vitiligo should be scheduled to minimize school absence and should focus on eradicating lesions that are most visible or symptomatic. In adolescents, even mild acne may trigger a great deal of anxiety, which can be controlled by physician counseling and appropriate medical management. Cystic acne should be treated early and aggressively to avoid permanent scarring.

Periodic reassurance from the practitioner should provide adequate support for many patients. Others may find participation in support-oriented groups, such as the National Vitiligo Foundation and the National Portwine Stain Foundation, to be particularly helpful. However, when normal relationships with family and friends are disrupted, psychiatric consultation and counseling may be necessary.

Psychophysiologic Disorders

Psychophysiologic disorders are also common in children. This term refers to a group of genuine dermatologic conditions that are triggered or exacerbated by emotional stress. Examples include atopic dermatitis, psoriasis, acne, hives, and hyperhidrosis.

Recognition of psychologic factors is the key to successful treatment of these disorders. Some patients may require specific stress reduction measures in addition to standard dermatologic therapy. Biofeedback training may be helpful in disorders such as hyperhidrosis and atopic dermatitis, in which stress or anxiety can trigger a worsening of symptoms within minutes.

Primary Psychiatric Disorders

In this category of psychodermatoses, the skin becomes the focus of a primary psychosis. In most cases either there is no true dermatologic disorder or minor findings are misinterpreted by the patient in accordance with his or her psychopathology. Although subtle symptoms may develop in childhood, most cases become manifest in adolescence or adulthood.

Individuals with obsessive–compulsive disease may develop trichotillomania. Unlike innocent hair pulling, trichotillomania is not self-limited and requires long-term psychiatric and medical therapy. In a related condition, acne excoriee, patients pick and gouge trivial

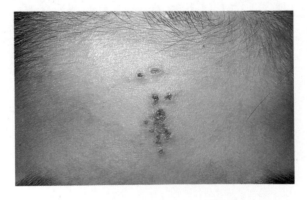

FIGURE 9.1 Acne excoriee. A 17-year-old girl compulsively picked at subtle comedones, creating punched-out ulcerations on her face.

acne lesions on the face, producing erosions and ulcerations which may heal with scarring (Fig. 9.1). Acne excoriee usually occurs in young women.

In monosymptomatic hypochondriacal psychosis, patients develop a false fixation that there is a serious disturbance in their skin. The most common presentation is delusions of parasitosis, in which the individual is convinced that the skin is infested with imaginary mites, worms, or insects. Other examples include delusions of bromosis (foul odor) and dysmorphosis (abnormal or ugly appearance). These patients have little insight into their disease, and usually refuse consultation with psychiatrists. Unfortunately, the prognosis is guarded, and symptoms may persist indefinitely. Recent studies indicate that a large proportion of patients will improve with pimoside, an antipsychotic drug of the diphenylbutylpiperidione group.

A subset of patients with self-induced skin disease, usually teenagers, develop lesions in association with situational stress (Fig. 9.2A and B). Disordered family dynamics, school phobia, lost love, and other acute or chronic psychosocial problems may lead to this form of attention-seeking behavior. When this diagnosis is suspected, lesions can be covered with occlusive dressings for several weeks to see if healing occurs (Fig. 9.3A and B). When confronted, the patients usually admit to the self-injurious behavior. Counseling and improvement in the psychosocial situation often result in an end to lesions.

Pseudopsychiatric Disorders

When patients develop bizarre symptoms with few or confusing clinical findings, a psychiatric source is often considered. However, careful attention to the course of symptoms and development of skin lesions may provide a clue to the true dermatologic diagnosis.

Dermatitis herpetiformis (DH) is a good example of a pseudopsychodermatosis. In DH, persistent, intense

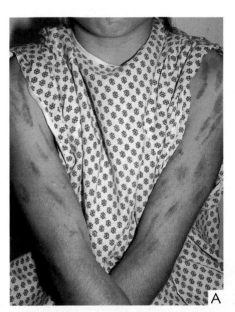
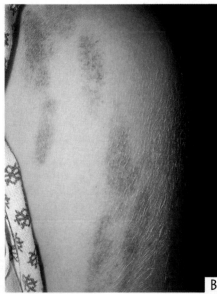

FIGURE 9.2 Factitial dermatitis. An emotionally disturbed adolescent developed symmetric linear bruises on her arms (**A,B**). During counseling she admitted to producing the lesions with a coin.

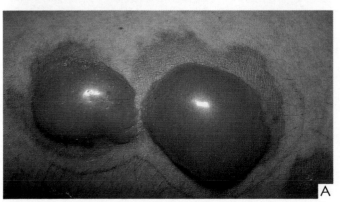
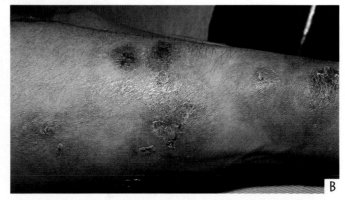

FIGURE 9.3 Factitial dermatitis. A 15-year-old boy would periodically return from the woods behind his house with large, tense bullous lesions on his arms (**A**). Under close observation in the hospital the lesions healed within several days (**B**). Later, in therapy, he admitted to applying a caustic liquid to the skin.

pruritus and subsequent excoriations that obliterate the primary vesiculobullous lesions make diagnosis difficult. Unless DH is considered and confirmed by skin biopsy, the patient may be mistakenly referred for psychiatric evaluation of "neurotic" excoriations. Scabies, folliculitis, urticaria, and other pruritic dermatoses may also be misdiagnosed as psychogenic pruritus.

Occasionally children with temporal lobe seizures present with pseudodelusions of parasitosis. Complaints of bizarre sensations in the skin should also prompt a search for medication overdosage (e.g., Benadryl) or illicit drug exposure.

CHILD ABUSE AND NEGLECT

Although the true incidence of child abuse is unknown, more than 2 million children are expected to be abused or neglected in the United States this year. This represents more than 40,000 severely injured children and 4,000 deaths. In many cases, affected children have been evaluated by practitioners who failed to recognize signs and symptoms suggesting the true diagnosis. Cutaneous findings frequently provide clues to acute or chronic abuse.

Risk Factors

This epidemic affects young children, almost two-thirds of whom are under three years of age. Premature, handicapped, and adopted children are also more likely to be abused. About 10 percent of cases involve sexual abuse, in which girls are victims three times as often as boys. Parental risk factors include a past history of being abused as a child, poor socialization, and limited ability

to deal with stress. Although families living in poverty have increased exposure to stresses that may result in abuse and neglect, families at all socioeconomic levels are affected. Alcoholism, addiction, and mental illness are often contributing factors. Families who move frequently and fail to develop support systems in the community are at particular risk.

Historical Clues

When the history of how the injury occurred is vague or is incompatible with the physical findings, abuse should be included in the differential diagnosis. Inconsistencies in the history when parents are interviewed separately and changes in the history when it is taken by different health workers should increase the index of suspicion. Delay between the time of the injury and the visit to the practitioner, inappropriate lack of concern for the injury, and abnormal interaction between the parent and child should also raise red flags.

A review of the primary care or emergency room medical records may reveal a large number of visits for accidental injuries, repeated fractures, and ingestions. Delayed immunizations and health maintenance visits may also serve as a warning. In infants and young children, poor growth or weight gain may be a sign of emotional abuse or neglect.

Clinical Findings

Every child suspected of being abused deserves a thorough physical examination. Care should be taken to peruse the entire skin surface including the anogenital area, mucous membranes, and scalp. All findings should be documented in the chart. Photographs of suspicious lesions should be labeled and dated. The inci-

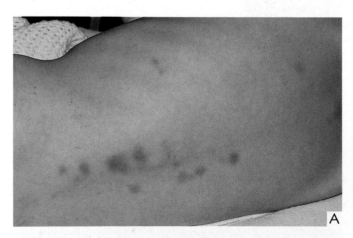

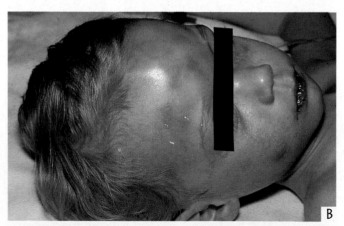

FIGURE 9.4 **(A)** Multiple ecchymoses are evident over the back and upper chest of this child who presented poorly nourished but with normal coagulation studies. **(B)** The same patient with multiple bruises on the face and forehead.

dent should be reported to appropriate authorities, including Children's Protective Services and the police, if necessary. Although the practitioner should play a role as advocate for the family, the primary responsibility is to ensure the safety of the child.

Cutaneous Lesions The distribution and shape of skin lesions may provide a clue to diagnosis. Innocent, play-induced bruises usually appear over bony prominences. Bruises suggestive of abuse occur on the inner and outer thighs, ears, groin, genitals, cheeks, and torso (Fig. 9.4A and B). Thumbprints on the chest and fingerprints on the back of a seizing or floppy infant point to the diagnosis of the so-called "shaken baby" syndrome, where shaking results in subdural hematoma with retinal hemorrhages.

Bruises appear purple and blue for the first three to five days and then evolve through greenish-yellow hues to faded brown at ten days. Multiple bruises of various ages suggest an ongoing problem, and the parent's history may not be compatible with the probable time sequence.

In many cases the configuration of bruises may conform to the imprint of the object used to induce injury. Linear lesions may result from injury by a wooden stick or metal wire. Circumferential bruises or erosions on the arms, legs, or neck may be caused by rope or wire ligatures (Fig. 9.5A and B). Lamp cords (omega-shaped loops), belts (U-shaped), belt buckles, and hands often inflict identifiable lesions (Fig. 9.6A and B).

Human bites also have a characteristic appearance. Animal-induced injuries usually produce puncture

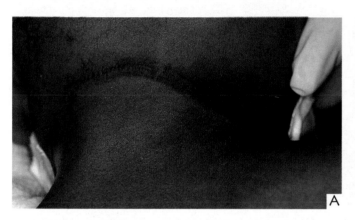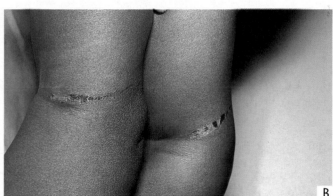

FIGURE 9.5 Physically abused toddlers had rope tied around the neck (**A**) and legs (**B**), producing circumferential bruising and erosions.

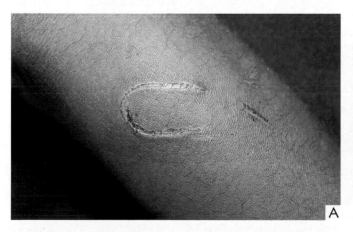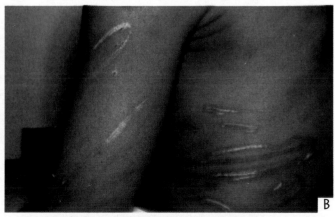

FIGURE 9.6 The shape of lesions often gives a clue to the object used to inflict injury. (**A**) The end of a belt produced the U-shaped cut on the leg of a five-year-old boy.

(**B**) Multiple scars produced by whipping with a looped cord are seen in this child.

wounds or tear the skin, whereas human bites cause crush injuries. Small bite marks may be inflicted by siblings. However, widths of greater than 4 cm occur with bites from adults.

Although burns are fairly common accidental injuries, the shape and distribution of lesions, inconsistent history, and delay in seeking medical care may point to deliberate injury (Fig. 9.7A and B). Hot water-immersion burns are a common presentation of abuse (Fig. 9.8A and B). Typical lesions include symmetric lesions on the hands, feet, and diaper area. Frustration with toddlers during toilet training is a common complaint. The tops of the feet and hands may be more severely involved because the skin on the palms and soles is thicker and may be relatively protected when the extremities are held against the bottom of the sink or tub. Burns from metal objects usually demonstrate the shape of the object (Fig. 9.9A and B). A triangular injury may indicate branding with a hot iron. A child held against a hot metal grate may show criss-crossing horizontal and vertical marks. Cigarette burns leave punched-out ulcers with dry, purple crusts (Fig. 9.10A

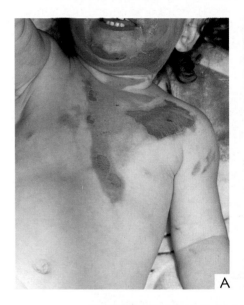
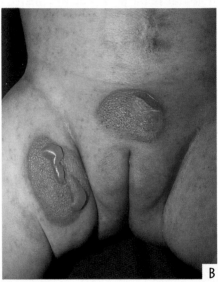

FIGURE 9.7 (A) A two-year-old accidentally spilled a teacup filled with hot water onto her face, neck, and chest. Note the irregular, asymmetric, but well-demarcated borders of the burn. (B) A babysitter was applying a caustic liquid to patches in this child's diaper area. The morphology and course of lesions were not consistent with the history provided by the sitter.

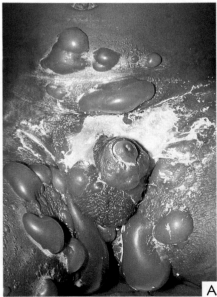
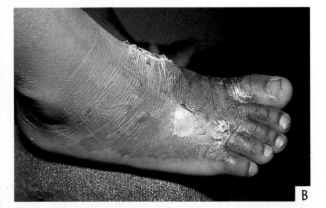

FIGURE 9.8 Hot water-immersion burns. (A) First- and second-degree burns are noted on the penis, thighs, inguinal, and suprapubic areas of a toddler who was held under a hot water spigot. His sacrum and buttocks were spared. (B) Symmetric, healing hot-water burns are seen on the top of the feet of another toddler. Note the sharp line of demarcation at the ankle and sparing of the sole.

and B). They can be distinguished from impetigo by their uniform size and dry, nonexpanding base. Repeated burns may be indicated by lesions at various stages of healing. Some lesions may become impetiginized. Widespread, untreated impetigo and poor hygiene are also signs of child neglect.

Sexual Abuse Patients evaluated immediately after sexual assault often demonstrate evidence of physical and genital injury (Fig. 9.11A and B). Bruises on the head, neck, torso, and thighs are commonly present. Genital examination may show erythema, bruises, or lacerations. In cases of molestation or incest that usu-

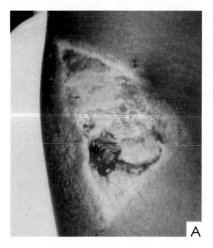

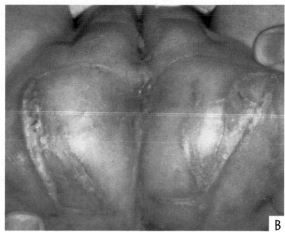

FIGURE 9.9 (A) The pattern of this full-thickness burn to the arm indicates that a hot iron was used on this patient.

(B) This infant received multiple, linear full-thickness burns when she was forced to sit on the hot grill of a space heater.

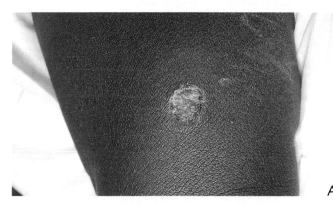

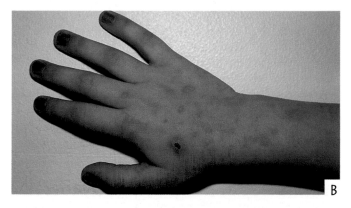

FIGURE 9.10 (A) A fresh cigarette burn occurred when this six-week-old allegedly walked into a lighted cigarette. Note the dry yellow eschar in the center with purplish,

peeled-back scale at the border. (B) Cigarette burns in various stages of healing are present on the hand and wrist of this abused five-year-old.

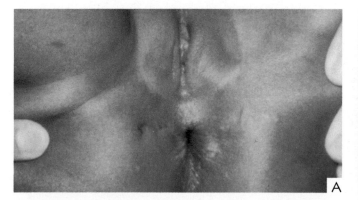

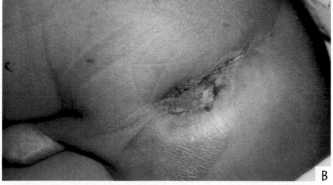

FIGURE 9.11 Physical signs of sexual abuse. (A) Abrasions, contusions, and punctate tears of the perineum and perianal area can be observed in this prepubescent girl.

(B) Severe perianal lacerations, contusions, and abrasions are apparent in this prepubescent boy subjected to sodomy.

ally occur chronically in a family setting, physical signs are subtle or absent (Fig. 9.12). Patients may present with chronic vaginitis, healed scars in the anogenital area, a patulous introitus, or reflex relaxation of the anal sphincter on perineal stimulation. About 10 to 15 percent of these children will have evidence of sexually transmitted diseases at the time of diagnosis. Consequently, evaluation should include cultures of the oral pharynx, rectum, and vagina for gonorrhea and *Chlamydia* and a serological test for syphilis. Children who have been sexually assaulted require a thorough examination and collection of forensic data in a medical setting equipped for the special needs of this evaluation.

Occasionally, dermatologic disease can simulate the findings of sexual abuse. Bullous pemphigoid and chronic bullous dermatosis of childhood have been misdiagnosed as sexually transmitted herpetic infection. Candidiasis and inflammatory bowel disease with labial involvement may also mimic sexual abuse.

Other Findings in Abuse Multiple unexplained fractures of various ages involving the long bones and ribs of an infant or young child are highly suggestive of child abuse. Often the bony injuries are noted as an incidental finding when the child is brought to the practitioner for a single injury or some other unrelated problem. When child abuse is suspected, a complete skeletal survey should be obtained to assess the full extent of the injuries. Blunt injuries may cause intraabdominal injuries, including duodenal hematomas, small intestinal or mesenteric tears, and lacerations of the liver and spleen. These childen may require hospital admission until their safety at home can be ensured. About 50 percent of children who are returned to the same environment are eventually killed by the abusive adult.

Innocent Mongolian spots should not be mistaken for bruises. Past documentation in the child's medical record or observation over several days will reveal the proper diagnosis. A bleeding diathesis which may present with increased bruising can be quickly excluded by a platelet count and coagulation studies. Insect bites may resemble cigarette burns, and, in rare instances, osteogenesis imperfecta or Ehler–Danlos syndrome can simulate child abuse.

GRAFT VERSUS HOST DISEASE

Graft versus host disease (GVHD) is an immunologic disorder resulting from injury induced by immunocompetent histoincompatible donor cells in a compromised recipient. Susceptible immunodeficient states include the normal developing fetus, congenital immunodeficiency, and acquired immunodeficiency.

GVHD that develops in utero in normal fetuses is caused by entry of viable maternal lymphocytes into the fetal circulation via spontaneous maternal–fetal transfusion. Affected infants usually show signs of chronic disease at delivery. In infants with congenital immunodeficiencies, particularly T-cell deficiencies and severe combined immunodeficiency, the development of GVHD may be the first symptom of the immunodeficiency, developing about seven to ten days after therapeutic blood transfusion. In many nurseries, sick infants receive irradiated blood, which eliminates the risk of accidental infusion of viable lymphocytes. The most common group of children at risk for GVHD includes patients with acquired immunodeficiencies resulting from chemotherapy, lymphoreticular malignancy, and bone marrow transplantation. Virtually every allogenic transplant patient experiences at least mild GVHD.

Acute disease usually begins with a widespread, symmetric, pruritic morbilliform rash within two to six weeks and up to 100 days after the introduction of donor cells (Fig. 9.13A and B). The face, neck, and the sides of the palms, soles, and digits are commonly involved. Hepatic involvement is evidenced by the presence of elevated liver enzymes, and gastrointestinal

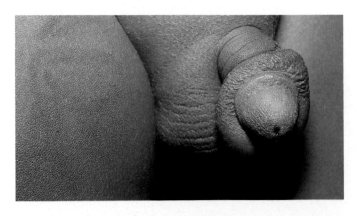

FIGURE 9.12 This three-year-old boy developed phimosis caused by a piece of hair tied around the foreskin.

symptoms include nausea and vomiting, often progressing to bloody diarrhea.

Chronic disease appears 100 to 400 days after the introduction of donor cells and may occur without antecedent acute symptoms. Chronic GVHD is a multisystem disease with autoimmune-like findings. Early in its course, the skin is involved with diffuse hypo- and hyperpigmentation, a lichenoid rash resembling lichen planus, and scaly patches. Occasionally patients develop a diffuse erythroderma. Untreated patients may eventually develop poikiloderma with atrophy, ulcerations, and progressive widespread sclerodermatous changes. Other findings include mucositis, cicatricial alopecia, vitiligo, dystrophic nails, Sjögren's syndrome, and chronic pulmonary, cardiac, and gastrointestinal disease.

Fortunately, in transplant patients aggressive immunosuppressive therapy with cyclosporine, prednisone, methotrexate, and other agents usually prevents the development of serious GVHD. Routine irradiation of blood products before transfusion can also reduce the risk of GVHD in transplant patients and other immunodeficient individuals. In infants with congenital immunodeficiency, mortality is high despite intensive supportive care.

ACQUIRED IMMUNODEFICIENCY SYNDROME

Although the prevalence of acquired immunodeficiency syndrome (AIDS) is relatively low in children, the recent epidemic, which has spread to heterosexual women of childbearing age, has already resulted in a rise in the number of pediatric cases. In some areas,

human immunodeficiency virus (HIV) seroprevalence among pregnant women exceeds 3 percent. The rate of transmission from these mostly asymptomatic mothers ranges from 15 to 35 percent. Other sources of infection in children include exposure to contaminated blood products, sexual transmission, and intravenous drug use.

Infected infants rarely develop overt disease during the first three months of life. However, before one year of age, nonspecific symptoms commonly include poor growth, generalized lymphadenopathy, hepatosplenomegaly, chronic oral thrush, and recurrent upper respiratory, middle ear, and gastrointestinal infections. At least 50 percent of infants show central nervous system involvement, with neurodevelopmental delay or loss of milestones, acquired microcephaly, spastic diplegia, and quadriplegia. Pulmonary disease is the most common manifestation of pediatric AIDS, affecting over 75 percent of children during the first several years of life. Interstitial pneumonitis caused by *Pneumocystis carinii* is reported in 60 percent of patients. Lymphoid interstitial pneumonitis associated with Epstein–Barr virus infection occurs in about half of patients who survive the first year. Other important opportunistic pathogens include cytomegalovirus, *Candida, Mycobacterium avium-intracellulare,* and *Cryptococcus neoformans.* Patients are also susceptible to bacteremia, severe soft-tissue infection, pneumonitis, and meningitis from encapsulated bacterial organisms such as *Streptococcus pneumoniae* or *Haemophilus influenzae.*

Skin Lesions

Cutaneous findings may provide an early clue to diagnosis (Fig. 9.14). Persistent diaper candidiasis and oral

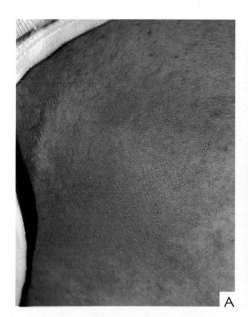

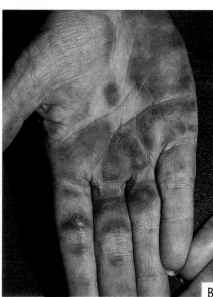

FIGURE 9.13 Acute graft versus host disease developed three weeks after an allogenic bone marrow transplant in a adolescent with acute myelogenous leukemia. **(A)** A widespread morbilliform rash became confluent in the skin creases and over the thighs. **(B)** Painful violaceous plaques appeared on the palms and soles.

thrush, recalcitrant to topical therapy, occur commonly and should prompt a search for HIV infection, especially in a child with growth failure or maternal risk factors. Many children are unable to localize common usually self-limited viral infections. Widespread, recurrent herpes gingivostomatitis and disseminated cutaneous herpes simplex, as well as chronic herpes infections, are a frequent problem. Recurrent localized herpes zoster and disseminated zoster have also been reported. Widespread, recalcitrant molluscum contagiosum may be the first sign of AIDS in an otherwise asymptomatic child. Persistent and widespread dermatophyte infections involving the skin, nails, and hair may occur. Disseminated deep fungal infections with cutaneous involvement, including cryptococcosis and histoplasmosis, have been described. Skin lesions produced by these fungi may simulate an indolent bacterial folliculitis or molluscum.

Crusted scabies infestations with thick, widespread scaly papules and patches require rapid identification to prevent spread to parents, teachers, and health-care workers. As in adults, the prevalence of seborrheic dermatitis, particularly widespread erosive lesions, appears to be high in children with AIDS. Cutaneous manifestations of nutritional deficiencies including zinc deficiency dermatitis, pellagra, and scurvy have been noted, particularly in children with chronic gastrointestinal disease.

An increased frequency of cutaneous drug reactions has been reported in adults and children with AIDS. This is a serious problem in patients who require chronic prophylaxis aganist *Pneumocystis* with trimethoprim–sulfamethaxozole. The incidence of morbilliform drug rashes in adults on this regimen approaches 75 percent.

Other cutaneous findings in children with AIDS include ecchymoses from idiopathic thrombocytopenic purpura and chronic leukocytoclastic vasculitis. Although cutaneous Kaposi's sarcoma is reported frequently in adults, in most of whom it is an AIDS-defining illness, it occurs only rarely in children.

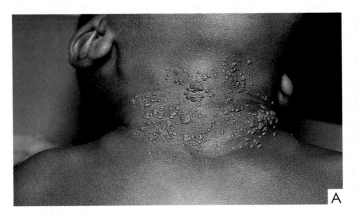

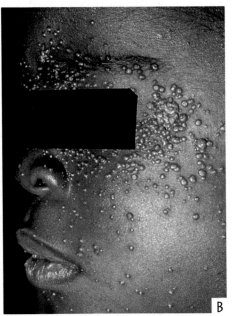

FIGURE 9.14 AIDS. **(A)** Multiple recalcitrant warts developed on the neck of this two-year-old with AIDS. **(B)** Severe molluscum contagiosum in a patient with AIDS. (Courtesy of Drs. G.B. Scott and M.T. Mastrucci, University of Miami School of Medicine.)

BIBLIOGRAPHY

Psychodermatology

Koblenzer CS. *Psychocutaneous disease.* Orlando: Harcourt Brace Jovanovich, 1987.

Koo JJM. Psychodermatology. *Curr Concepts* (Upjohn) 3–45, 1989.

Koo JJM, Smith LL. Obsessive-compulsive disorders in the pediatric dermatology practice. *Pediatr Dermatol* 8:107–113, 1991.

Child abuse and neglect

Davis HW. Child abuse and neglect. In Davis HW, Zitelli BJ, eds. *Atlas of Pediatric Physical Diagnosis.* New York: Gower Medical Publishing, 1987: 6.1–6.14.

Helfer RE, Kempe RS, eds. *The battered child,* 4th ed. Chicago: University of Chicago Press, 1987.

Krugman RD, ed. Child abuse and neglect. *Pediatr Ann* 21:471–511, 1992.

Wald ER. Gynechologic infections in the pediatric age group. *Pediatr Infect Dis J* 3:S10–S13, 1984.

Graft versus host disease

Anderson KC, Weinstein HJ. Transfusion-associated graft-versus-host disease (review article). *N Engl J Med* 323:315–321, 1990.

Berger RS, Dixon SL. Fulminant transfusion-associated graft-versus-host disease in a premature infant. *J Am Acad Dermatol* 20:945–950, 1989.

James WD, Odom RB. Graft-versus-host disease. *Arch Dermatol* 119:683–689, 1983.

Paller AS. Disorders of the immune system, graft-versus-host disease. In: Schachner LA, Hansen RC, eds. *Pediatric Dermatology.* New York: Churchill Livingstone, 1988:119–123.

Acquired immunodeficiency syndrome

Italian Multicenter Study. Epidemiology, clinical features, and prognostic factors of pediatric HIV infection. *Lancet* 2:1043–1046, 1988.

Kaplan MH, Sadick N, McNutt S, Meltzer M, Sarngadharan MG, Pahwa S. Dermatologic findings and manifestations of acquired immunodeficiency syndrome (AIDS). *J Am Acad Dermatol* 16:485–506, 1987.

Modlin JF. Infectious disease, human immunodeficiency virus. In: Jones MD, Gleason, CA, Lipstein SU, eds. *Hospital Care of the Recovering NICU Infant.* Baltimore: Williams & Wilkins, 1991:91–93.

Prose NS, Mendez H, Menikoff H, Miller HJ. Pediatric human immunodeficiency virus infection and its cutaneous manifestations. *Pediatr Dermatol* 4:267–274, 1987.

INDEX

triggering factors in, 3.18–3.19, **3.32**

Auspitz sign, in psoriasis, 3.4, **3.5**

B
acterial infections
secondary, in atopic dermatitis, 3.18, **3.30**
vasculitis in, 7.20–7.21, **7.28–7.29**
vesiculopustular eruptions in, 2.21–2.22, **2.45**, 4.7–4.8, **4.9–4.11**

Barrier properties of skin, in infants, 2.2

Basal cell carcinoma, 5.8, **5.13**

Basal cell nevus syndrome, **5.2**, 5.3, 5.8, **5.14**

Bazex syndrome, **5.2**, 5.3

Becker's nevus, 6.5, **6.7**

Berloque dermatitis, 6.6

Betamethasone
benzoate, topical, **1.10**, 1.12
dipropionate, topical, **1.10**, 1.12
valerate, topical, **1.10**, 1.12

Bites, human, wounds from, 9.5–9.6

Blackheads, 8.13
neonatal, 2.8

Blistering
in mechanobullous disorders, 2.23–2.27, **2.47–2.50**
morphology of bulla in, **1.4**, 1.6
Tzanck smear in, **1.9**, 1.10, 1.11
in vesiculopustular eruptions, 4.2–4.16
neonatal, 2.20–2.23, **2.43–2.46**

Bloom's syndrome, **5.2**, 5.4, **6.2**, 6.3
photoreactions in, 2.4, 7.28

Blue nevus, 6.10, **6.16**

Blueberry muffin lesions, 2.37, **2.74**, 7.9

Bulla, morphology of, **1.4**, 1.6

Bullous dermatosis of childhood, chronic, 4.10, 4.11–4.12, **4.14–4.16**

Burns
in child abuse, 9.6, 9.7, **9.7–9.10**
in intensive care nursery, 2.5

Buschke–Ollendorff syndrome, 2.34

C
afe-au-lait spots, **6.1–6.2**, 6.2, 6.3

Calcifying epithelioma of Malherbe, 5.10–5.11

Cancer-associated genodermatoses, **5.2**, 5.3–5.4

Candidiasis, 3.30, 3.31, **3.51–3.52**
diaper dermatitis in, 2.16–2.17, **2.37**
disseminated, neonatal, 2.22–2.23
paronychia in, 8.19, 8.20, **8.31**

Carcinoma, basal cell, 5.8, **5.13**

Catagen, 8.3

Catheters, arterial, complications in infants, **2.3**, 2.4, 2.5

Cellulitis, 7.25, **7.36**

Charcot–Marie–Tooth disease, palmoplantar keratoderma in, 3.8

Chediak–Higashi syndrome, **5.2**, 5.4, 6.14–6.15, **6.25**

Chest tubes, complications in infants, 2.4–2.5

Chicken pox. *See* Varicella

Child abuse and neglect, 9.4–9.8
cutaneous lesions in, 9.4, 9.5–9.6, **9.4–9.10**
differential diagnosis of, 7.20, 7.35–7.36, 9.8
sexual abuse in, 9.7–9.8, **9.11–9.12**

Clobetasol propionate, topical, **1.10**, 1.12

Clothing-covered sites, rashes in, **1.2**, 1.4

Clubbing of nails
congenital, 8.17
in systemic disease, 8.22, **8.38**

Coagulation, disseminated intravascular, 7.17–7.18, **7.24**

Cockayne's syndrome, photoreactions in, 2.4, 7.28

Coffin–Siris syndrome, nails in, 8.19

Cold exposure
panniculitis in, 7.24–7.25, **7.35**
pernio in, 7.15, **7.21**

Collagen vascular disorders, 7.29–7.36
antinuclear and anticytoplasmic antibodies in, 7.31, **7.44**

Collodion baby, 2.11, **2.25**

Comedones, 8.13
neonatal, 2.8

Compression solutions, 1.11

Condyloma acuminatum, 5.5

Connective tissue nevi, 2.34, **2.68**

Conradi's disease, 2.14, **2.28**

Contact dermatitis, 3.9–3.11, **3.14–3.16**
allergic, 3.9–3.11, **3.14–3.16**
in diaper area, 2.16
differential diagnosis of, 3.19, 3.21

of feet, differential diagnosis of, 3.30–3.31
id reaction in, 3.10
irritant, in diaper area, 2.15–2.16, **2.34**
photosensitizers in, 3.10, 6.6

Corticosteroids, topical, **1.10**, 1.12, 1.13
toxic effects in infants, 2.3

Coup-de-sabre, 7.34, **7.50**

Cowden's disease, **5.2**, 5.3

Coxsakie virus infection, hand, foot, and mouth syndrome in, 4.7, **4.8**, 7.12

Cradle cap, 2.17, **2.38**, 3.21

Creams, 1.11

CREST syndrome, antinuclear antibodies in, 7.31, **7.44**

Crohn's disease, differential diagnosis of, 7.36, **7.54**

Cross syndrome, 6.14–6.15, **6.25**

Crust, morphology of, **1.5**, 1.7

Cutis calcinosis, in dermatomyositis, 7.33, **7.48**

Cutis marmorata
in newborn, 2.6, **2.7**
telangiectatica congenita, 2.6, **2.8**

Cysts
dermoid, 2.35–2.36, **2.71**, 5.11
inclusion, epidermal, 5.10
trichilemmal, 5.10
vellus hair, 5.11, **5.17**

D
actylitis, blistering distal, differential diagnosis of, 4.5

Darier's disease, 3.5–3.6, **3.8**

Darier's sign, in mastocytosis, 2.28

Dennier's lines, 3.16

Dermal melanosis, 6.2, 6.7–6.10, **6.10–6.17**

Dermatitis
atopic, 3.11–3.21, **3.17–3.33**
blistering in, 4.14–4.15, **4.20**
contact, 3.9–3.11, **3.14–3.16**
diaper, 2.15–2.19, **2.34–2.41**
endogenous, 3.9
exogenous, 3.9
herpetiformis, 4.12, 4.13, **4.18**, 9.3–9.4
perioral, 3.21–3.23, **3.36–3.37**
seborrheic, 3.20, 3.21, **3.34**
in AIDS, 9.10
differential diagnosis of, 3.19, 3.21

Dermatofibromas, 5.14, **5.23**

Yeast-related infections,
   3.30–3.32, **3.51–3.54**
   potassium hydroxide preparation
      in, **1.6**, 1.8–1.9
Yellow nail syndrome, in systemic
   disease, 8.22, **8.38**

Zinc deficiency, acrodermatitis
   enteropathica in, 2.19
Zoster, 4.6, **4.7**